¡BUEN CAMINO!

BUEN CAMINO!

A father–daughter journey from
Croagh Patrick to Santiago de Compostela

NATASHA MURTAGH AND
PETER MURTAGH

Gill & Macmillan

Gill & Macmillan
Hume Avenue, Park West, Dublin 12
with associated companies throughout the world
www.gillmacmillan.ie

978 07171 4843 1

All photographs have been supplied by the authors, unless otherwise stated.

Typography design by Make Communication
Print origination by Síofra Murphy
Cartography by Design Image
Printed in Sweden by ScandBook AB

This book is typeset in Linotype Minion.

The paper used in this book comes from the wood pulp of managed forests. For every tree felled, at least one tree is planted, thereby renewing natural resources.

A CIP catalogue record for this book is available from the British Library.

5 4

Peter: For Moira and Patrick
who were with us every step
of the way.

Natasha: For my Dad.
Thank you for being my Camino
and my inspiration.
I love you.

The walking pilgrim

With scarce belongings on your back
And enormous heritage in your soul.
Free from material things,
You greet many people
And love even more,
Free from material things,
You smile to all,
And give away good wishes.
This is how you will climb and climb,
Feet firmly on the ground,
Walking to your dream.
Pilgrim, walk in freedom,
Walk without your belongings;
Pilgrim, always towards your destination,
But never alone.
You encounter many in your way,
And they remain forever in your heart.
You carry them in your rose-scented hands,
With which you give not only objects
But also joy.
Pilgrim, may God remain forever
Wherever you transit.

POEM IN A CHURCH ON THE CAMINO

CONTENTS

ACKNOWLEDGMENTS

PETER: My interest in the Camino began when my motor biking partner, Tony Sullivan, suggested in 2007 that we ride two BMW 1200 Adventures across France to Vezelay and from there, follow the Camino to Santiago to arrive on 25 July, St James's Day. The people I met along the way, their stories and motivations, interested me greatly, and so the following year Natasha, my then 16-year-old daughter, and I walked some 300 kilometres, from León to Santiago. That enriching and uplifting experience in turn prompted both of us to undertake the entire journey from St-Jean-Pied-de-Port and to write this book. So, thank you, Tony, for giving me something from which I have derived extraordinary pleasure, and will continue to do so for the rest of my life. Thanks also to my colleagues at *The Irish Times*, particularly the Editor, Geraldine Kennedy, for facilitating the time off necessary to do the walk and write my part of this book. My thanks to Fergal Tobin for running with the idea and for his encouraging comments as we made our way across Spain, writing daily and dispatching material to him. And thanks to everyone at Gill & Macmillan, especially Deirdre Rennison Kunz for her light touch editing, photo researcher Jen Patton and Ciara O'Connor for co-ordinating all the visuals, and Teresa Daly for helping get the book noticed. Thanks to Elaine Byrne for persisting in Samos and eventually succeeding (with the help of Padre Augustine). Thanks also to Elaine and to my friend Elizabeth Carnes in Virginia Beach in the United States for reading the manuscript and giving me the benefit of their observations. Thank you to my brother and sister, Nigel Murtagh and Jane Brickenden, for tolerating my plundering of our family history and exposing bits of it for all to see. Finally, thank you, Moira, for putting up with all this! I could not do it, and much more besides, without your support, encouragement, advice and tolerance.

NATASHA: For me, the Camino was brought to me by Dad. You told me about it, and asked me if I wanted to do it with you. So thank you for giving me the most wonderful experience of my life so far, and endless memories to carry throughout my life. Also, thank you for the opportunity to write this book. Without you I would have never had this given to me. With that, I too would like to thank Fergal Tobin for supporting both Dad and me with our book. Thank you to our Camino family. My experience wouldn't have been the same without you. Thank you for all the laughs and all the memories, and the stories to write about you gave me. Thank you to all my friends who cared and showed interest in what I was doing. Thank you, Mum, for all your texts along the way about the cats falling in the pond that gave me something to write about. And thank you for all your encouragement in this whole project. You were brilliant.

Natasha and Peter Murtagh
Greystones, Co. Wicklow
January 2011

INTRODUCTION

The Camino de Santiago is a pilgrimage to the reputed tomb of St James, whose shrine is in the great cathedral named in his honour in Santiago de Compostela in Galicia, northwest Spain. The Camino is over 1,000 years old and is rich in Christian history and heritage, and indeed in pre-Christian history as well. It attracts people of all faiths and, increasingly, people of none.

Like all pilgrimages, the Camino is a journey. It is an actual physical journey in the sense that it is a walk (or a cycle) from the Pyrénées in France, across Navarra and into Pamplona, then on to the Rioja and across the great Meseta Alta, the high plateau of central northern Spain, home to the cities of Burgos and León, and finally over the mountains of León into Galicia and to the beautiful city of Santiago. The distance is a little short of 800 kilometres, and for those so inclined there is a further 85-kilometre Camino to Finisterre, to the end of the earth, where the sun sets beyond the horizon in the Atlantic Ocean.

For some pilgrims, the Camino is a journey intimately connected to their faith, or perhaps faltering faith, in God, and a quest for renewal. But the appeal of the Camino is very broad, and for many who undertake it the pilgrimage is a journey of a different sort. It may be a journey of examination of one's life to date, taking slices of time and events from a shelf of one's memory and examining them. It may be a journey taken in remembrance of a recently departed loved one, a time to process feelings and raw emotions, a way of saying goodbye. It may be a journey away from something, the pressures of contemporary life perhaps, which turns into a journey towards something else, a changed life. It may be a journey that is quite simply the pressing of a pause button, time out to take stock.

In all cases the Camino is an opportunity for contemplation and reflection, and many people who undertake the journey find that this contemplative aspect of the pilgrimage has a strongly spiritual side to it.

The history of the Camino is intimately connected to the growth of Catholicism in Spain and the re-conquest of the country from the Moors. Religion can be very much part of the Camino for those who want it. But nothing is forced and many non-Roman Catholics, such as ourselves, feel perfectly at home, and are welcomed, when they choose to participate in Masses or other purely religious aspects of Camino life.

There are several different Camino routes in Spain, some starting in France and indeed elsewhere in western Europe. We walked the Camino Francés, the so-called French Way which is the main Camino and goes from St-Jean-Pied-de-Port in the Pyrénées to Santiago and on to Finisterre. We began our Camino by climbing Croagh Patrick in Co. Mayo on Reek Sunday to make a special connection between our home in Ireland and our pilgrimage in Spain. We did the Camino simply because we love it and wanted to write a book about it—a book about ourselves and the people we met on the way—and to do it as father and daughter; spending time together, having fun together. Because we walked part of the Camino before, 300 kilometres from León to Santiago, we knew what to expect. We love the people we meet, the friends we make, the places we see and stay in, and the fun and challenge of it all. We love the countryside through which we walk and the altered perspective on life that comes from living simply when you turn away, even for a short time, from the pressure and demands of contemporary, urban living.

This is not a guide book, though we hope it will prove helpful to anyone contemplating doing the Camino. You don't have to walk nearly 900 kilometres to experience the Camino. You can do it in stages over several years. But if you do decide to do it, and however you do it, you are highly likely to have an experience that will be with you for a long time and that you will find enriching and uplifting and very rewarding. We certainly did.

And as you move, unhurried, savouring the experience, people along the way will greet you by saying *Buen Camino!*—which means, in effect, "Enjoy it."

MAPS

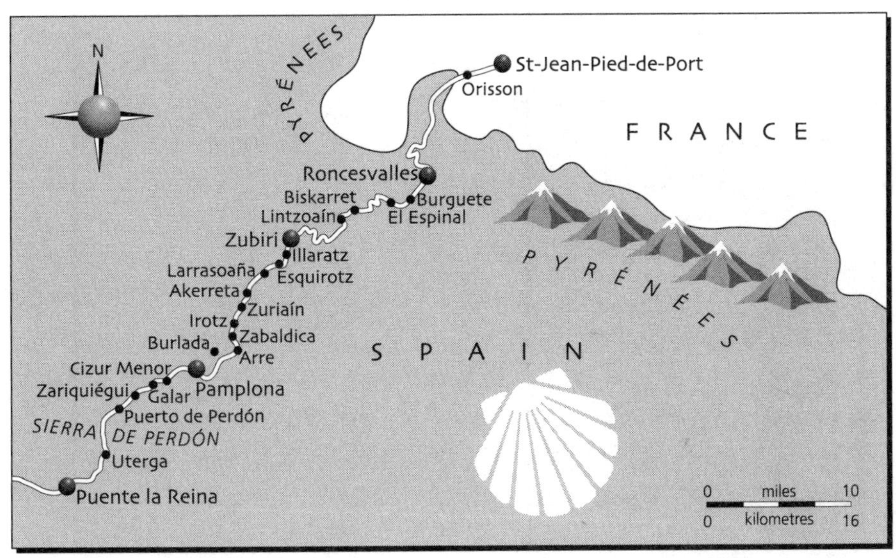

MAP 1
(pages 12–42)

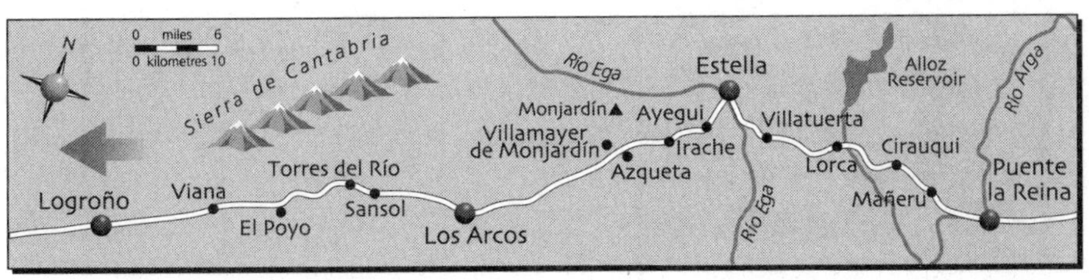

MAP 2
(pages 42–61)

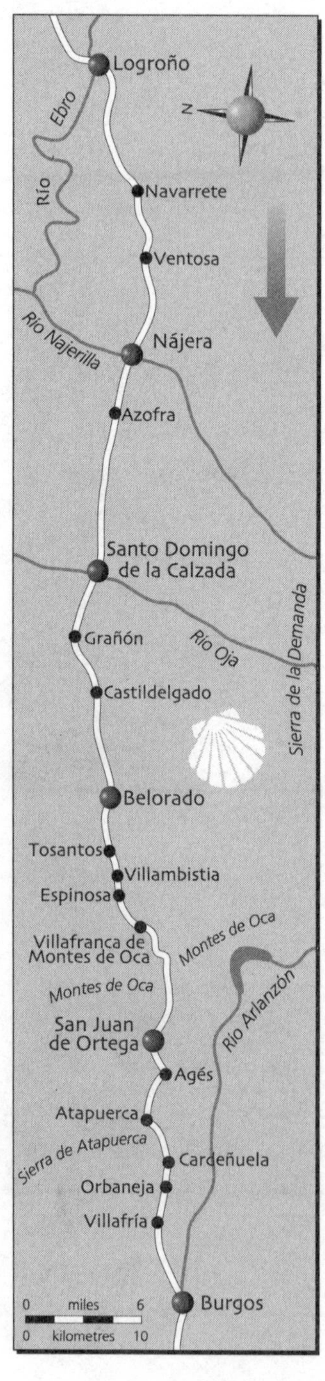

MAP 3
(pages 61–96)

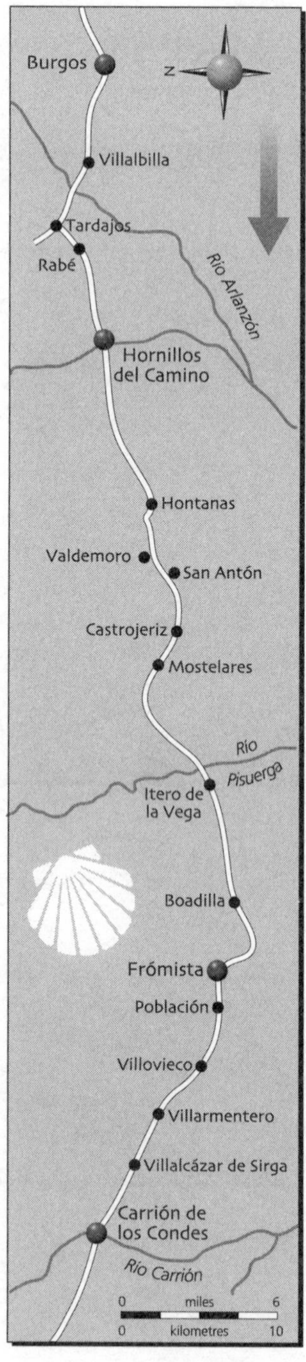

MAP 4
(pages 96–108)

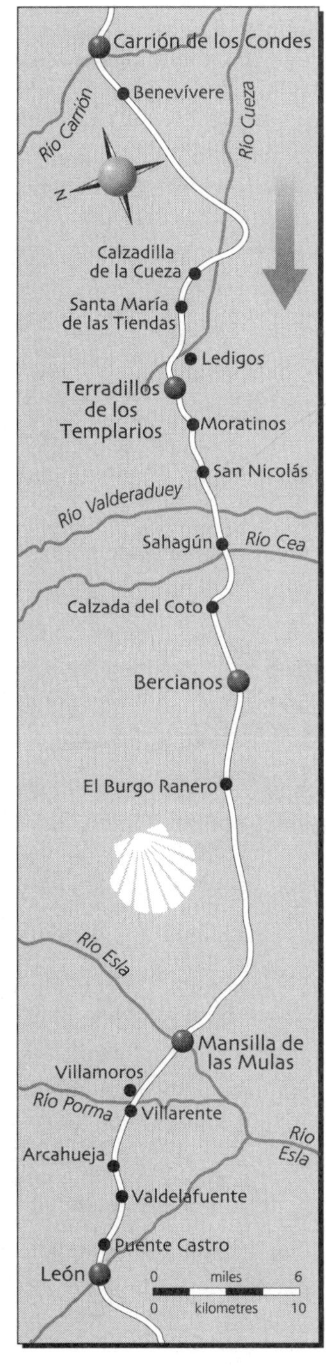

MAP 5
(pages 108–35)

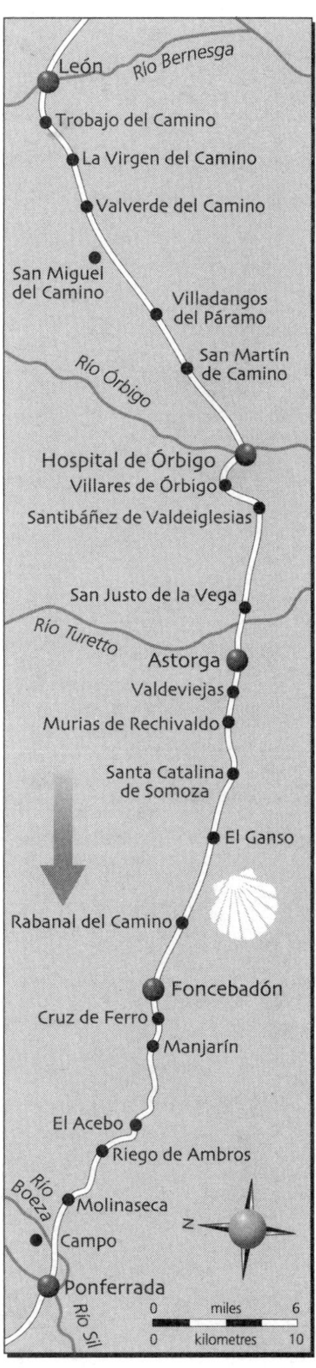

MAP 6
(pages 136–50)

Río Sil
Ponferrada
Compostilla
Columbrianos
Fuentes Nuevas
Camponaraya
Magaz
Carracedo
Cacabelos
Pieros
Villafranca del Bierzo
Pereje
Trabadelo
Portela de Valcárcel
Abasmestas
Ambascasas
Vega de Valcarce
Ruitelán
Sierra de Ancares
Herrerías
Hospital
Sierra de Courel
La Faba
O Cebreiro
Liñares
San Roque
H. de Condesa
Padornelo
Alto do Poio
Fonfría
Biduedo
Filloval
N
As Pasantes
Ramil
Triacastela
San Cristobo
Renche
San Xil
Montán
Samos
Furela
A Balsa
Pintín
Calvor
Aguiada
S. Mamede
S. P. de Comiño
Sarria
Vilei
Barbadelo
Rente
Mercado da Serra
Mouzós
Peruscallo
Xisto
Río Sarria
Lavandeira
Brea
Ferreiros
Río Miño
Mirallos
Pena
Rozas
Parrocha
Vilacha
Portomarín
0 miles 6
0 kilometres 10

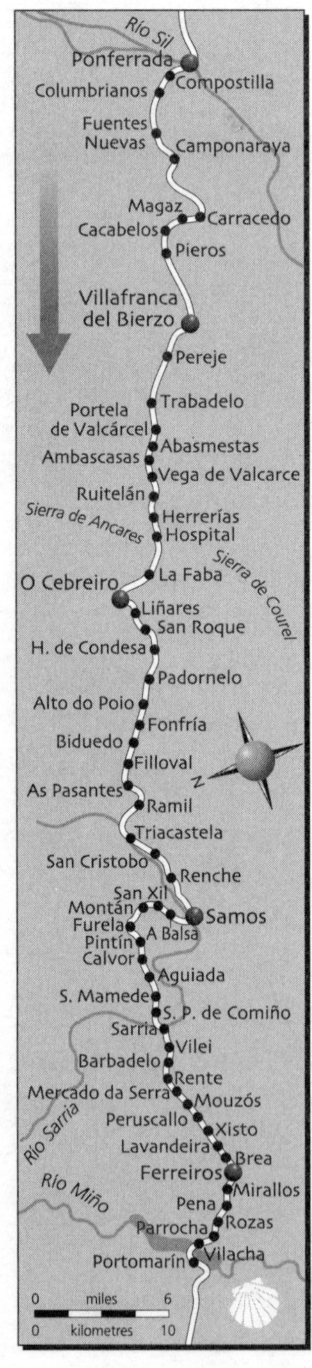

MAP 7
(pages 151–85)

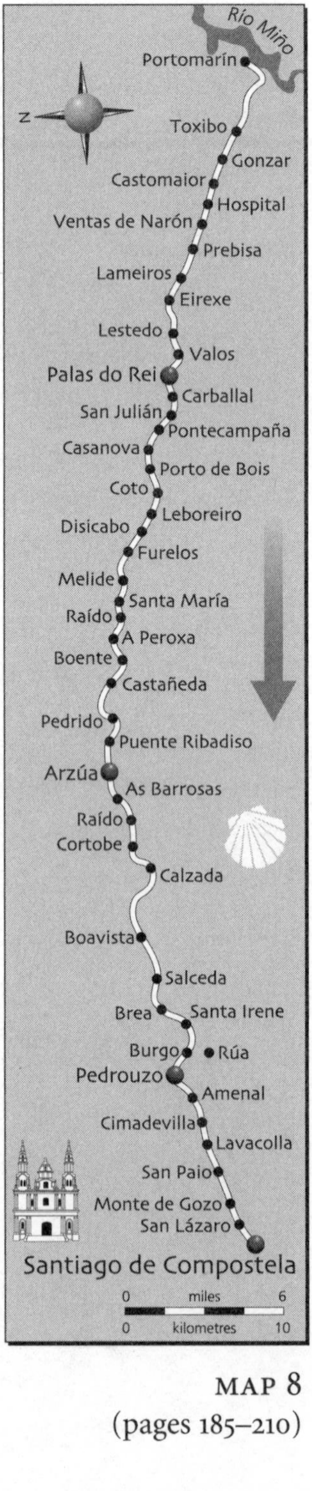

Río Miño
Portomarín
N
Toxibo
Gonzar
Castomaior
Hospital
Ventas de Narón
Prebisa
Lameiros
Eirexe
Lestedo
Valos
Palas do Rei
Carballal
San Julián
Pontecampaña
Casanova
Porto de Bois
Coto
Leboreiro
Disicabo
Furelos
Melide
Santa María
Raído
A Peroxa
Boente
Castañeda
Pedrido
Puente Ribadiso
Arzúa
As Barrosas
Raído
Cortobe
Calzada
Boavista
Salceda
Brea
Santa Irene
Burgo
Rúa
Pedrouzo
Amenal
Cimadevilla
Lavacolla
San Paio
Monte de Gozo
San Lázaro
Santiago de Compostela
0 miles 6
0 kilometres 10

MAP 8
(pages 185–210)

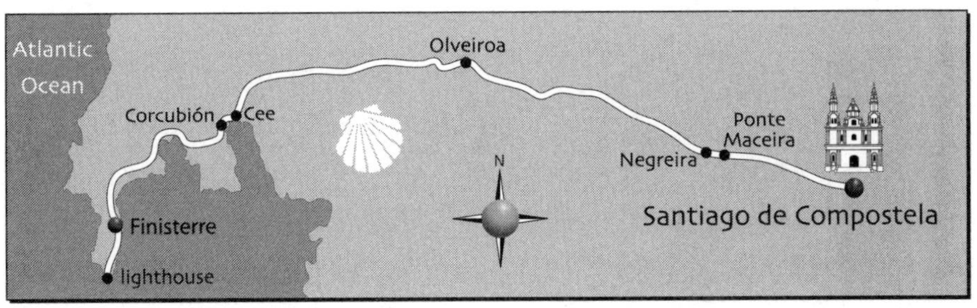

MAP 9
(pages 210–29)

1 | IRELAND

I

Sunday 25 July 2010
Reek Sunday in Mayo
St James's Day in Santiago de Compostela

PETER: We began the ascent at 3.35 am. In the dark. And the mist. And the drizzle, the almost always present Mayo drizzle.

That was the way we wanted it. Do Croagh Patrick in the night and aim to be at the summit for the sunrise.

Reek Sunday, 25 July—St James's Day. *The* big day in Santiago de Compostela. A convenient symmetry with the Galician city, destination of all Camino pilgrims; a couple of countries and just two flights away. And because of that symmetry, we—Natasha, my 18-year-old daughter, and I—decided to begin our Camino by scaling the Reek, Ireland's Holy Mountain overlooking Clew Bay in Co. Mayo.

It seemed like a good idea, one that was challenged at 2.45 am when the alarm went off telling us to get up and out of bed in the pitch dark. My brother Nigel and sister Jane agreed to come with us; so too did a neighbour, Austin O'Malley, a veteran of the Reek and of many other hill walks in and around Louisburgh. Just before we left our house in the dark, word came that our immediate neighbours, Gerard and Margaret O'Malley, were also up for it. In fact, they were up for the entire night: first the Daniel O'Donnell concert in Castlebar which gave way to a wedding in Westport and dancing into the small hours. Sure why bother with bed at all? It's great to be young.

The Reek looked bleak, inasmuch as we could see the Reek at 3.35 am. But after a while, it's surprising just how much the human eye can detect in the dark. The rocky, gravelly, slippery and in places very, very steep path was quite passable, even in the half light.

NATASHA: Things are looking great already as I zip up my rain coat to shelter my face from the cold wind and spitting rain. As I do so, I think of my Mum and Aunt Dolly who are curled up in their beds back at the house, along with the majority of the country as normal people would be asleep at this hour.

The bottom of the mountain is quite steep, but manageable. It involves a lot of hopping over large rocks and avoiding small streams. Like always I walked ahead and alone. I'm not very talkative when it comes to walking. I'm happy to walk by myself and to just think. Also, as I looked at the vast mountain, which was disappearing behind darkness and mist, I thought I'll never make it to the top with these oldies dragging me down. I had to ditch them as a matter of survival.

I followed the light of a torch from the person in front of me. From looking at the other torch lights dotted along the path, there seemed to be only a couple of hundred walking at this time. I had a jumper on and was beginning to get warm. As the gradient steepened, I got a call from Uncle Nigel telling me not to go too far ahead. I perched on a rock in the darkness and waited. Once we had all grouped again, I was off.

The trail doesn't stay manageable for long; after 20 minutes you find yourself panting and needing small breathers. I was now really warm.

PETER: The key is to pace yourself: don't rush it. It's not a race but it is a test of endurance and stamina. In 2009 some 28,000 people scaled the 764-metre high mountain on Reek Sunday, the final and most important of several annual summer pilgrimage days.

When we began our ascent in the early hours, the pilgrims were numbered in dozens. A motley collection that included young people out for a laugh, all talk, cans of beer and mobile phones; early birds of one persuasion or another; and the devout who, despite the hour, nonetheless paused at each of the stations and observed their religious duties.

Austin, who was 70 in March, loves the climb. "I'm addicted to it," he says. "I'm all the time thinking about the next time I'll do it. I love it. I love the walk and the people you'll meet on the way."

The Camino de Santiago is made for Austin. He has a deep spirituality and a love of the world about him. A tall, handsome man with striking blue eyes, Austin sees flowers, shrubs, trees and aspects of the landscape that pass others by. He loves poetry and has a deep appreciation of Irish culture. Austin can sit on the sand dunes above his local beach in the early morning and marvel at the light of the sky and the tone of the colour it gives the sea. He will describe the sight of a wave breaking on the beach and then washing back into the sea to meet a fresh, incoming wave and for the two to collide, in a knife edge of spray, ripping along the length of the strand. He will describe this with the wonder of a child, as though he has just seen it for the first time, even though he has been watching it all his life.

A year ago I met Austin on the Reek and he invited me to join him a week later for a walk up Mweelrea, Connacht's highest peak, just a few kilometres away. We scaled it in glorious sunshine. I was thrilled he could come to the Reek with Natasha and me for our special climb.

At Tochar Patrick, the point where the ancient pilgrimage route from Ballintubber Abbey via Aughagower joins the path up from Murrisk on the shoulder of the Reek, Austin peers down at a lake below, an almost perfectly circular pool of water some hundred metres beneath us. He picks up a stone, spreads his feet and stands side on to the lake. And then, in the manner of a handball player, he flings the stone underarm with one strong, graceful sweep into the air. Seconds later, there is the sound of a perfect 'plop!' as it lands in the centre of the lake.

"God, how did you do that?" I exclaimed.

"It has to be a good flat one," he advised as I bend down to copy. "Astride now," he said, "and underarm."

I flung the rock and it vanished into the heather well short of the lake.

I'm not going to be beaten by a man with 13 years on me, I thought. And so I picked up another rock, a bigger one and no worries about the shape either, just a lump of Croagh Patrick quartz. I flung it over arm as hard as I could and, sure enough, there is a satisfactory splash.

"Isn't it great to be daft!" exclaimed Austin as we both laughed and moved on up the Reek.

The higher we go, the amount of airborne water in the mist increases and the wind starts to drive it through almost any covering you have on.

It's getting lighter now and just before the summit, at about 5.30 am, the sun rises—not that you can see it clearly for the swirling, driving mist. The final stretch of the climb, the awful, hideously steep scree slope below the summit, is taken foot by careful foot, the wind getting ever stronger. And then the summit opens up, a high vista lashed by the wind and the driving, dripping mist. Visibility can't be more than 50 kilometres. So much for witnessing the sunrise! The place seems godforsaken: how St Patrick stayed here for 40 days and 40 nights, and sorted out the demon blackbirds, not to mention those snakes and poisonous reptiles, I'll never know.

NATASHA: The mist is incredibly thick and low. I could only see about 50 metres in front. The climb was getting very steep, very quickly, and the muddy path soon turned to scree, which is very difficult to walk on. The people passing me on their way down looked tired and wet and had pale faces. Yet they seemed to hold a sense of accomplishment and satisfaction.

I was really near the peak now. The gradient was at its most challenging and I found myself using my hands to pull myself up. The jingling of falling stones would cause my head to rise and avoid the person coming down towards me. Everyone around me was groaning and cursing for the top to appear. People on the way down would smile and say: "Only 10 minutes now." Well, those 10 minutes were taking about half an hour! With frustration I would burst out in sprints and then stop for a minute. Then sprint again.

Finally, as though God himself tapped me on the shoulder, I looked up and saw a tiny little greyish church. From the bottom of the mountain on a clear day it looks like a magnificent white temple fit for Zeus himself. Nonetheless, it was a church, on Croagh Patrick, at 5.20 am, and I was in front of it.

PETER: People are huddled in the lee of the tiny chapel, sipping hot tea sold from tarpaulin-covered stalls. Some suck on cigarettes, others slug beer. A Jack Russell named Oscar busies himself about the place. Everyone shivers; it's bitterly cold. The faithful walk devoutly around the church the required number of times. Gerard and Margaret are there first, up the Reek like a pair of whippets. Gerard stands me a welcome cup of hot tea. Then comes Nigel; sadly, the climb was too much for Jane. Finally Austin emerges through the mist, smiling, happy, acknowledging friends along the way.

And all of us, 50 people maybe, stand there in the half light in utterly foul weather, mist and rain swirling around, gusts of wind whipping our backs. And then, just for an instant, the mist parts on the eastern horizon and the sun breaks through. For one or two glimpses it is a blurred haze, then shining bright, then blurred again, then swallowed once more in dense mist. But it's the sun, minutes after the sunrise, on the summit, on Reek Sunday, on St James's Day—just as planned. Just as requested.

The descent comes easy; the flow of pilgrims going up has grown from dozens to hundreds—a steady stream of men and women and children, many of them country folk from all parts of Ireland. Their numbers will grow to more than 20,000 by the time the sun sets. And none will be deterred by the weather. Friends passing on the path greet each other and pause for a chat.

"See you next year," many say, the annual ritual observed as it has been for centuries.

And we head home. Home for a feed of bacon and eggs and sausages and boxty and toast and jam and coffee and warmth and chat with wonderful neighbours.

And after all that, Gerard and Margaret finally get to bed.

II

PETER: Today's pilgrims to Croagh Patrick walk in the footsteps of their ancestors. Long before the early Irish Church, through St Patrick, embraced the Reek, our pagan predecessors had no doubt but that the mountain was a special place. Evidence for this abounds in the landscape around the south shore of Clew Bay.

A few kilometres south and east of Croagh Patrick on a patch of scrubland sandwiched between a cottage and some ugly, breeze-block sheds, there is a rocky outcrop. This is the Boheh Stone upon which are inscribed a mass of swirls and so-called keyhole shapes. The Boheh Stone is one of the most important examples of prehistoric rock art in Britain or Ireland and the only one west of the Shannon. It dates from sometime between 4000 BC and 2500 BC. 4000 BC was the infancy of the

Neolithic, the New Stone Age; 2500 BC was the Early Bronze Age. Archaeologists who have examined the stone in detail estimate that it dates from between 2000 BC and 3000 BC—that is, four to five thousand years ago. To put those dates in perspective, when our ancestors in Mayo were grinding their thoughts onto the surface of a rock, Homer was composing the *Odyssey*; in Egypt, the first pyramids were being erected; in England, Stonehenge was taking shape.

When the sheet ice of the last great Ice Age retreated from Ireland over 7,000 years ago, secreting from beneath itself as it melted a string of muddy hillock clay and boulder drumlins across the country, our ancestors were able to move onto the land thus exposed. The drumlins are there still, stretching in a line east–west across Ireland from Cavan to Mayo and out into Clew Bay. Semi-submerged there, they are the islands that give the bay its distinctive character. The people who gradually colonised the 'new' land freed of ice were hunter gatherers, people who caught, killed and ate what they could, and picked wild fruits when they couldn't. Such people are believed to have lived in Mayo between 5500 BC and 3500 BC.

Fossil pollen analysis, indicating changes to plant life prompted by human activity, suggests that the first farming, that is, the systematic cultivation of crops and rearing of animals, began near Croagh Patrick some 3,500 years ago.[1] This way of life gradually replaced hunting and gathering, and with it grew an appreciation and awareness of the seasons: the ebb and flow of the year, the weather and the importance of the sun, the giver of life. The Boheh Stone appears to be an acknowledgment of this. Our ancestors could have crawled out of wherever it was they slept and carved their thoughts onto any rock, of which there is an abundance in Mayo. But they didn't; they chose the Boheh Stone, from where one has a commanding view of the Reek, its cone standing proud into the sky, higher than anything immediately around it.

The possible significance of the stone was noticed first in the modern era by an amateur archaeologist living in Mayo, Gerry Bracken, who was a retired agricultural scientist. He began a prolonged study of the rock in 1987, and on the evening of 24 August 1991—

1. Morahan, Leo, *Croagh Patrick, Co. Mayo—archaeology, landscape and people*, p. 15.

St Bartholomew's Day—he saw something magical: for a period of about 20 minutes, the setting sun seemed to roll down the north face of the Reek's almost perfectly formed cone before disappearing out of sight behind the ridge. The Rolling Sun phenomenon, as it has become known, happens twice a year, on 18 April and on 24 August, the day Gerry Bracken first saw it. These two dates plus 21 December, the Winter Solstice, divide the year into three roughly equal parts equating to the sowing, growing and harvesting seasons, April being associated with sowing, August with harvest.

Bracken was dazed and exhilarated by his discovery. As he noted later, to stand at the Boheh Stone, and to observe its relationship with Croagh Patrick, is to be in no doubt but that ancient man regarded this place as somewhere special, somewhere almost certainly sacred in his mind.[2]

The Boheh Stone's so-called cup-and-ring markings seem to confirm this. They are strikingly similar to markings more widely associated with the swirling circle carvings in Newgrange. The stone is "the most comprehensively-worked example of its type in Ireland and distinctive in style from similarly marked stones in Britain or on the Atlantic seaboard of the European Continent," according to Maarten van Hoek, a Dutch geographer and expert in prehistoric rock art, who has made a detailed study of them.[3]

"What the special meaning of the keyhole-pattern has been is unknown and may always remain a mystery and a matter of subjective speculation," according to him. "It has often been suggested that cups and cups-and-rings are symbols of celestial bodies. Just possibly the keyhole pattern is a symbol of a tailed phenomenon once visible in prehistoric skies—a comet possibly. The areas where keyholes are found could be parts of the country where the weather conditions allowed prolonged opportunities to observe this phenomenon." But that, as he acknowledges, is just speculation.

The Tochar Patrick ancient pilgrimage route passes the Boheh Stone. Today the stone is more commonly known as St Patrick's Chair, an

2. *Cathair na Mart*—Journal of the Westport Historical Society, No 12, 1992; article by Bracken, who died in December 2007, and the late Patrick Wayman, director of the Dunsink Observatory, pp 1–12.

3. *Cathair na Mart*, No 15, 1995; pp 15–25.

example of early Christianity embracing pre-Christian culture and practices, making them its own. Another is Lughnasa, the pre-Christian Irish festival honouring the Celtic god Lugh and rooted in Celtic mythology. Lughnasa marked the start of the harvest season and was an occasion for funeral feasts and games in honour of Lugh's mother, Tailtiu, who died of exhaustion after clearing the land for farming. The gathering of the seed to make bread and the ripening of the season's first fruits, usually wild berries, became a time of community gatherings, market festivals, horse races and reunions with distant family and friends. When Lughnasa was absorbed into Christian ritual among the peoples living on the southern shores of Clew Bay it became known as Domhnach na Cruaiche—or Reek Sunday, then as now a quintessentially rural rite and the most popular pilgrimage day to Ireland's Holy Mountain.

The Mayo landscape is littered with examples of pre-Christian and Christian practices, blending into a seamless narrative, if one wishes to see it that way. Scattered around the land between Clew Bay and Killary Harbour are megalithic tombs, cairns, standing stones, some of them in rows, others isolated but, viewed from one vantage point, seeming to have a relationship with the Reek and Caher Island, a small island in the Atlantic peppered with early Christian graves.

In 1994 archaeological excavations were carried out on the Reek, at St Patrick's Oratory, a few metres to the east of the current church on the summit.[4] Among the items found were three flints, animal bone, a fragment of iron and one possibly of stone; shards of medieval pottery, two corroded bronze pins, two worked pieces of flint, and fragments of iron. There was some modern glass and iron, modern coins and religious medals. There was charcoal which was carbon dated as originating between 430 AD and 890 AD. Glass beads were found, dating anywhere from the Iron Age to the early medieval period, that is, between the third century BC and the fourth century AD. The Reek is also home to several pre-Christian cairns.

St Patrick came to the Reek in 441 AD. He was on his second visit to Ireland. The first was when he was 16 after he was kidnapped in his native England and made a slave. He escaped after six years, went home and became a priest, returning to Ireland in 432 AD on a mission to

4. See Morahan.

bring Christianity to the island. He is said to have travelled west, to Mayo and to Aughagower, near Westport, from where he climbed the Reek, spending 40 days and 40 nights, suffering the attention of those demon birds.

Patrick understood the importance of the sun but he ascribed to it a significance markedly different to the pagans surrounding him. "… For that sun, which we see," he wrote in his *Confession*, "by God's command rises daily for our sakes, but it will never reign, nor will its splendour endure; but all those who worship it shall go in misery to punishment." And he went on to extol the value of faith in God and to refer to "Christ the true Sun".

The pagans believed him. Patrick brought Christianity to Ireland and the sun worshippers passed, leaving in their wake the likes of the Boheh Stone and other archaeological debris that helps define the landscape. A millennium and a half of Christianity has brought its own heritage. In the 11th and 12th centuries, Irish devotion to St James saw many pilgrims make the arduous journey to Galicia, many of them in wine ships returning empty to Bordeaux. Those that came back to Ireland (many pilgrims died going to, or coming from, Santiago) brought souvenirs. During 1996 excavations at the former Priory of St Mary in Mullingar, for instance, the remains of several monks were exhumed. On each was found a scallop shell, the symbol of St James and a fair indication (though not conclusive evidence) that each had journeyed to Santiago de Compostela to pay homage to James the Great, one of Christ's inner circle of Apostles. St Mary's Priory was founded in 1227 and lasted until 1539. An etching in the *Dublin Penny Journal* of 1836 shows it in poor condition but still standing. However, it fell into greater and greater disrepair and vanished … until the foundations were rediscovered in 1996. The site is now host to a supermarket.

Another link comes from the early Christian settlement at Illaunloughan Island in Co. Kerry, a tiny place between the mainland coast and Valentia Island. Once again, during recent excavations of graves dating back to the eighth century, fragments of scallop shells were found.

But the most exciting find in recent times was made at Ardfert Cathedral, one of a cluster of churches within a walled burial ground in the village of Ardfert, near Tralee in Co. Kerry. The cathedral may be dated variously from the 11th to the 17th centuries. Between 1989 and 1998 archaeologists excavated parts of it as a restoration programme carried out by the National Monuments Service.

Ardfert comes from *Ard ferta* in Irish, meaning high burial ground, but may also be derived from *Ard Ferta Breanainn*, suggesting a link with St Brendan. In an echo of the bird story involving St Patrick on the Reek, Brendan, said to have been born around 484 AD making him a contemporary of the national saint, decided to build a monastery at Killeacle. As he surveyed the area, a bird swooped on him, snatched the plans from his hand and flew off, dropping them at Ardfert and prompting Brendan to build there. In truth, there is no contemporary evidence to support assertions that Brendan founded Ardfert, but the tradition endures.

During the excavations Ardfert yielded up one of the most delightful pieces of evidence of the draw of Santiago de Compostela during the late Middle Ages. In the nave of the cathedral, in a stone-lined grave where two people had been buried, one directly on top of the other, archaeologists found a tiny pendant, a scallop shell of pewter with a gilded figure attached to it. The shell measures approximately four centimetres across and the same from top to bottom. The moulded, gilded figure, who is about three centimetres tall, is soldered onto the front of the shell and looks forward. He is a pilgrim, a man wearing a long cloak and a pilgrim's hat. In his left hand he is holding a walking staff; his right hand clutches the strap of a satchel which is slung across his shoulder and rests on his hip. His features are clearly visible: nose, eye sockets, hands and fingers. The figure could be St James, who, uniquely, is often portrayed as a pilgrim to his own shrine, or it could simply be a representation of the archetypal pilgrim. But cleaned and polished after conservation, this 500-year-old trinket looks exactly like hundreds of others on sale today in souvenir shops in Santiago.

It's a fair assumption that one of the people in the grave had made the pilgrimage to Santiago and wore the pendant as a badge of devotion to the saint. Or perhaps this person was given it as a present by someone else who had been to Santiago. Either way, the trinket was treasured sufficiently to be buried with its owner—the scallop shell and pilgrim figure clearly had meaning and was of importance.

At the foot of Croagh Patrick on the shore of Clew Bay there is a place known locally as Murrisknaboll. It is a peninsula surrounded by the sea on three sides; the water is shallow, a good place to land fish from small boats. On a north-facing part of the shore, where the bank joins the beach, there is a shell midden, the remnants of an ancient dump used by fishermen. Archaeologists have estimated that the midden could date from the Mesolithic era, making it among the earliest repositories of evidence of settlement around Croagh Patrick.[5] Thousands of years ago, fisherman in dug-out canoes possibly came ashore at this spot and landed their catch, a catch that included shellfish which were eaten and the shells then discarded. When the midden was examined in the 1990s, the archaeologists noted that it contained various shells, mainly oyster and scallop. The sea then was lapping the bank and the archaeologists warned that it was likely to be eaten away, its contents falling back into the sea from whence they came. Since then, a landowner has built up the bank to protect it from further erosion and the midden is now hidden.

A few days before we climbed the Reek at the start of our Camino, I went to the ancient midden. Some scallop shells were visible among the mud and rocks supporting the bank. Could they be from the midden itself, disturbed as the protective earthworks were set in place? It is possible—unlikely, perhaps, but possible nonetheless. The area is littered with oyster shells, debris from a nearby oyster farm. There are scallop shells too, modern ones for sure, further down the shoreline, away from the midden. I took the two scallop shells from among the rocks protecting the midden—two Mesolithic (maybe) scallop shells. They are now attached to our backpacks, proclaiming Natasha and me to be pilgrims on the way to Santiago de Compostela, in the manner of a tradition going back more than a thousand years.

And so we are off. Breakfast eaten; hugs, kisses and goodbyes exchanged, we're away to Knock airport, and then Gatwick, and Bordeaux for one night before we head into the Pyrénées. A scallop shell on our backpacks and a little silver box in my pocket.

5. See Morahan, p. 30.

| FRANCE

PETER: The contrast between the TGV and the little train could not be greater. The TGV—smooth, slick and modern, the pride of French railways—glides silently on unbroken tracks, making hardly a sound. We have flown from Knock to Gatwick and from there to Bordeaux where we spent the night. Now we ride the TGV to Bayonne; it is a flawless, technological performance. There is nothing wrong or flawed about the little old diesel train that chugs from Bayonne to St-Jean-Pied-de-Port, the start of the Camino in the Pyrénées. It is just from another era. It has a comforting, old-world rhythm—clunkedy-clunk, clunkedy-clunk, clunkedy-clunk, clunkedy-clunk; and, when it passes over points, clunkedy-clunkedy-clunkedy-clunkedy, before it settles down again to the more familiar clunkedy-clunk, clunkedy-clunk, clunkedy-clunk.

The little engine heaves its way high into the mountains, the land and vegetation changing as we pass. Wide, flat fields with maize give way to a patchwork of smaller fields, each one on a slope and most playing host to dairy cattle. The flat fields that remain are in bends of a river valley and most are used to grow vegetables. It is all very lush, very pastoral and Alpine in appearance.

St-Jean is a medieval citadel town built of old red sandstone. There must be a local authority ordinance that directs everyone to paint the outside walls of their properties white and the woodwork a deep, dull red because they are all like that. The town is pretty and touristy. Geraniums sprout from window boxes; shops cater for the pilgrim market—or, one suspects, those who want pilgrim memorabilia but without actually doing the walking.

The pilgrim office, from where one must obtain one's pilgrim passport, the *credencial del peregrino*, is on rue de la Citadelle, a cobbled street inside the old town that runs parallel to the city walls, right down to the river. The office is manned by volunteers from Les Amis du chemin de Saint-Jacques Pyrénées-Atlantiques. Only bona fide pilgrims may enter here; it is not a tourist office. The walls are covered with pictures of the Camino and practical advice to starters: what to wear, where to stay, weather reports, and some statistical information as well. Religious music wafts gently from a CD player. There are four desks, behind which sit *les quatre volunteers*. The whole place exudes an unhurried but efficient calm.

"Ga'day, mate! How can I help you?"

It's Peter from Australia, a 77-year-old (as of 29 July) retired civil engineer from Colac, a place about 250 kilometres from Melbourne. Like so many other people, Peter came upon the Camino by chance. And like them, he was seduced and it is now a significant part of his life. It began when he was in Brittany in the late 1990s chasing ancestral family links and, with his civil engineering skills, finding himself helping a local archaeological dig. St James figured prominently and, curious as he learned more of the links between France and the Apostle, Peter walked part of the Camino, from León to Santiago, in 2002. The following year, he did another section, and another in 2004, still another in 2008. Now in 2010, he's working in the Camino office in St-Jean.

"I haven't met anybody who hasn't said after doing the Camino that it changed their life in some way," he explained. And what impact did it have on him? "I had fallen out with my sister many, many years ago. It was awful: her family didn't speak to me and mine and we didn't speak to her or hers. So the first thing I did after my Camino when I went home was go around to her and apologise. 'Whatever it was', I said, 'sorry, it was my fault and we should never have let it get to this.' And now we're fine. I also got rid of a lot of garbage in my life after my Camino. I resigned from a whole lot of things and now I do a lot of voluntary work.

"The Camino's not religious for me, it's spiritual. The ambiance of the Camino is fantastic. I like nature, I like walking, I like to go walkabout back home. After the Camino, after walking, you realise that in civilisation you are dealing with a lot of bullshit."

Peter is a self-evidently happy, balanced, cheery man who takes pleasure in helping people and engaging with them and their lives. A survey of pilgrims' motivations carried out by the office until 2002 used to include a multi-optional question about motivation. But it was dropped when they ran out of options that seemed to match the reasons: at the time, a mere 20 per cent of pilgrims filling in the form gave religion as their motivation for doing the Camino. More and more people simply wanted time to opt out of their everyday life at home for a multiplicity of reasons: it might be needing time to process feelings after the death of someone close; or it might be an inchoate but irresistible desire to escape from technology.

The relatively minor place accorded to formal religion as a motivation for doing the Camino is evident from a glance through the office visitor book to which pilgrims are invited to contribute their thoughts before setting off. "Charming village," noted a couple from England; "It's so hot! Happy Canada Day!" wrote Robert Ring; "In memory of [name indecipherable] on her birthday," wrote Jill and Thomas Payne; "Everything is done. Forget everything and start new," advised someone who signed themselves St-Jean; "My spiritual vacance [sic]," wrote Anna from Seoul; "For our friends and family. May God send down His grace upon us all,"—JMS; "A journey individually, together, and as a community," was the hope of Jennifer; "10-year anniversary of our first Camino. Back in 2010!" enthused Jean and Jim.

And for Natasha and me? "May this Camino be as enriching and uplifting as my first," was my wish.

We present ourselves to another of the assistants and get our pilgrim passports which are essential for staying in the *albergue*s, the hostels that dot the entire Camino all the way to Santiago. These cater especially for pilgrims and charge peppercorn rates for bunk beds, usually between €4 and €8. You cannot book; you just turn up from around mid-day on; preference is given to foot pilgrims; cyclists have to wait their turn. The man who fills out our pilgrim passports misreads my Irish passport. Instead of transcribing my surname, he transcribes my nationality. Camino statistics will show that a 'M. Éireannach'—Mr Ireland—received his Camino passport on 26 July 2010!

And so to bed in the *albergue* up the street—a bunk bed in a room with 10 others, in an 18th-century stone house with incredible views ... and all for just €8 each.

| OUR CAMINO

St-Jean-Pied-de-Port to Roncesvalles: 27 km in 6.5 hours

NATASHA: Walking out of the *albergue*, the streets of St-Jean are empty. The evening before, they were bustling with life. Tourist families were floating up and down the cobble-stone surfaces, children running in and out of doors; pilgrims marching like soldiers, eager to register in the Camino office and receive their passports.

The same street is very different at 7.00 am. A thin darkness covers the buildings; nearly every shutter on every house is closed. The only noise that disturbs the sleeping town is the light tinkle of walking poles hitting the cobbles as the pilgrims set out for the mountains. As Dad and I walk down the street in the old town, the air is filled with a light smell of fresh breads and pastries. These are the first real steps of our Camino, which will bring us over the Pyrénées and west across Spain, all the way to Santiago de Compostela.

St-Jean ends abruptly and we are immediately surrounded by lush green fields and the noises of distant farm animals. The walk begins tough; the road out of St-Jean is very, very steep. It slithers between fields, leading us higher and higher. The countryside is rather like Ireland, as a girl from Belgium, another pilgrim on the way to Santiago, remarked.

I was expecting the sun to burst through as soon as the night sky had gone completely, but it didn't. Instead, a heavy white mist remained. I was grateful, as the climb alone was making me sweat. The road was bordered with delicate little flowers of purples and yellows. As we got higher there were spits of gorse that had been ambushed by vast amounts of what looked like little silver bowls. These turned out to be spiders' webs that sat flippantly on the plants, catching little dew beads and bouncing in the breeze. I leaned a little closer to examine one of these impressive works of art, but was turned away quickly by the threatening stare of the occupant, perched at the side.

At the top of each hill we take a breather and listen to the faint ringing of cow bells coming from the vanishing valley below. The higher we get, the colder it gets. At one stage I lost Dad. I didn't notice when it happened, but after making it to the top of a long, sheer road, I took a breather at the side, to wait for him. But he didn't come. I was thinking he was just struggling with the gradient. Feeling rather pleased with myself, I took my bag off and sat on the side of the road and waited and waited. I began to think I had taken a wrong turn when two cyclists appeared through the mist. Exhausted and out of breath, one of them said in Italian: "Natasha, indietro!" or something along those lines. I laughed and nodded, pretending I understood what he was saying. But really, I was confused: how did he know my name? Then I thought it must have been Dad. I turned my phone on and rang him; I had gone the wrong way. Brilliant! So I began my trek back down the way I had come.

PETER: After two hours we reached a place named Orisson, little more than a bend in the road but with a welcome café. It is 790 metres up—higher than Croagh Patrick—and it has taken a hard, two-hour slog to get here. Coffee and bread was never more welcome and a chance to replenish our water bottle. The café owner says the rest of the gradient for the remainder of our trek across the Pyrénées will not be as steep. He gestures with the palm of his hand, showing a more gentle climb. Nonetheless, we have another 600 metres to surmount.

NATASHA: The café owner said there was nothing from now on until we got to Roncesvalles. The road ahead wasn't as steep as before, but it was still challenging. We began to get very high, very quickly. Stopping had made me cool down and the sweat from my clothes had turned cold. The mist was still very heavy and low, and walkers that were ahead of us were sucked in and would disappear from vision, like a pirate ship at sea. We cross a cattle grid and are now in upland commonage—no fences, no hedges and very few trees. But lots of grass, lots of sheep and some horses. The edges of the road are sprinkled with crowds of what look like sea holly and nettles. Only the noise of a car would make us move to the side, as seeing it was impossible until the headlights poked through the mist.

PETER: There's a refrain in the film *Local Hero* in which a noisy motorcyclist zips through a Scottish seaside village at the precise moment the main character, a hapless American oilman, tries to cross the road to use the phone box. No explanation is ever offered as to why the motorcyclist whizzes by; he just does. Near the top of the Pyrénées, there's a small white Renault van that keeps emerging from the mist. We hear it first—a high-pitched engine, somewhere out there, somewhere in the mist, unsure whether it is in front of us or behind. And then it appears, always in front. And always driven by what looks like the same middle-aged farmer. There's a big dog in the rear that snarls and yaps at us through the back window as the van disappears once more into the mist. Twenty minutes or so later, the van's back. Same routine, same driver, same yapping dog and always coming at us from the front. Weird. But funny too. They're probably still up there, tootling about in the mist, yapping at pilgrims …

Suddenly there's a break in the mist and out of it emerges Jan, standing behind a table which he has set up under a lean-to canopy in front of his white Citroën transit van. He is surrounded by sheep and pilgrims, who have plonked themselves on the grass and are eating and drinking.

"Hello," says Jan with excessive cheeriness. "Where are you from?"

"Ireland," I say.

"Ah! My first today."

And with that he turns to the side of his van, takes out a felt tip pen and adds me to the list of nationalities that he has written down the outside of the driver's door. There's information written all over the side of the van: we are 1,200 metres up, with 11 kilometres to go to Roncesvalles. Jan dispenses Lidl-sourced chocolate bars and juices; everything seems to sell for €1. Clever Jan offers the only respite for kilometres in either direction and just about everybody walking past gives him their custom.

NATASHA: Soon after Jan, the mist cleared for good as we rose through it and welcomed the much missed warm sun. For the first time in ages, we can see in the distance the beautiful countryside we had been walking through. In front of us in a great panorama—Spain! The sky is a magnificent, completely clear blue. The path now has signposts, each with the scallop shell in yellow and blue, the colours of the Camino. The signs tell us we have two hours and 15 minutes until we reach Roncesvalles. We are feeling every muscle in our legs but we're sure we can make it.

The path gradually makes its way down towards the treeline, to hedgerows and small trees and then a beech forest—a small one at first after which we emerge into scrubby fields and then into another beech forest, a vast, enormous wood than seems to go on forever, and forever downwards. My legs start to wobble like jelly; Dad's were the same. Walking down can be just as hard as going up. We had to be very careful not to let our knees bend too much and just collapse down hill.

Though difficult, our path is extremely beautiful. We are enveloped in gigantic green forest where the floor is cool and sheltered from the sun, dappled light dancing on the path. Where there are gaps in the trees, beams of light hit the forest floor and there are explosions of ferns and grass and berry bushes.

And then a sign telling us Roncesvalles was less than a kilometre away. Ahead of us as we emerge from the forest onto a broad, open path, there are two women walking. One has no backpack and seems to be struggling. The other, walking in front of her, carries two bags. As we pass them, the bag-less girl is in tears and seems to be in a lot of pain. She is Italian. The other girl is Austrian. They met this morning, and coming down the mountain the Italian girl fell and hurt her leg. She is devastated, in pain and angry with herself. She thinks her leg is broken. Dad gets a man in a car to bring her to the *albergue* and an ambulance is called. I felt so sorry for her; her Camino is over before it has really begun.

RONCESVALLES

PETER: Roncesvalles is a very substantial religious settlement at the foot of the Pyrénées in Navarra and is the first major point of departure on the Camino in Spain. There are two routes to Roncesvalles from France: one is the Cize Pass, up and over the Pyrénées, which is the one Natasha and I took, like almost all other pilgrims; the other is via Valcarlos, a way that follows much of the modern road into Spain from St-Jean-Pied-de-Port and which derives its name from the fact that Charlemagne's army suffered a great defeat there, or thereabouts, in 778 AD.

History, myth, legend and lies all combine in and around Roncesvalles. They do so to such an extent that it is almost impossible to disentangle the story of the development of the Camino from the 9th century on and the great French/Spanish drive simultaneously against the Moors, the Reconquest of Spain. They have become part of the overall story. On the one hand, there was the secular political imperative on the part of the French and the dispossessed rulers across northern Spain to regain territorial control from the Moors. On the other, the Catholic Church wanted to rid Iberia of Islam. In this, the church's great driving force was the Benedictine abbey at Cluny in France, which had imperialistic ambitions to extend its rule far and wide. To this end, it funded the building of religious communities in France and Spain, and the means to move between them.

It was good luck indeed that in 813 AD, the Galician hermit Pelayo heard music and saw lights above a place known as *campo stella*—the field of stars. Stars were already an established part of life across much of northern Spain: the Milky Way, whose stars seems to 'flow' west, directed pagans to a place they knew as the end of the earth, *finis terra*, where they saw the sun, their giver of life, disappear into the sea beyond the horizon only to return the next day, reborn. They traversed an east/west road or path which opened the way to and from the mineral-rich areas of Asturias and Galicia and which the Romans then used as a template for much of their road across northern Spain, the Via Traiana. In northern Spain as elsewhere in the Northern Hemisphere, the sky at night can be filled with shooting stars, in the summer months in particular. But the ones Pelayo said he saw directed him to a particular spot on Mount Libredón. And there he found the graves of three people whom the bishop on the Galician port city of Iria Flavia, Bishop Teodomiro, quickly 'confirmed' were the remains of St James the Greater and two of his disciples, Atanasio and Teodoro. James was no ordinary saint: of the 12 Apostles, he was one of the three closest to Jesus Christ and may even have been related to him through his mother, who was related to Mary, the mother of Jesus.

No one knows how James came to be buried in Galicia. Medieval assertions have him preaching there after Christ's edict to his disciples to spread his Word. It was claimed that James went to 'western places', said to be Galicia. He preached and recruited seven followers but returned to Jerusalem where he fell foul of King Herod and was beheaded in 44 AD. Somehow his body was returned to Galicia (in a stone boat without oars or sails, according to one version) and was buried in secret ... until Pelayo the hermit came along at a most politically and religiously opportune moment. Between James's death and the discovery of his remains, the Romans had left Iberia and were replaced by the Visigoths, who were themselves displaced by the Moors. But the Moors never quite got all of Iberia and, in the north, small groups of Visigoth Christians remained. Their ultimate reconquest of Spain took all of 800 years. The Moors rode into battle with relics of the prophet Mohammed. The Christians had no such inspiration to steel their nerves; but the finding by the hermit Pelayo gave them a powerful, and locally based, talisman.

Over the succeeding decades and centuries, a church and eventually several cathedrals were built in the *campo stella*, which soon became Santiago—Spanish for Saint James—of Compostela, hence Santiago de Compostela. The relics of the saint were kept inside the holy shrine and were fought over many times. Miracles began to be attributed to the saint and James himself appeared, at one time riding to war as Santiago Matamoros, St James the Moor Slayer, smiting Saracens all about him and making a decisive intervention that turned a major battle into a Christian rout of their enemies. On another occasion, a horseman was said to have fallen into the sea off Galicia and James appeared to save him, pulling the man from what would have been a watery grave. The rider emerged from the sea festooned with scallop shells. These quickly become the enduring symbol of the saint and are today worn by almost every single pilgrim who makes the journey to Santiago de Compostela.

But there is reason to suspect that, like so much else in Christianity, the story of the scallop shell may be deeper, richer and more complex. The scallop has been associated with notions of fertility, and hence birth and re-birth, since at least the 8th century BC when the Greek oral poet Hesiod explained the birth of Aphrodite, the goddess of sexual love. She was said to have emerged from the sea off Cyprus floating on a scallop shell. The motif turns up in a Christian context around 245 AD in a painting above the Torah shrine in a synagogue in Dura Europos, a city on the eastern bank of the Euphrates in modern-day Syria. And we find it also in a poem by the Christian Sophronius, who was born in Damascus in 550 AD and became Patriarch of Jerusalem in 633 AD. One of his compositions is *The Anastasis*, which in ancient Greek means resurrection, in which there is a claim that Christ's tomb was surrounded by shells (conches), also suggesting rebirth.

Let me walk thy pavements
and go inside the Anastasis,
where the King of All rose again,
trampling down the power of death.
I will venerate the sweet floor,
and gaze on the holy Cube,[6]
and the great four …
… like the heavens.
Through the divine sanctuary
I will penetrate the divine Tomb,
and with deep reverence
will venerate that Rock.
And as I venerate that worthy Tomb,
surrounded by its conches
and columns surmounted by golden lilies,
I shall be overcome with joy.

None of this detracts from the validity of people's faith or devotions, in my view. It just makes it all more interesting—richer, deeper, more layered and colourful. Symbolism was an enormously powerful force in the Middle Ages and a powerful tool in the hands of those promoting devotion to St James and also those who saw securing Spain for Catholicism as part of the one battle against Islam. (For similar reasons, the dictator Franco invoked Santiago Matamoros as he sought to entrench Catholicism in Spain following his Civil War victory in 1939.)

In the late 8th century, the Moors were fighting among themselves. The Muslim rulers of Barcelona, Zaragoza, Girona and other parts of

6. The tabernacle, similar to the kaaba, the cube-shaped building in Mecca, holiest shrine in Islam.

northern Spain were under threat from Abd ar-Rahman I, the all-powerful emir of Córdoba. They sought help from Charlemagne, the strongly pro-Catholic Carolingian King of the Franks who, during a life of war, would unite much of western Europe under his rule and eventually be crowned Emperor of Rome on Christmas Day, 800 AD. As ruler of France, it was in Charlemagne's interest to have compliant Muslim allies just over the Pyrénées in northern Spain and so he invaded Spain to support them, encouraged no doubt also by the promise of booty by the Muslim ruler of Barcelona. Charlemagne conquered Girona and Pamplona and laid siege to Zaragoza but without success. On returning to France through modern-day Roncesvalles and the subsequently named Valcarlos, the rear of his army was set upon by Basque bandits on the afternoon of 15 August 778 and he suffered a great defeat.

Charlemagne's biographer, Eginhard, in his *Life of Charlemagne* written around 830, records how the trapped soldiers were all slaughtered without mercy and the Basques made off with much of the loot from their Spanish campaign. The battle is commemorated by a monument, a giant lump of rock, on a grassy area by the road in the centre of Roncesvalles. A few metres away is the Silo of Charlemagne, the oldest building in the village. It is an unusual structure—square and low lying, it is surrounded by iron railings and looks a little as though it might be a communal wash-house. When you enter, you climb stairs to a sort of altar-like seating area; below is a walkway, a bit like a cloister, that circumnavigates a pit. You can peer into the pit—into the mass of skulls and other human bones that are reputed to be the remains of those massacred in 778, including 12 of Charlemagne's most noble knights and closest warriors, one of whom was Roland, Duke of the Marches of Brittany. Excavations in 1982 found the pit was several metres deep in bones, some of them dating indeed from Carolingian times. But it is likely that many of the bones are from other graves, disturbed over time (by weather and bandits) and removed to the pit out of a sense of respect for the dead.

For the next almost 400 years, the memory of the Battle of Roncesvalles (or Ronceveaux, as it is known in French) marinaded gently in French consciousness. It re-emerged in the middle of the 12th century as the fully formed *Song of Roland (La Chanson de Roland)*, the earliest surviving major work of French literature. A significant work for sure but one in which the Basque bandits have been transformed into blood-thirsty Muslim Saracens, and Charlemagne's army, far from scurrying north to escape the ambush, nobly turns around (on hearing Roland's olifant, or horn, calling for help). Christian warriors to a man, they reinvade Moorish Spain and avenge the deaths of their comrades.

The key to this propagandising is the Camino and the parallel imperatives of re-establishing Catholicism throughout Spain and repelling the Moors back across the straits of Gibraltar into north Africa. The *Song of Roland* draws the two together in a seamless narrative that propagandises the cause in epic poetry through 4,002 lines in 291 verses. The rearguard of Charlemagne's army is given as 20,000 strong; the Saracens, sometimes referred to as *paynims* (an old French word for Muslims or pagan) are 100,000 strong. The imbalance suits the need to portray one side as noble and fearless.

Charlemagne is portrayed as seeking an honourable peace after an offer comes from Marsilion, the Muslim ruler of Zaragoza, to convert to Christianity if Charlemagne will only leave Spain. Marsilion

… Promise him lions and bears and hounds galore,
Sev'n hundred camels and a thousand mewed [i.e. non moulting] hawks,
Four hundred pack mules with gold and silver store,
And fifty wagons, a wagon train to form,
Whence he may give his soldiers rich rewards …

And the Moor says he will follow Charlemagne to Aix in France and there … *submit unto the Christian law, / And be his man of faith and fealty sworn …*

Charlemagne is convinced eventually of the Moor's good intent and he leads the main part of his army through Valcarlos and back into France, leaving his rear guarded by a force led by Roland and some of his, Charlemagne's, bravest knights. But as Charlemagne crosses into France, Roland hears a great hubbub bearing down on them from behind—*One hundred thousand stout Saracens … each one afire with zeal to do great deeds …* Roland seeks to rouse and inspire his men for battle.

… 'Here must we stand to serve on the King's side.
Men for their lord's great hardship must abide,
Fierce heat and cold endure in every clime,
Lose for his sake, if need be, skin and hide.
Look to it now! Let each man stoutly smite!
No shameful songs be sung for our despite!
Paynims are wrong, Christians are in the right!
Ill tales of me shall no man tell, say I' …

The battle rages; the slaughter is great. Roland uses his olifant to summon Charlemagne's return. He fights mightily with his trusty sword, Durendal, and when overwhelmed, falls on top of both it and the horn to prevent them falling into Saracen hands. (Legend has it that Durendal came from Hector of Troy, that it contained a tooth of St Peter and a piece of the raiment of Mary and that, today, a sword plunged into a rock in Rocamadour, in Lot in southwest France, is the very same Durendal of Roland.) But all Durendal's powers cannot save the brave knight.

… Now Roland feels death press upon him hard;
It's creeping down from head to heart.
Under a pine-tree he hastens him apart,
There stretches him face down on the green grass,
And lays beneath him his sword and Olifant …

He makes his peace with God.

… On the steep hill-side, toward Spain he's turned his head,
And with one hand he beats upon his breast;
Saith: 'Mea Culpa; Thy mercy, Lord, I beg
For all the sins, both the great and the less,
That e'er I did since first I drew my breath
Unto this day when I'm struck down by death' …
… 'Father most true, in whom there is no lie,
Who didst from death St Lazarus make to rise,
And bring out Daniel safe from the lion's might,
Save Thou my soul from danger and despite
Of all the sins I did in all my life.'

His right-hand glove he's tendered unto Christ,
And from his Gabriel accepts the sign.
Straightway his head upon his arm declines;
With folded hands he makes an end and died …
… Roland is dead, in Heaven God hath his soul.
The Emperor Charles rides in to Ronceveaux …

Too late of course … but not for revenge against the Saracen army—*Sons of the desert, a wild and godless clan; / You'll ne'er hear tell of such repulsive scamps*—which he pursues to the banks of the Ebro, killing tens of thousands before taking Zaragoza.

… All Saragossa lies in the Emperor's might.
Some thousand French search the whole town, to spy
Synagogues out and mosques and heathen shrines.
With heavy hammers and with mallets of iron
They smash the idols, the images they smite,
Make a clean sweep of mummeries and lies,
For Charles fears God and still to serve Him strives …

This was stirring stuff indeed, sufficient to inspire faltering pilgrims on their way to Santiago de Compostela. The pilgrimage to Santiago grew by leaps and bounds through the 8th, 9th and 10th centuries to the point where it was one of the three most important shrines in Christendom, along with Rome and Jerusalem. Roncesvalles was founded in 1132 as a religious community and hospice, the main aim being to protect pilgrims from wolves and propagate devotion to the Virgin Mary. Over subsequent centuries, many other buildings emerged—a colegiata church with an abbot and both monks and secular canons, a cloister, a chapel to Santiago, an ossuary for the bones of pilgrims who died crossing the Pyrénées (now the Silo of Charlemagne) and a granary that today is a museum containing many fascinating items. One of them is Charlemagne's Chessboard, a square frame collection of relics set in rows of beautifully presented gold, silver and cobalt-blue enamel boxes. The relics of those believed to have been closest to Jesus are at the top. Women are at the bottom. At the height of their power, the Order of St Maria of Roncesvalles had estates in Spain, France, England, Germany and Portugal and the head of the community was second in authority in Navarra after the Bishop of Pamplona.

It fell to a 12th-century French monk, Aymeric Picaud from Poitou in France, to produce the first pilgrim's guide to the Camino. It was titled the *Codex Calixtinus* or the *Liber Sancti Jacobi.* He made the pilgrimage on horseback and brought a determinedly French perspective to all he surveyed. He is very much part of why the main Camino from St-Jean to Santiago is still called the Camino Francés, the French Way. The first reference you will find to the good monk is on a viewing plaque not far from Orisson as you scale the Pyrénées. From where you have come, and what lies ahead, according to his guide, you may not find encouraging.

According to him, St-Jean-Pied-de-Port is a place where "there are evil toll-gatherers who will certainly be damned through and through. In point of fact, they actually advance towards the pilgrims with two or three sticks, extorting by force an unjust tribute. And if some traveller refuses to hand over the money at their request, they beat him with the sticks and snatch away the toll-money while cursing him and searching even through his breeches. These are ferocious people; and the land in which they dwell is savage, wooded and barbarous. The ferociousness of their faces and likewise of their barbarous speech scares the wits out of those who see them. Though according to the rules and regulations they should not demand a tribute from anybody but merchants, they unjustly cash in from pilgrims and all sorts of travellers. Whenever they ought to receive, according to the usage, four or six coins or a certain service, they cash in eight or twelve, that is to say, double."

At the top of the mountain, history and myth collide. Remember, when Charlemagne was verifiably in Roncesvalles, the alleged remains of St James had yet to be found in Santiago.

"In the Basque country," writes Picaud, "there is on the road of St James a very high mountain, which is called Port-de-Cize ... On the summit of this mountain there is a place called the Cross of Charles, because it was here that Charles, setting out with his armies for Spain, opened up once a passageway with axes, hatchets, pickaxes and other implements, and that he first erected the sign of the cross of the Lord and, falling on his knees and turning towards the land of St James, use to offer there a prayer while each planted his own cross of the Lord like a standard. Indeed, one can find there up to a thousand crosses; and that is why that place is the first station of prayer of St James ... Near this mountain, to be sure, towards the north, there is a valley called Valcarlos where Charles himself encamped together with his armies after his warriors had been slain at Roncesvalles … in descending from the summit, one finds the hospice and the church with the rock that Roland, the formidable hero, split with his sword in the middle, from top to bottom, in a triple stroke. Next one comes to Roncesvalles, the site where, to be sure, once took place the big battle in which King Marsile, Roland, Oliver as well as forty thousand Christian and Saracen soldiers were slain …"

According to Picaud, once beyond Roncesvalles and into Navarra, the pilgrim must beware!

"This is a barbarous nation, distinct from all other nations in habits and way of being, full of all kind of malice, and black colour. Their face is ugly, and they are debauched, perverse, perfidious, disloyal and corrupt, libidinous, drunkard, given to all kinds of violence, ferocious and savage, impudent and false, impious and uncouth, cruel and quarrelsome, incapable of anything virtuous, well-informed of all vices and iniquities.

"In malice they resemble the Getae [a people living in Thrace, near the lower Danube] and the Saracens, and are in everything inimical to our Gallic nation. If they could, the Navarrese or the Basque would kill a Frenchman for no more than a coin. In certain of their regions, namely in Vizcaya and Alava, when the Navarrese warm up, the man shows to the woman and the woman to the man their respective shame. The Navarrese also make use of animals for incestuous fornication. It is told that the Navarrese affixes a lock to the behind of his mule or horse, so that no one else but he may have access to them. Also, he kisses lasciviously the vulva of women and mules.

"That is why the Navarrese are rebuked by all who are prudent. Notwithstanding the above, they are valorous on the battlefield, inept in the assault of fortresses, reliable in the payment of the tithe, and assiduous in making offerings on the altar. Every day, in effect, when the Navarrese goes to church, he makes an offering to God of bread or wine or wheat or some other substance.

"After this land, one traverses the forest of Oca, to be sure in the direction of Burgos. There follows the land of the Spaniards, that is to say, Castilla and Campos. This country is full of treasures, of gold and silver; it abounds in fodder and in vigorous horses, and it has plenty of bread, wine, meat, fish, milk, and honey. On the other hand, it is poor wood and full of evil and vicious people.

"Thence, having crossed the territory of León and cleared the passes of Mount Irago and Mount Cebrero, one arrives to the land of the Galicians. This country is wooded, provided with excellent rivers, meadows and orchards, and with plenty of good fruits and clear springs; on the other hand, it is poor in cities, towns, and cultivated fields. Bread, wheat, and wine are scarce, but rye bread and cider abound, as do livestock and beasts of burden, milk, and honey. The sea fish is either enormously large or small. The land abounds in gold and silver, fabrics, the fur of wild animals and many other goods, as well as in Saracen treasures.

"The Galicians, ahead of the other uncouth nations of Spain, are those who best agree in their habits with our French people; but they are irascible and contentious."

Onwards to Galicia! But I better keep a careful watch over Natasha lest those disgusting Navarrese set their eyes on her …

THE APPEAL OF THE CAMINO

NATASHA: When I try to think of why I'm doing the Camino, my mind runs loose on thoughts. It's the most commonly asked question by people you meet along the way, and by people at home, some of whom have never heard of it. There is a curiosity behind the walk and the people who do it. Many presume people walk for religious reasons, and this is often the case. People often find doing the Camino will help them find their religion, or at least help them understand why they believe in the religion they do. Or perhaps people do it to connect further with their religion because it's a very ancient, religious and spiritual pilgrimage. In nearly every town we pass, there is an old church, and often a Mass on in the evenings to which one can go.

But many do it because they can. Because it's there, and because they want to get away from it all. The Camino is the Camino. There are no complications or snags here such as there might be at home. In

Roncesvalles, Dad and I met a family of four from the Netherlands. The parents were saying goodbye to their two teenage daughters who were starting their journey from there. The dad was telling us that one day he just got up and closed the door of his house in Holland and started walking. He walked all the way to Santiago, from April until July.

When you're walking, it's just you and your surroundings. Your mind goes wandering to places you never thought possible. You have time, with no distractions; time to think about a particular issue in your life that needs action. There is nobody here to influence you. The decisions made here are completely yours, and you will never doubt them, because you have had so much time to make them. The people you meet and the places you go to will make you re-evaluate things in your life. You will start to reconsider what's genuinely important to you and what's important in general. The Camino acts as a cleanser: it clears your mind, releasing all the stress that has kept you lying awake at night worrying. The walking brings you freedom of mind, and with that freedom you can make the decision you need to.

There are many reasons why I'm doing this. But yet I find it difficult to explain when asked. This is my second time doing the Camino, so the thought of another journey was always there. I suppose, to begin with, it was never my idea—it was my Dad's. Perhaps one of the reasons I'm doing it is because it was offered to me. But the more I thought about it, the more I liked the idea. It interested me; I didn't quite understand the idea of walking on a specific trail that was made for the pilgrims. I saw it as a sort of treasure hunt. And our treasure was Santiago and infinite rest. Another reason it appealed to me was because it was an athletic challenge. Exercise is something I enjoy, and so this also drew me in. But the biggest and most important reason I wanted to do this was, it meant time with my Dad, time with him that will be remembered and appreciated forever, particularly when I'm old.

I've noticed from last time I did this, and this time, that often we won't speak for an hour, yet we will be beside each other. Both our minds are thinking about different things, and the only noise is the tapping of our feet walking, together.

I often think about my Mum and brother Patrick, and what they might be doing. Mum usually sends me a ridiculous text that sums up her day, and sometimes signs it from one of our dogs or cats. I also think about my best friend, Andrea, and what news I'm missing out on. My curiosity is often satisfied with a gossipy text, which usually arrives from her around evening time.

The Camino is also an opportunity for me to see my Dad flourish in his interesting choice of holiday wear. As I stand and observe him taking a photo for a couple underneath the sign for Santiago in Roncesvalles, I think: "How embarrassing!" He stands up straight, his right leg a little forward, and leaning ever so slightly backwards. He wears a pair of beige cargo shorts that have zips on the ends where you can add on the end of a leg to turn them into long trousers. He has his self-proclaimed 'rather cool' Velcro sandals on and a mini-hip fanny pack, where our camera sits. His T-shirt is grey and has a huge baseball glove on it with writing across the chest spelling: 'American Baseball league'. And to finish things off, he has a cream fishing hat with a couple of badges perched on his head. He says, other than it being "really cool", it protects his bald patch from getting burnt.

Those are the sort of things that make Dad, Dad. Along with ridiculous jokes at 6.30 am, which is when he seems to be at his liveliest, and his continuous 'wannabe poet' comments like: "Don't you just love the peace of the woods and the crunching of our footsteps". And changing him would be changing my Camino, because he is what really makes the Camino special for me, and he makes up the biggest reason for doing this.

Roncesvalles to Zubiri: 21 km in 6 hours

PETER: When we arrived in Roncesvalles, almost the first thing we did (after getting our pilgrim passports stamped and unloading our backpacks in the *albergue*) was have a cold beer. Nothing tastes as good as a well-earned, cold beer. Except perhaps another. Sitting in the shade of the only café in the village and watching the world go by we met two other pilgrims, Paul and Eva from Sweden.

"Do you know Burguete?" asked Eva.

"No," I replied.

"Only we were thinking of going there tonight and not staying in Roncesvalles."

"Why? After such a long trek over the mountains, have you not had enough for one day?"

"Yes, but we want to see the piano on which Hemingway wrote his name."

"The vandal! Surely not," I said.

"Yes, I think it is so," said Eva before explaining that Ernest apparently used stay in some fancy hotel in Burguete.

For a period when I was about 18, I was sure I was going to be Hemingway. I got over it soon enough but not before ploughing through many of his books, starting with *Fiesta—The Sun Also Rises*, a part of which is set in Pamplona, and moving on to *A Farewell to Arms*. Like him, I fell in love with his Italian nurse, and I too would live a dissolute life in Paris, roam the world making love and having adventures. It would be life on the edge, and I would write about it and make a fortune. A year or three later, I guess, reality got in the way …

Eva and Paul headed off on their Hemingway pilgrimage and, as we set out from Roncesvalles in their wake next morning, I wondered had they found the hotel. At 6.00 am, the moon was still huge in the sky; the sun but an ochre tinge behind the ridge of the Pyrénées. Tash and I walked through the woods in silence, listening to the dawn chorus. Soon there was a group of Spanish people behind us, one of them insisting on talking at full volume. We sped up past the Cruz de Peregrinos, a 14th-century cross just outside Roncesvalles, and made good our escape.

Burguete is a pretty little village with both the Camino and the main road running in unison through it. 'Ruta Hemingway' proclaims a large poster at the entry to the village. It shows a picture of the great man and some of the locations in Navarra associated with him. A little further on in Biskarret, there is a welcome café with a table outside. Paul and Eva are there before us.

"So?" I said, "did he?"

"What?" asked Eva.

"Write on the piano!"

"Oh. We didn't stay there. It was €45 and we didn't want to spend that much, but it looked like a nice hotel."

Forty-five euro seems a paltry sum to satisfy one's Hemingway interest. The occasion demanded crisp, clean sheets in a boutique hotel at a minimum. A bottle of Margaux, surely …

Paul operates a lathe in a small engineering firm in Örebro in western Sweden. He is slim and tall, wears a baseball cap over salt-and-pepper hair and is rather serious, in a Scandinavian sort of way. Eva is a youth worker and a trainer of other people who want to work with young people. She is shorter than Paul, stocky and has a round face which regularly breaks into a warm smile. At a guess, I'd say they are both in their early 50s. They have three children: two of their own, a boy and a girl; and the third, an unofficially adopted Serbian woman from Bosnia. Boka was 15 when her parents sent her to relatives in Örebro, away from her home near Banja Luka because of the war then raging in Bosnia. The relatives, however, had reared their own children and, it seems, didn't fancy second helpings. Relations didn't work out, all of which became known to Eva through her youth work.

"We chose her and she chose us," Eva explains with a smile.

There was no official adoption; Boka simply moved in with the family and has spent the rest of her life in Sweden. She is now in her 30s, is married to a Swede and is expecting a baby, a source of joy to Paul and Eva. She is going to be a youth worker like Eva. Paul's son works with him but is about to go to college in Stockholm to study engineering. Their other daughter is training to be a pastor.

Paul and Eva are practising Lutherans. They take their faith seriously but wear it lightly. They hope to be in Santiago on 25 August, their silver wedding anniversary. The family is flying down from Sweden to join them. Eva likes what Natasha and I are doing.

"You know, in Sweden," she says, "one in five young people in ninth grade has done self harm. There is really something wrong today. I do not know what it is but there is something wrong."

I say that Swedish society has always seemed to me to have a lot of things sorted out. "Yes," says Paul, "but you know in Sweden if you are not in the system, if you fall out somehow, you really don't exist any more."

Paul and Eva are typical of the people you meet on the Camino.

A village shop yields up salami and cheese and nectarines and apples and a stick of bread plus a penknife to attack it all. It takes the pain away from the disappointing municipal *albergue* in Zubiri. Built between 1939 and 1940, when Franco was settling in for the duration and the Spanish church was entering its period of greatest influence in the 20th century, it has all the architectural charm of a telephone exchange. Or maybe an ESB sub-station. It is painted white with green windows, which is fine. Perhaps it was the metal grills over the windows or the rural national-school lino on the floors and glossy painted dormitory walls inside that did it. Either way, it is a place devoid of charm.

Zubiri itself is not much better. It straddles either side of the Roncesvalles to Pamplona road and the largest employer in town is a huge magnesite factory just outside. The plant is on the floor of the lush, tree-lined Esteribar Valley where it makes its presence felt, belching stuff into the atmosphere. There are huge, inert tailing ponds further along the valley floor, and dust, lots of dust.

Pilgrims enter and leave Zubiri by crossing a steeply arched medieval bridge over the Río Arga. The central pillar holding it up is said to contain a relic of St Quiteria. According to local lore, cows that walk around the pillar three times are protected from rabies.

But not from the magnesite plant.

Zubiri to Pamplona: 21 km in 6 hours

PETER: Today's walk promises not to be stressful. The gradient is mostly down, ending in our first major city, where we must stop for two days to catch up with writing. The Camino winds its way along the side of the valley, through woods of dappled light and welcome shade. The villages are mostly tiny; some have even ceased to be villages as such. At one, Illaratz, the church has been incorporated into a house, to the evident absence of benefit to either structure: both look like they are about to fall down. There is a scattering of other houses, sturdy looking buildings on the side of the valley, leaving the valley floor, with its rich soil, free for farming. The houses are three or four storeys high, the bottom floor in times past being used for animals. An enterprising young boy has taken over the basement of his family home and sells soft drinks and biscuits to passing pilgrims.

At Zabaldica, a sign urges pilgrims to visit the 13th-century church of St Stephen. It is a tiny building perched at the top of a steep slope but it has to be worth a visit …

NATASHA: We are welcomed by an old lady. She is standing outside the church and asks us to come in. "Where are you from?" she inquires in accented but perfect English. I tell her I'm Irish, to which she replies: "Ah yes, of course you are; you have freckles and red hair!"

The church is built of dressed stone. A leaflet in English says it is Romanesque and that its barrel-vaulted dome is pointed. It has a delicate, subtle beauty, which is not intimidating and makes one feel welcome. The inside is tiny, with room for only five or six pews on either side of the aisle. But what really caught my eye was what was immediately in front of me through the entrance door: a statue of Jesus Christ on the crucifix, and around him, hundreds of green post-its in the shapes of arrows. Written on them were visitors' messages. There was so many, they were almost swallowing the statue. They were overlapping one another, and some were in a basket on the floor. As I got closer, I could see that almost every language was there. Even small children had written messages and drawn little pictures to go with them. I scanned the green sea for English ones that I could read. Among them I found one that read: "For my grandson, Juhl Bengard, and for his health. Watch over him." Another: "Dad, this is for you. I want you to get well. God bless John, Rosie, Jean, Damien and all our friends."

They were wonderful to read. I hope their wishes come true, and somehow, I felt that there was something special about this board of notes, and that I should write my own. Mine read: "Thank you for everything I have; my Mum, my Dad, my brother and all my friends. Thank you for my loved ones I have lost; please give them my love."

I thought of my Granddad. As I walked away, I somehow believed that Nanna, Granfa, Granny, Uncle Mike and Granddad were all sitting there reading my note.

PETER: The altarpiece is typical of many one sees in Spanish churches, even ones as tiny as this, supported by a community of just eight homes and 29 residents. Even in centuries gone by, there cannot have been many people living here. At the top of the altarpiece in the centre is Mary being assumed into Heaven. On either side of her are Engracia of Zaragoza, Catherine of Alexandria, Mary Magdalene and Barbara. In the middle row there's St Stephen, pride of place in his own church; Michael the Archangel, his foot firmly holding down an ugly looking, cloven-hoofed demon; the Apostle Bartholomew; a depiction of the martyrdom of St Sebastian; and St Francis of Assisi. The bottom row shows John the Baptist, Bishop Stanislaus from Poland (for no reason that is apparent); John the Evangelist; and, of course, St James himself. Zabaldica straddles the Camino, the church on one side of the path, the village on the other. In the altarpiece James is shown as a pilgrim to his own shrine, a common depiction and one apparently unique to him.

"Where are you from?" asks the old lady who welcomed us in and I tell her Wicklow; very near Dublin, I add. "Monkstown," she says. "I have been to Monkstown."

"Really?" I say.

"Yes. And Drumcondra as well. We have a house there."

"So does the Archbishop," I add.

"And we have a school also. Mount Anville. I am with the Sacred Heart. My name in Mariasun. Buen Camino!"

And she gives me and Natasha a short printed note, headed El Camino and written a few years ago by a Jesuit, José Antonio Garcia Monje. This is what it says:

> *The journey makes you a pilgrim. Because the way to Santiago is not only a track to be walked in order to get somewhere, nor is it a test to reach any reward. El Camino de Santiago is a parable and a reality at once because it is done both within and outside in the specific time that [it] takes to walk each stage, and along the entire life if only you allow the Camino to get into you, to transform you and to make [you] a pilgrim.*
>
> *The Camino makes you simpler, because the lighter the backpack the less strain to your back and the more you will experience how little you need to be alive.*
>
> *The Camino makes you brother/sister. Whatever you have you must be ready to share because even if you started on your own, you will meet companions. The Camino breeds community: community that greets the other, that takes interest in how the walk is going for the other, that takes and shares with the other.*
>
> *The Camino makes demands on you. You must get up even before the sun in spite of tiredness or blisters; you must walk in the darkness of night while dawn is growing; you must just get the rest that will keep you going.*
>
> *The Camino calls you to contemplate, to be amazed, to welcome, to interiorise, to stop, to be quiet, to listen, to admire, to bless … Nature, our companions on the journey, our own selves, God.*

PAMPLONA

PETER: The Camino enters Pamplona the way cities should be approached—slowly so they reveal themselves bit by bit, layer by layer. In Pamplona's case there are first modern outer suburbs, as might be expected. But then, unlike a modern road slicing its way through virgin territory and attracting development in its wake, the Camino, because it is ancient and set in its way, veers this way and that, taking one through scrubland, rows of old cottages and tiny farms and then, without warning, one is at the beautiful Puente de la Magdalena, a medieval arched bridge over the Río Arga. The city is built strategically on a bend in the river, high on one bank. The Camino winds its way through a gap in the 16th-century fortifications, up a cobble-stoned street and into the cathedral area, part of what is known as the city's historic quarter.

The streets are narrow and all pedestrianised. The buildings front immediately onto the streets and are all four and five storeys high. The façades are not in great condition; in fact, it all looks a bit dingy but it's alive with character and charm. There are old-world shops, family-run affairs; old-style drapery stores and suchlike. And yes, of course, there are tourist shops and restaurants and all of what a visitor would expect. But at the same time it seems genuine, not so cutie-pie perfect. The municipal *albergue* is incredible: it is inside a refurbished, early 17th-century church, the Church of Jesus and Mary, which belonged to the Jesuits. In 2007 the city authorities opened it as a pilgrim hostel. The inside of the building is now ultra modern, all wood panelling and subdued lighting. There are 112 beds set out in dormitories in the side aisles on the ground floor. The same layout is repeated above, on a suspended glass floor. There are communal showers and toilets, internet connections, a courtyard for the smokers and, at the very top of the building, an ultra-modern kitchen. You stay here (but only if you are a *bona fide* pilgrim) for €4 a night, plus €2 for a sheet and pillow case.

Ernest Hemingway used to stay at the Hotel la Perla on the edge of the Plaza del Castillo and if it didn't cost him an arm and a leg in the 1920s and 1930s, it sure would today. Just opposite is 'his' café/bar, the Iruña, now a very chi-chi place altogether. The experience of sitting there in the sun having a beer, scribbling in my Moleskine notebook and pretending ... is spoilt by having to listen simultaneously to the most boring Austrian on the planet. I feel I now know the blisters on his two little toes probably as well as he does ... and everyone else he has met in the past two days. The city makes the most of its Hemingway heritage, something which apparently depressed the old man when he returned in the late 1950s and saw what his writing had spawned. The running of the bulls, about which he wrote in *The Sun Also Rises*, had become a monster fiesta. The shops all along Estafeta, the main street through which the running takes place all the way down to the bull ring, have photographs of the fiesta in years gone by and it is clear that in the 1920s just a handful of men, several dozen maybe and mostly in suits, diced with the bulls by running ahead of them. By contrast today, tens of thousands crowd into the city for the running in early July, and hundreds of runners (mainly but not exclusively men; I nurture a yearning to have a go one day) do their thing wearing 'traditional' Basque garb of white trousers, red scarves and carrying what look like rolled-up newspapers. Not much of a defence against a raging bull …

They enter the bull ring by a bust of the great man, a magnificent bronze head sticking out of a polo-neck sweater and mounted on a suitably monumental plinth of granite. He looks strong, noble even. Ernest Hemingway, it proclaims, Nobel laureate, friend of Pamplona, admirer of fiestas. There is precious little nobility on show when the bulls eventually get into the ring. I went to a bull fight once in Mallorca. It was ghastly; horrific. No grace under pressure, no death with dignity. Just cruelty and butchery and degradation of man and beast. Man is not made for defeat, Hemingway once wrote. But there is something fundamentally defeating about watching a creature slaughtered for ritual human pleasure. It doesn't seem like winning to watch a bull fight. Poor old Hemingway. It all ended miserably for him too—with a double-barrelled shotgun in a hunting lodge in Ketchum, Idaho. For many, his best work (and the one he felt should have won him the Nobel Prize for Literature instead of *The Old Man and The Sea*) was *For Whom The Bell Tolls*, his novel set against the backdrop of the Spanish Civil War. It's one of the best titles of a novel, ever. It comes from one of John Donne's poems, a poem whose central message chimes with the Camino, a place and a state of mind, where you meet people from all corners of the world and we look out for each other …

No man is an island entire of itself; every man
is a piece of the continent, a part of the main;
if a clod be washed away by the sea, Europe
is the less, as well as if a promontory were, as
well as any manner of thy friends or of thine

own were; any man's death diminishes me,
because I am involved in mankind.
And therefore never send to know for whom
the bell tolls; it tolls for thee.

As it happens, the Camino and the route of Pamplona's bull run intersect, at Plaza Consistorial. Had Hemingway paid more attention to the Camino he might have had a happier time of it and a less bloody exit.

There's a market hall not far from Estafeta (best tapas, by the way, is to be had in the incredibly cool Bodegón Sarria on Estafeta—to hell with Café Iruña!). The market hall is filled with displays of fresh fish and meat, fruit and vegetables, cold meats and cheese. For the princely sum of €8.91 we get: 10 slices of salami, six of parma ham and about 25 centimetres of chorizo; four thick slices of local cheese and a wedge of brie; a whole baguette; a bruiser of a tomato and a whole garlic; two apples, two peaches, two nectarines and a litre-bottle of ice tea. We picnic like royalty.

Pamplona turns out to be a two-day affair—too far behind with our writing, so we need to catch up. As pilgrims are allowed stay just one night in each *albergue* (unless injured), we have to move. Just outside the old city, beside the Puente de la Magdalena, is the Casa Paderborn, a pretty two-storeyed stone and stucco house backing onto the river. Its window boxes are overflowing with geraniums. A tiny garden to the side is a little oasis of perennials—daisies, more geraniums and day lilies all hemmed in by privet hedging—and a dining table under the shade of a vine-covered pergola. Here a pilgrim may stay for €4 (plus €2 more for breakfast if desired!) in the lea of the city walls and cathedral, two minutes walk from everything.

Casa Paderborn sleeps 26 and is run by the Freundeskreis Der Jakobuspilger (rough translation from German: the association of friends of St James) from Paderborn, which is about 100 kilometres east of Dortmund. Katrin, a smiley 33-year-old volunteer, is on duty when we arrive. She ushers us inside, over beautifully polished floors into what has all the appearance of a family home. Katrin is a Roman Catholic. She walked the Camino in 2008 because 'something was wrong' with her life. "I knew something was wrong and I wanted some free time, time on my own."

Katrin had left school at 16 and trained to work with mentally disabled people—helping them in a non-medical way; how to get in and out of bed, how to wash and dress; look after their financial affairs and deal with the authorities. She worked long hours and every weekend. When her sister had a son, Katrin found there was no time in her life for the little boy and she knew this was wrong. So what did the Camino do for her?

"I found I could reach my goal, which was coming to Santiago on my own and with not too many fears about [what was going on back] home. I was totally on my own, with foreign people, alone as a woman in a foreign country; maybe it was a little dangerous. But I was fine! The Camino teaches you that you don't need special things in your life—only a bed, some *café con leche* … you can have life with little things."

Katrin is now self-employed, doing exactly what she did before but working for herself this time. The Camino gave her the confidence to take charge of her life and change it.

Our dormitory bedroom is shared with two German men, two quiet, friendly fellows. We overlook the river and leave the window open for air. Lights out at 10.30 pm … and we are all fast asleep in no time at all. And wide wake again at about 1.30 am. The frogs in the river are holding a convention and noisy debate is in full flow. While hundreds seem to be croaking at the same time, there are, nonetheless, distinct voices. Conversation ebbs and flows and ceases every 10 minutes or so. And explodes again a few minutes later. The ducks do their best, quacking away at the frogs but to no discernible effect …

At 6.00 am the Aristophanean chorus dies away and is replaced by softly sung Gregorian chants wafting into every bedroom. It's the Paderborn Cathedral choir telling us it's time for breakfast … and a walk to Puente la Reina.

Pamplona to Puente la Reina: 25 km in 6.5 hours

NATASHA: It was 6.30 am and there was complete silence walking along the river by the Casa Paderborn on our way out of Pamplona. I loved it there. It had life I hadn't seen in a town before and I could have stayed longer. The city was still very much asleep as we walked up the steep street towards the cathedral. The sun was creeping up behind the horizon at our backs, casting a yellow/white sari along the silhouette of the mountains. As we came closer to the outskirts of the city, a bass seemed to beat in the cobbles. Then there was the loud chat of Spanish, and we could soon see that a nightclub was still very much alive. People were pushing out of a tiny door and spilling out onto the street. Drunk and tired, they watched us walk by, on our journey out of the city.

It was going to be a hot day, we could tell already. The sky was crystal clear—white baby blue; the colour of a hot sky. It took us half an hour to get out of Pamplona, and almost immediately we were directed to a dusty, stony path, and remained on it almost the whole way. The scenery was beautiful until the very end. We were ambushed by sunflower fields right, left and centre. They dominated the mountains and swept across the land. They had their heads down, but when the sun was high in the sky their little faces lifted, almost like they were waking up.

At times the path would grow narrow and steep and was bordered by spiky green bushes and cut wheat fields. I would often stop walking and look around me. It was just beautiful. The land below us looked like a patchwork quilt of greens, yellows and browns. There were no trees around; we were completely exposed to the sun, apart from the odd high bush that covered us for a minute or two. Tired pilgrims were visible in the distance, plodding along, sweaty and struggling. One clever man had an umbrella hat on, as comical as it looked. I was a little envious.

It had been about six kilometres and Dad and I both were in need of a drink. We came to a village. We were sure there would be a café, but soon enough we found ourselves at the edge of the small town, drinkless. We asked some pilgrims who were walking out of the town if there was a café around. They said no, and just then, we heard a squeaking of Spanish from above. We looked up to see an old lady who had popped her head out of her window with the word *café*, and was throwing a bunch of words at us, one of them being *café*, and swinging her arm in the direction out of the town. Ah, there must be one just over this hill then. "Gracias!" we shout, and were off in search of our promised café, but to no avail. Maybe the old lady just wanted shot of us talking under her window!

We carry on walking on a gradual slope; beads of sweat are streaming down my face and stinging my eyes. Wiping does nothing; there's no part of your body that doesn't sweat in heat like this. I wasn't very chatty this morning; my mind was spinning, rather like the row of massive white windmills that danced on the hilltops around us. I was thinking of many things, and after about half an hour I realised I was having full-blown conversations with myself, on the various topics. I began to think the Camino was making me crazy. Perhaps it was just the heat.

I turned to Dad and said: "I can't stop thinking about my exam results."

Dad replies: "The Camino will bring us no worries."

"Or maybe it only brings me more time to worry," I say.

No matter how hard I tried, everything was going back to them. They come out in a couple of weeks or so, and I can't bear the thought of opening my results over the computer and having to add them up in order to determine my future for the next few years. I suppose the Camino is exactly what I will need *after* I do know what I have got. It will give me time alone. That's exactly what I fear I'm going to want.

After reaching the top of the hardest gradual slope we have come across yet, there on the top, looking over the bowl that holds Pamplona, sits a sculpture. One I have seen before on brochures and that. It was made of some sort of iron, and showed a cut-out trail of pilgrims walking in a row, and animals with them. It was lovely. At that moment, something that was even lovelier was a little white van perched 100 metres away. I could make out a price list on the side. €1.50 poorer, but a can of cola happier, Dad and I carried on, on the last eight-kilometre leg of our journey, downhill. There was a small village in the distance, but unfortunately it was too near to be Puente la Reina, which was where we had planned to stop. Eventually we pass through one last village before Dad speaks the words that kill me every time: "Tasha, let's just have a quick look at this church?"

Like I just bit a lemon, I twisted my face up, but said nothing, and swayed in the direction of the church. Like Dad always reminds me, his suggestion turned out to be quite cute. The little church was decorated with flowers for a wedding taking place later that morning.

PETER: The village was Uterga, an unremarkable little place on the Camino, medieval in origin but distinguished mainly by 19th- and 20th-century housing. The Church of the Ascension was pretty and had some scenes from the life of Mary and there was also a pilgrim depicted. Outside the entrance door an area of flagstones was bathed in dappled light and shade from some plane trees. A lovely place to get married; for all its ordinariness relative to other churches one sees on the Camino, later that day it will be for a time the most special place for two happy people.

NATASHA: Finally, after a good old sweat, we see Puente la Reina in the distance. Dad spots the top of the church poking through the hills. It's about five kilometres away. I'm tired, smelly and in no mood for a cheery conversation and *bang!* one hits me in the face.

"You are red!" a foreign voice shouts at me from behind. Presuming it's a comment about my hair, I turn around to see a hairy German man. "You want some cream? Your shoulder is red!" he exclaims.

I look down at my shoulder, and for once, I'm actually not burnt. I look back up at the German and realise he is wearing red-tinted sunglasses. To avoid further conversation I reply: "Oh goodness, yes I am," and take out my bottle of sun cream and squirt it on my shoulder. "Thank you," I call, thinking that's the end of that. How naïve of me.

"Where are you from? What country?"

Shit, I think. "Ireland, and you?"

"Germany," he says. "I am so tired, I walk so hard yesterday and now it's not so good on my feet and I just want my arrival to come now or I will just die."

And there it was. I was trapped. He had begun the never-ending conversation of: "It's not so good on my feet." Both Dad and I have learned *never* to ask foreigners how their feet are. After the longest 15 minutes of my life, I say: "Okay, see you later," and walk as fast as I can. It is 12.45 pm when we arrive in our *albergue* for the night. I shower and settle into my Hemingway book, *Fiesta*, which Dad bought me in Pamplona. Comfy and satisfied, I lift my head to the sun for a moment. And there he is! The German, and he's coming my way. I nosedive to the grass and pretend to sleep. He walks over, he looks, and he walks away. Relieved, I move my head, to which is followed: "Ah! You're awake, great! Oh, I'm so happy for my arrival here. My feet are tired ..."

Caught, by the German.

Puente la Reina to Estella: 22.5 km in 5 hours

PETER: Just before Puente la Reina, one of the other Camino routes from France—one that includes several other routes that have crossed the Pyrénées in the centre of the range—meets the main Camino route from St-Jean and Pamplona and merges with it. Thus, since the development of the Camino in the 11th and 12th centuries, Puente la Reina has been a place of some importance—the first significant stop on the expanded Camino. It was then a place of some difficulty for pilgrims because of the width of the Arga River. Numerous ferrymen exploited pilgrims heading west. One of the queens of Navarra, Doña Mayor or Doña Estefania, which is unclear, decided to finance the construction of a bridge.

It is a magnificent structure. Cut-stone pillars sunk into the water support graceful arches holding up a narrow, cobbled road. Like almost all the medieval pilgrim bridges, it is quite steep but a pleasing combination of elegance and strength. Natasha and I ate well, sitting on the grass on the river bank beneath the bridge, feeding on bread and cheese and salami and garlic and lemon tea and fruit. A French pilgrim caught 40 winks in the shade on the grass beside us.

Puente la Reina developed as a large village essentially on the eastern bank of the river. The main street runs straight through it right down to the bridge. There is virtually nothing on the other side. This main street is dominated by the Church of Santiago which is dedicated to St James. It has the most beautiful floor of any church I have seen: fat, wide planks of what looks like oak, half a metre wide at least, polished and varnished to a high gloss. The *retablo* behind the altar is a huge Baroque structure from the late 17th century. Panels tell James's story, from the apparition of the Virgin Mary to James, to his execution by Herod, in rather theatrical, over-the-top style. At the moment of his execution, he even has a scallop shell on his shoulder—odd, seeing as the scallop shell part of his story didn't really emerge for another 800 years or so. And there's yet another depiction of James as a pilgrim to his own shrine.

The other feature dominating the centre of Puente la Reina is the plaza, still decked out for the village bull-fest. Unfortunately, the Christian message preached in James's church was somewhat lost on the community in 1345. Two Jews, who happened also to be gay, were burned alive in the plaza for sodomy. All over northern Spain the Jews got a fairly raw deal from the 12th to the 15th centuries (mostly at the hands of Christians); gay Jews didn't stand a chance ...

Over the bridge and out of Puente le Reina next morning, the beauty of the Navarrese countryside unfolds again. Arable farming dominates: all the grain has been harvested even though it is only early August and some of the fields have even been ploughed in preparation for the next sowing. Vineyards start to multiply and there are clusters of olive trees and some almond and walnut trees. All the land is used and well tended.

Leaving a village named Cirauqui, suddenly we are walking on the best-preserved piece of the ancient Roman Via Traiana of perhaps the entire Camino. In the near distance is a motorway and flyover but we are walking on a paved stone road that is around 2,000 years old. It is edged with large cut slabs and the stones of the road itself are polished. I am mesmerised by the thought that the shine and smoothness of the stones has been caused by the feet of millions of pilgrims, among others, walking to Santiago, a procession of people that I have now joined. The Via Traiana snakes around and down a slope outside the village to a small valley and a Roman bridge, itself partly restored. In the distance, lorries swoosh along the modern highway and, not for the first time, I am struck by the parallel worlds of the Camino, the one in which we now exist, and the other from which we have escaped, albeit temporarily. These are the moments when you are most conscious that your life on the Camino operates to a different, altogether more natural, rhythm. You rise as the day begins and move through it at a pace that seems in tune with nature. You have time to think, time to examine the countryside, time to notice life.

At Lorca, a small village with a single east/west street that dominates the high ground on the road from Puente le Reina to Estella, a sweaty, unshaven, fat man sits outside his café with special offerings for pilgrims—breakfast and such like and free internet access. We stop for coffee. Fat man has some great old music on. The Crystals were belting out *And Then He Kissed Me*, with that great, all-embracing 'wall of sound' effect created by Phil Spector, now serving 20 years minimum for sticking a gun into the mouth of a sad and rather unsuccessful actress whose brains were then blown out. Spector said his wall of sound was meant to recreate Wagner for the early 1960s pop generation. Thinking of him and all that went wrong in his life got me thinking about two American lads Tash and I met at the German *albergue* in Pamplona and about whom I had been wondering how, and what, to write.

We met them mid-evening, the best time in a hot climate—the time when there's breathing in the air, the temperature is down a little and a glass of something lubricates reflective chat. The two Americans, who were aged about 23, were sitting under the vine arbour talking with David, a former British Army officer with experience in Northern Ireland. We joined them. David and I talked a bit about the North and I could tell from what he said (and didn't say), plus the sort of unit in which he served, that David had a lot of stories about the North. But like most people, David has moved on and now writes a lot of poetry and studies the effects of conflicts on those who participate in them, with particular emphasis on the effects a person's actions have on themselves. Interesting area.

The two American lads were from the mid-West and were studying, in the case of one, English, and of the other, English and film studies. The film studies one was a dead ringer for the actor Jake Gyllenhaal; same dark features, same long face, same slightly hangdog look. He also has a close-cropped black beard and long black hair. "He looked like Jesus," observed Tash. Indeed he did, did Jesus Jake. The other one has a more round face, fair hair but equally long. He was more what you'd expect to find clutching a surfboard somewhere on the coast in California. Our Irish nationality emerges early in the conversation.

"Awesome, man," says Surf Boy. "Awesome."

"Yeah," says Jesus Jake, rather longer than the word actually required.

"I'm so, like, really into your literature," says Surf Boy. "You know a guy named Sing?"

"Yes," I reply. "John Millington Synge. Wrote plays and was an important person in what we call the Celtic literary revival led by Yeats the poet."

"Yeats!" Surf Boy exclaims. "Aw man, he's just so cool. I, uh, really like Beckett and Joyce. Read him twice."

And he pulls up his sleeve to reveal a Joyce tattoo. And another of Marcel Proust. Jesus Jake smiles a silly smile at nothing in particular.

So what have you guys been doing? I ask. Aw, this an' that, comes the reply. They've been to Paris and Madrid. And then walked a bit. And then went to Santiago. Then Finisterre where they slept rough. Then back to Madrid, or was it France? And then walked some of the Camino (backwards). Now they were trying to get to Logroño, or maybe León, to get to Madrid, from where they'll fly to Amsterdam, for a 13-hour wait ("But that'll be cool," they giggle) before flying back to the States.

This prompts a conversation about the idiocy of airports and the questions you are asked by the US authorities. Last time I was in the US, three years ago, I had to fill in a form that included the query along the lines: 'Do you plan to engage in any terrorist activity while in the United States?' The lads giggle. Yeah, they say, and they also ask you have you done any drugs while abroad? "Like, wo-ho man, you want the whole list?" they tell the imaginary security guard at the airport and giggle.

It's all a bit sad, really. Two otherwise personable fellows, intelligent and well mannered, and all they seem to have done for weeks and weeks is mooch about large tracks of Europe getting stoned. Tash is deeply unimpressed. I'm glad about that …

FIESTA—THE PILGRIM ALSO RISES

I

PETER: We arrive in Estella hot, sticky, tired but glad to have started so early and to have reached our destination before the sun gets punishingly hot. Outside the town's municipal *albergue*, a three-storey-high former pilgrim hospital on a pretty, cobble-stoned street, two other walkers are waiting. It's 11.30 am and the *albergue* won't open until 12.30. But there's no question of walking further—we've done enough for today and the wait will be worth the rest it delivers.

And then, unexpectedly, the door to the *albergue* opens. Out comes a small, elderly man who walks with a slight stoop. He might be 60; he might be 70. He has close-cut grey hair, a lined, weathered face and a kindly smile. He's a wiry sort of fellow, full of beans and delighted to see some pilgrims. He's wearing a white shirt and trousers, a red scarf Boy Scout style around his neck and shoulders, and a red cloth belt, worn like a crios, tied at the side and hanging down the outside of his left leg. On his feet are a pair of white canvas espadrilles with extravagant red laces tied like a bow. Behind him is a younger man, similarly dressed, and another older man emerges from the *albergue*, also dressed in this manner.

NATASHA: I was too tired to move, budge or show any signs of a reaction. I sat hunched on the bench, squinting my eyes at these mad people. Dad thinks this is great. In his usual, peculiar manner, he gets down on one knee in front of the three men, shouts, "Oi!" to attract their attention and starts taking photos of them.

PETER: What happened next is the sort of thing that central casting could not advance as a story line because no one would believe it. But it is true and it is what makes travel in general—and the Camino in particular—truly wonderful.

NATASHA: Dad is in fits of laughter. Then the unimaginable happens; Dad starts to put his boots back on. I don't understand and I look at him, puzzled, then I look at my poor little feet, naked and in my nice open flip flops. "Come on! Put your boots on!" Dad exclaims excitedly. "You must be joking. No way," I refused.

"They want us to join the parade! Come on!" he pushes. I can see I'm unfortunately not going to win this one. So I slowly start to get up, a face of disgust. I couldn't want to do anything less. But it was just as well I did, because what we saw, and took part in, was unbelievable.

PETER: It is fiesta time in Estella. The fiesta is in honour of the town's patron saint, St Andrés. There's all the usual stuff going on for a week: the daily running of bulls, bull fights, street music and bunting, things especially for children, exhibitions and a bit too much food and drink will be had by all. Today, however, it's time for the annual procession, which includes parading through the town a relic of St Andrés, along with sundry other participants—devotees of other aspects of faith (adherents to Mary, for instance), traditional Navarrese dancers, bands of musicians (both traditional in a general sort of way, and some that are very particularly Basque). The relic is held in a gold and glass case and is carried shoulder high on a special platform, held aloft very carefully by four volunteers. Two other statues of Mary are carried similarly, shoulder high and decorated with bouquets of quivering, fresh flowers.

Meanwhile, back outside the *albergue*, "Come! You take this," the smiling elderly man, who turns out to be Pablito, says in Spanish. The younger man, who turns out to be named José and who used to work on logistics with Cirque du Soleil, translates for Natasha and me. We are coming? You are invited! "Eh?" "Yes, come on; you can be part of the procession." All we have to do is carry traditional pilgrim staves which Pablito has made and adorned with scallop shells and a gourd, just like the ones medieval pilgrims used as water carriers. But then out comes the banner: a tabard-style, silk cloth banner hanging from the top of a pole and cross piece, and with white silk cords and tassels hanging down the side. Los Amigos del Camino de Santiago de Estella is embroidered onto it, along with various Camino symbols including the scallop shell and the cross of St James. We, it seems, are to be the real deal—exhibits straight from the Camino, live pilgrims walking in the procession with Los Amigos. As we cross the steeply sloped medieval bridge just outside the *albergue* and walk to the tree-lined gravel square area in front of the Church of St Michael perched high above the whole town, José hands me the banner. "Can you carry?" he says. Well, what the hell! In for a peso ... as they say.

Only when we are in front of the church does the scale of what we are involved in become clear. There are some 30 groups taking part, about 500 people in all. Me and Tash and a German pilgrim (whom we have nicknamed Oddball because he is a dead ringer for the character played by Donald Sutherland in the film *Kelly's Heroes*) and the three Los Amigos—Pablito, José and the other man, who is Luis—are ushered to the front and told to lead off. To lead off the whole show, no less! The streets are lined with thousands upon thousands of people—Mums, Dads and children, all the men dressed in the traditional Basque red and white—and they want us to lead this? My father used to claim that he once took a wrong turn in the centre of Dublin on St Patrick's Day and found himself in the parade. Well, Dad, I and your granddaughter *led* the Fiesta of St Andrés procession in Estella! Thankfully, around the few bends as we got down into the town proper, more suitable leaders—giant *papier-mâché* Macnas-style figures and Basque musicians—were wheeled in at the head of the procession and Los Amigos were more appropriately located somewhere back around the middle.

And so we proceeded. Up and down and around just about every one of the old town's narrow main streets and squares. All were lined with excited local people having a great day out. Others watched from balconies. Los Amigos and the real deal pilgrims, dusty hiking boots and dirty sweaty T-shirts as proof positive that we had just breezed into town, were led by three musical Amigos playing drums and txistus, Basque flutes. We aroused great interest. Mums and Dads pointed us out to their children; the local press photographers made detailed studies. José, who had excellent English, and Natasha chatted away like old pals. Me and Oddball and a Spanish pilgrim, also, and a little confusingly, named Luis, took turns with the banner. Every 50 metres or so the procession stopped. The dancers and bands would entertain the bystanders to cheers and applause. Everyone, absolutely everyone in the whole town, knew Pablito and clapped and cheered and smiled lovingly at him.

NATASHA: People everywhere shake hands with Pablito and shout his name. As we walk along the streets, he bows his head in acknowledgment, squints his eyes kindly and shakes hands, saying a few words. Laughs are often exchanged. He reminded me very much of my Granddad. They had similar faces but their actions were even more similar. Every Christmas, at home, the whole of our family goes to the carol service in St Patrick's Cathedral in Dublin where Granddad was a choir boy when he was young. At the end of the service we walk back down the aisle towards the exit. As we move slowly, Granddad was often approached by people, like the little celebrity that I think he liked to believe he was! And like Pablito, he would bow his head and exchange a few words. Granddad would put on a modest front, but on the inside, I knew he was thrilled to be recognised. As this was happening with Pablito, I was thinking he must be famous. And he is. José told me that he is in nearly every Camino guidebook and has made thousands of the iconic Pilgrim walking staves.

PETER: Walking along with Javier, in-coming president of Los Amigos, he told me all about Navarra's recent history, about the percentage of children learning Basque (40% he says), about how everyone pays their taxes via the Navarrese authorities and not directly to Madrid, about the instruments and the music … The procession clearly for many, Javier included, was about a lot more that the relic of an old saint. This was a great family-oriented people's day out during which several layers of identity were on display. They were not saying "We're Spanish and proud." Spain they see as Castile. They're Navarrese for sure but it was not clear to me whether all of them regarded themselves also as Basque. They were saying they were different and to some degree separate from Spain. How separate they saw themselves, or wanted to be, was not clear.

As the procession turned into the Plaza de los Fueros, the town's main square, the bells rang out above the Church of San Juan Bautista, which occupies one whole side. The huge base bells and their wooden counterbalances swung in and out of the bell-tower, generating great bongs! Fireworks were launched skyward—Whoosh! Bang! Fiesta! The dancers and musicians now had more room to move about and display their talents. Everything stopped in the crowded cafés and restaurants around the square as customers and staff watched the spectacle.

NATASHA: … drums banging and guitars strumming, crowds on their tippy toes to see the parade, and opening the closed shutters of the houses along the streets … I feel like I am hallucinating as I am swallowed into a sea of white and red, and filled with cheering and music. It was like the climax scene in a dramatic thriller, where the James Bond character is racing through a rowdy crowd, chasing the baddies.

The sun is belting down on the city, poking through down to the street at lower buildings. José tells me that the people on either side of us are turning to their children and whispering, "They are the pilgrims." I walked with José the whole way. He was lovely, and very interesting. He was a lover of travel, and no follower of 'plans'. He had a sense of pathos about him; a yearning for adventure and exploration. He had done the Camino two months ago and passed through Estella and fell in love with its aliveness and character. He says we are very lucky to have come to the town on such a special occasion, the day of the parade. As he spoke to me about Estella, his face began to light up and his body filled with energy. He was truly in love with the place. He was also filled with knowledge on the city's traditions and beliefs, which he was filling me in on, as we walked along. The moment where it hit me that this was really special to the people of Estella, was when one of the men, who was friends with Pablito, turned to me.

"Spanish, English or German?" he said over my shoulder, asking what I speak.

"English," I replied.

"Where are you from?" he asks in perfect English.

"Ireland, just outside Dublin."

With this, he says: "Thank you for taking part in this," and kisses me on the cheek.

I looked in his eyes. They were full of happiness; I could see that this really meant a lot to him. I was so happy to have taken part in it.

PETER: And then, suddenly, we were back in front of St Michael's and it was all over and the banner came down and there were smiles and expressions of great satisfaction and commitments that it will be done again next year for sure.

Beer was ordained to be appropriate and as Los Amigos and the pilgrims sat in a nearby pub drinking, a three-piece guitar group walked in. A man stood up and apparently asked the Navarrese equivalent of "Lads, do yous know *The Fields*?" And they were off—measured, simple strumming of the guitars but the singer launching himself into some very passionate verses with notes at the end of lines that are held long and high and wrung for all they are worth. The singer won strong applause and the awe-struck approval of the musicians. The music is *jota*, Javier tells me, music from southern Navarra, and the musicians are part of the *aurora* tradition, strolling minstrels who used to busk in the cities at sunrise but who now emerge only on special days.

And boy, was this a special day!

Back at the *albergue* Pablito had knocked up a vast paella for all the pilgrims now arriving, for the banner carriers from the procession and just about anyone who happened to drop by. Oddball, who started walking from Marburg in central Germany two and a half months ago, wolfed down several plates and then said he was off looking for some monks he heard about who had two fountains—one with water, the other with wine—10 kilometres down the road. He wasn't really sure if the wine fountain was still working but he felt that, on balance, it was worth checking it out. And, as he himself noted somewhat enigmatically in an earlier conversation with me: "Everything is possible if you walk the whole way."

Tash and me? Tomorrow they're running the bulls at 8.00 am and again at nine. Two shots at that then ...

II

PETER: Next morning, Estella has a slight hangover. As pilgrims leave the *albergue* (to the strains of Bob Marley's *Redemption Song*—great!) and strike out for Los Arcos in the half light, revellers roam the streets, dodging mechanical road sweepers and early morning bread delivery vans. Young men the worse for wear, but held vertical by adoring young women, saunter uncertainly about the narrow streets, all the time threatening to fall over into a sleepy heap. Bands of other young men, invariably without women, walk the streets talking too loud but completely oblivious to the consequences of their condition, and are up for the next challenge … whatever it might be. It is the morning after the night before, but for them yesterday is still going strong and tomorrow, well, tomorrow is just another day and they'll deal with that when it comes around.

We re-acquaint ourselves with the layout of the town; the direction from which the bulls will come, the turns they will take, whether they are likely to hug the inside of the curve of the street, or the outside (upon which judgments will rest possibly matters of life and death). We note the best vantage points along the route, all the way down a corral for the bulls which is near the *albergue.* We pick our spot and are joined by two lads from Northern Ireland, Gary and Andrew.

NATASHA: It's only been a week, and the things that we have experienced along the way are almost indescribable. I don't know how I can write everything with the emotion and effects they had on me.

It's 7.00 am in Estella, and we're downstairs having breakfast in our *albergue.* We are sitting around a long table shared with all the other pilgrims. Out of nowhere I hear a voice beside me say: "So where in Ireland are you from?" in the sweet sound of an Irish accent. We have finally met fellow Irish pilgrims, something I have been waiting for. I'm thrilled.

It's Gary McCartan, a 21-year-old from Newcastle in Co. Down. He has just finished his second year studying nursing at Queen's University in Belfast. With him is Andrew Lee, a 20-year-old from south Belfast, also studying nursing. There was a third member to their gang, Reece, but I didn't get to know him as well because he walked ahead to get to the next stop early. Dad and I told Gary and Andrew that we were going to stay on for the 8.00 am running of the bulls, Dad adding that he was thinking of running. They seemed very interested and declared they would too. We departed the *albergue* separately at 7.30 am, knowing we would bump into each other later.

For the half hour we had to wait, Dad and I slowly walked along the quiet street. The further up we went, the louder it got. There were drunken youths spilling out of the side streets and onto our paths, singing and swaying with one another. Temporary wooden gates and barriers were being set in place at junctions and side streets to prevent the bulls straying off course. Gary and Andrew were sitting on a fence at one of the main junctions. I joined them while Dad sat on top of the fence opposite, his camera out. Clearly he wasn't going to run. Andrew and Gary had been saying they were going to run but they weren't standing in the middle of the narrow street, waiting with the other men for the bulls to arrive.

PETER: The bulls are released from the bull ring, which is at the upper end of the town, and forced to run down a series of narrow streets to the corral. An hour later they are released to run back to the bull ring where, later in the afternoon for each day of the fiesta, bull fights are held and they meet their fate.

NATASHA: At exactly 8.00 am there are two loud bangs, explosions that signal to everyone that the bull run has begun. About one minute later, we hear the thundering hooves. Like a cloud of black, the angry beasts come haring round the bend. With excited eyes we watch as they get closer to passing us. Suddenly, out of nowhere, Andrew slips under the fence 15 metres ahead of the bulls, and starts to run. Gary and I watch as he careers round the bend of the street, a bull 10 metres behind him, big handlebar horns and all.

"What just happened?" said Gary, looking to where Andrew had been on the fence. Ten minutes passed and Andrew had yet to reappear. "Well, it was nice knowing him," I thought to myself, sure he was lying dead somewhere. With that, the brave madcap came trotting towards us, clearly pleased with himself. He was ambushed by questions from his envious friend.

"Right, I'm doing the 9.00 am run then," Gary said, eager to hold the adrenaline rush Andrew had.

"Okay, if you are doing it, I'm doing it," I promised. And so we waited.

PETER: Me too! I strolled down the street to the corral to inspect the enemy. There were eight of them, one seriously big fellow, three or four medium-sized ones and three or four not much larger than calves. They were mainly black, although the big one had a large white patch on his back, and there was also a brown one. Several of them had bells around their necks which somewhat diminished their ferocity. But they all had well developed horns.

The streets of the bull run are thronged with people once more; the wooden barriers have been slid out of their sockets and normal life has resumed, sort of. A brass band with drums has emerged out of nowhere and marches jauntily up and down playing breezy little tunes, kind of Herb Alpert meets Um-pah-pah. It is a little like a musical jeer at the

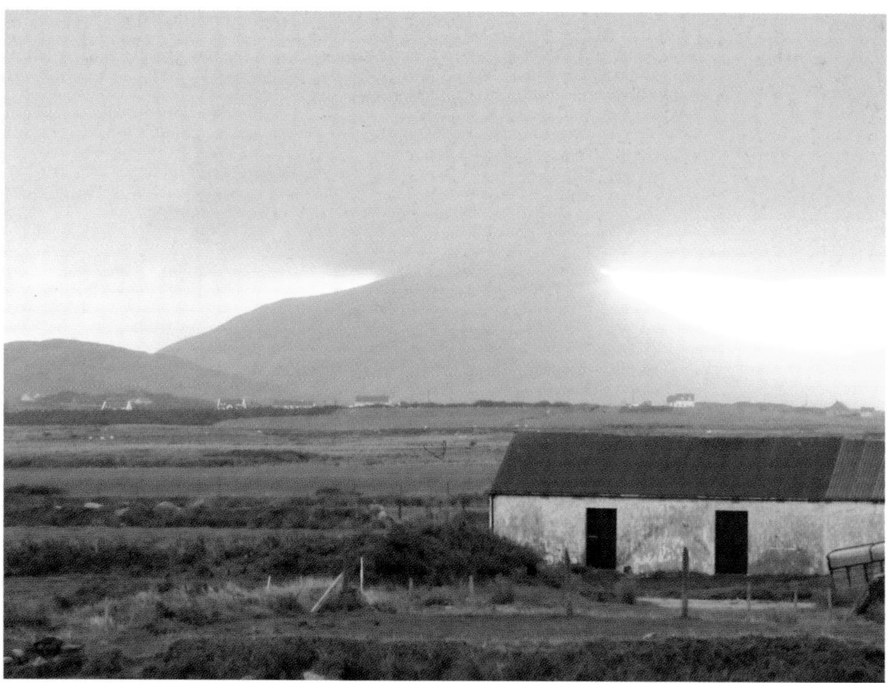

Croagh Patrick in Co. Mayo seen from the west, silhouetted against the dawn sun.

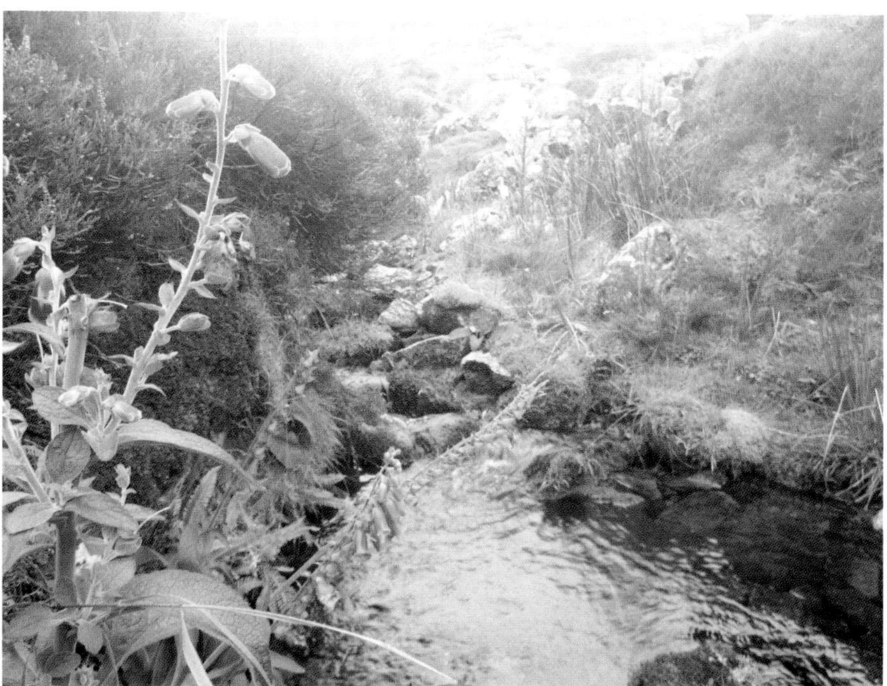

Foxgloves by a stream flowing off Croagh Patrick.

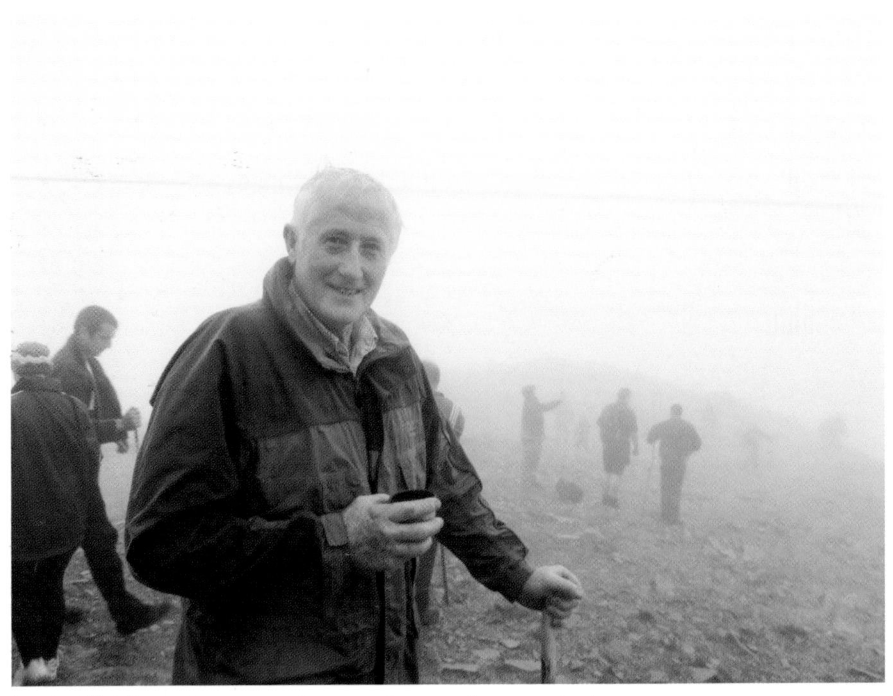

Austin O'Malley enjoys a warming cup of tea on the summit at 5.30 am.

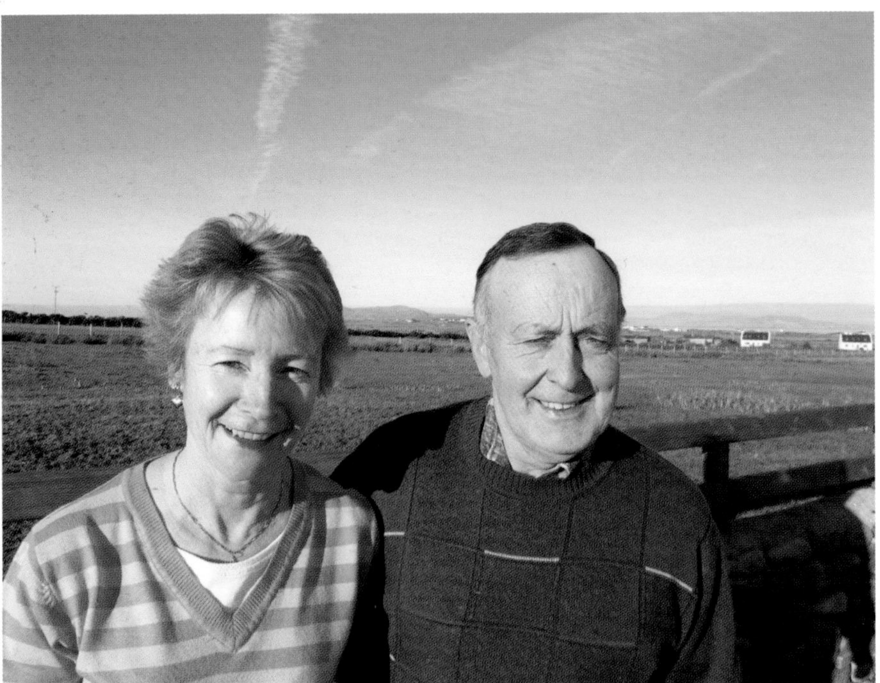

Margaret and Gerard O'Malley.

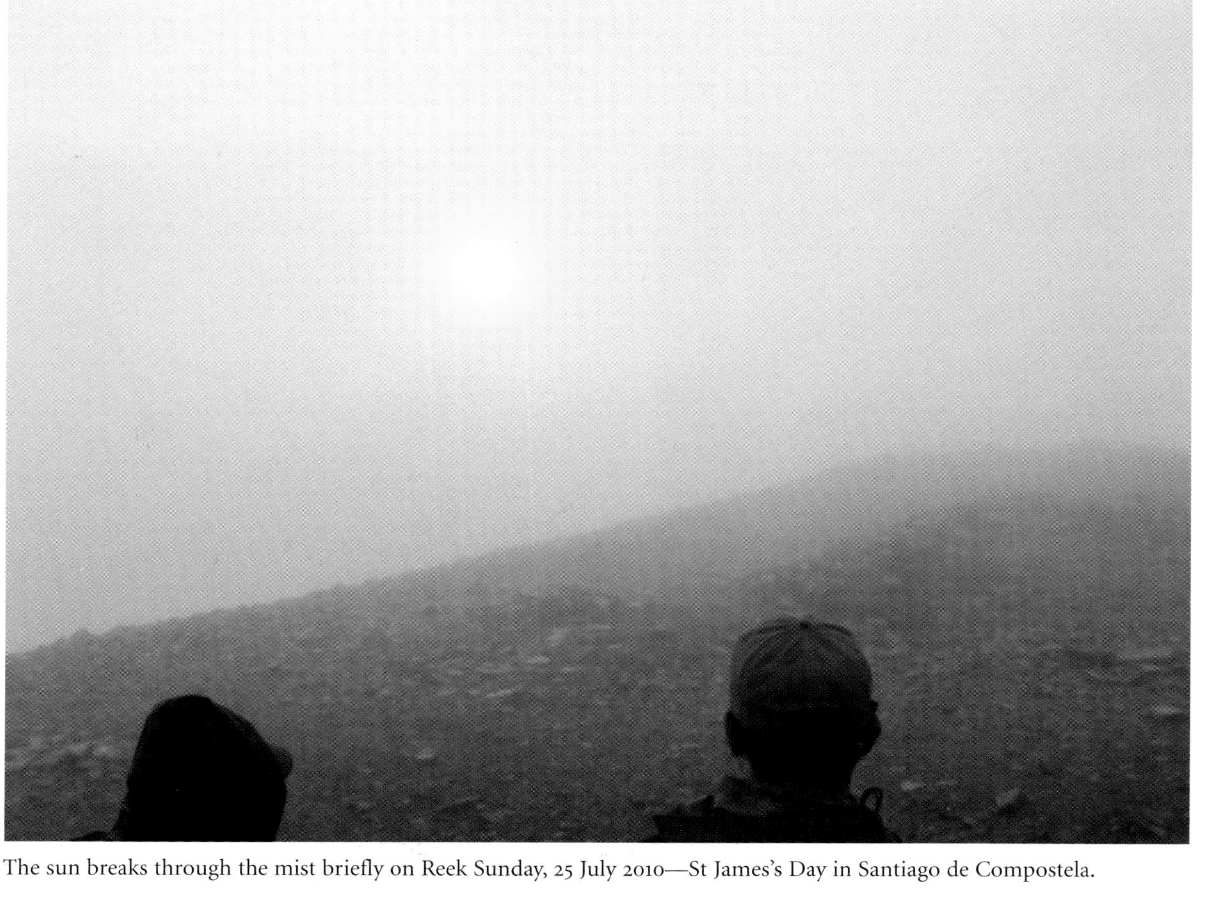

The sun breaks through the mist briefly on Reek Sunday, 25 July 2010—St James's Day in Santiago de Compostela.

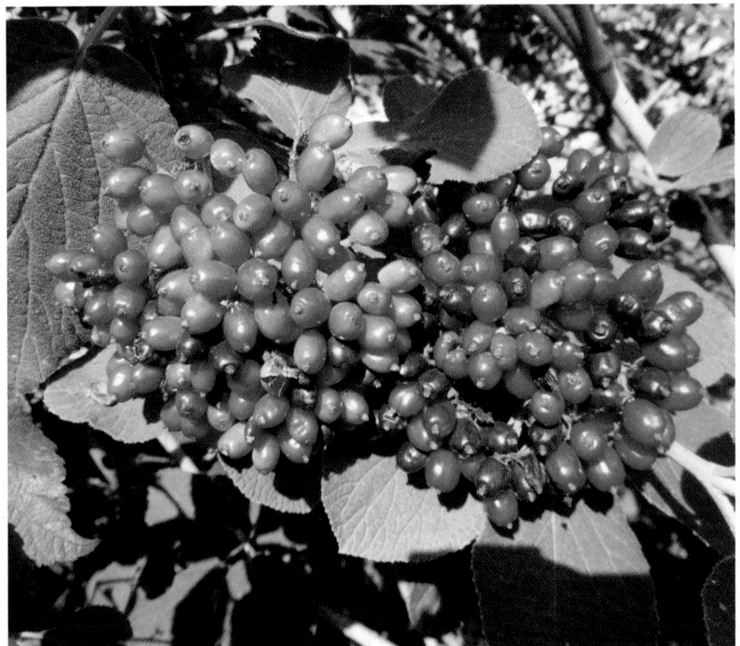

Hedgerow fruits on the Camino.

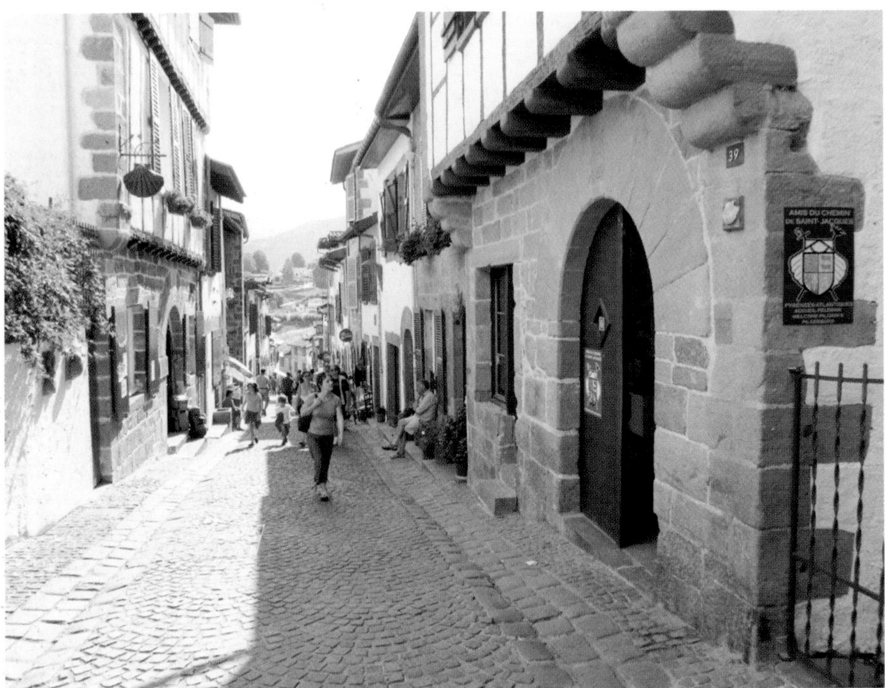

The start of the Camino in St-Jean-Pied-de-Port in the French Pyrénées. The pilgrim office is on the right.

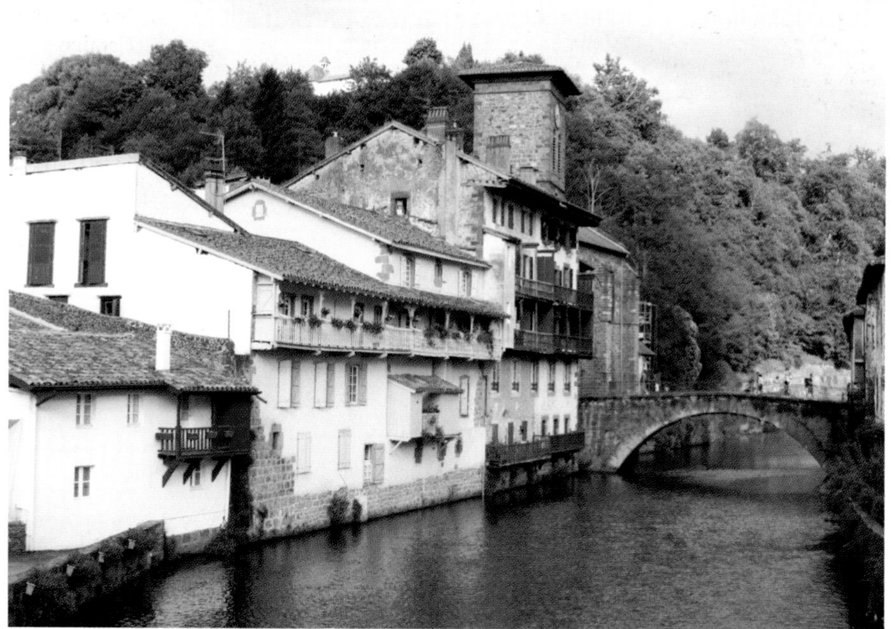

The pilgrim's exit from St-Jean.

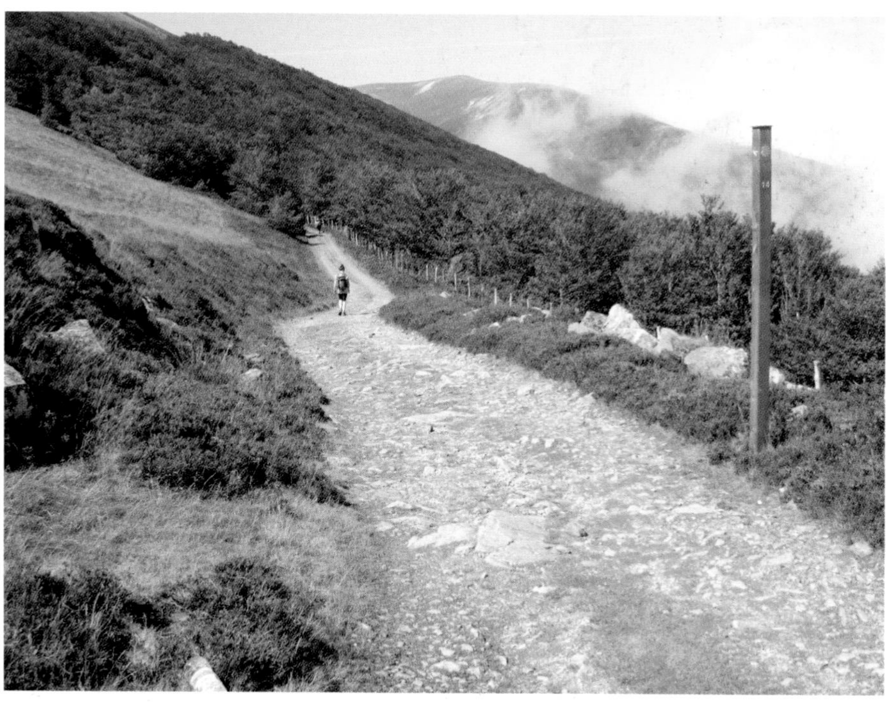

Across the top of the Pyrénées—Navarra beckons … and Santiago, 800 kilometres away.

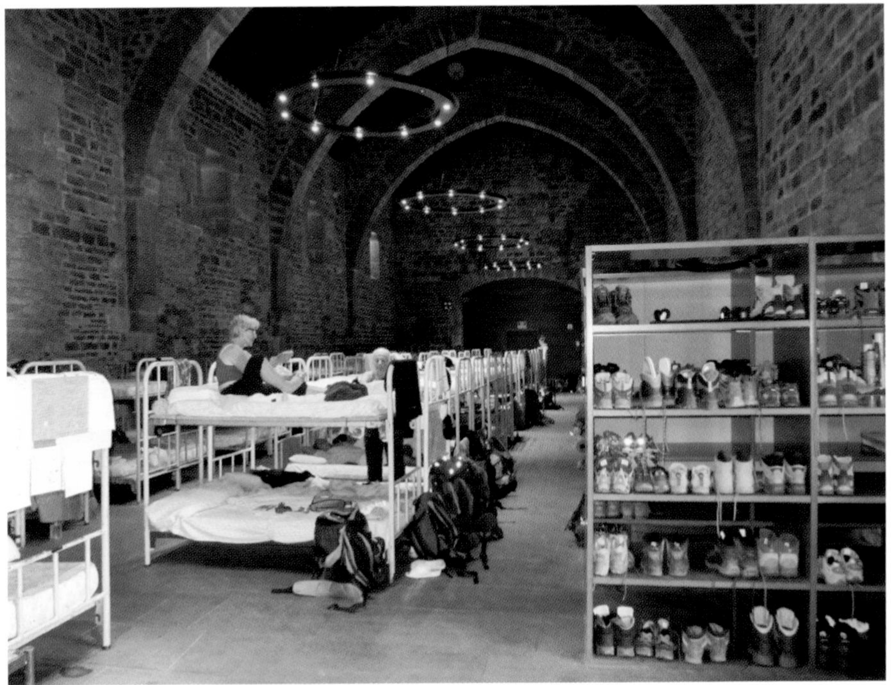

The pilgrim hostel in Roncesvalles, with dormitory bunk beds typical of almost all *albergues* along the Camino.

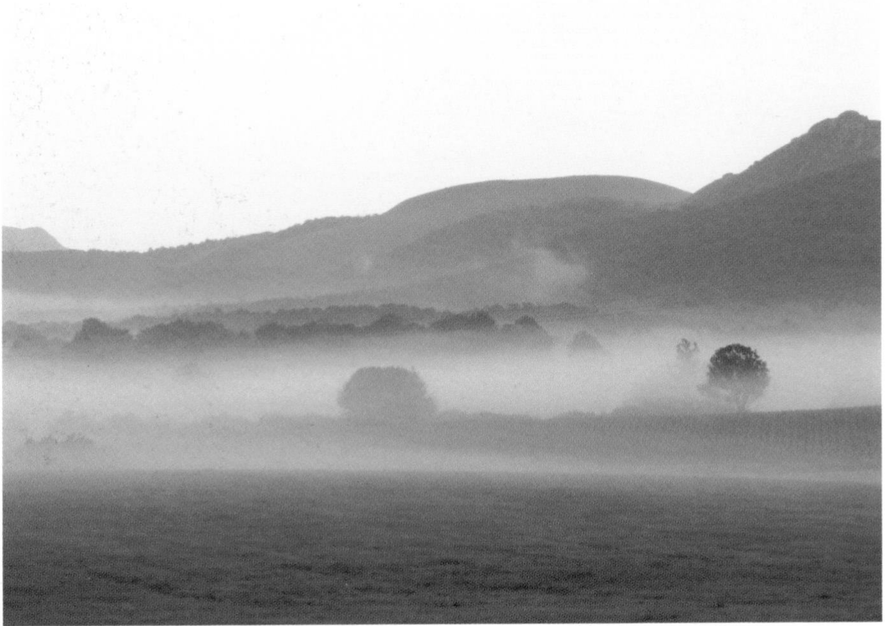

Early morning mist cloaks the Navarra countryside.

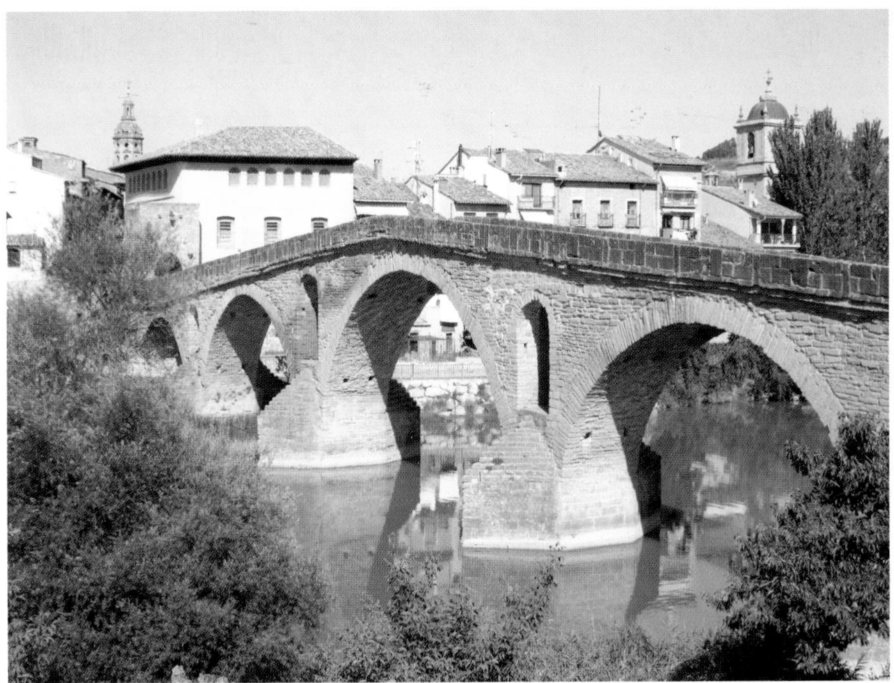

The beautiful, five-arched medieval bridge leading west out of Puente la Reina.

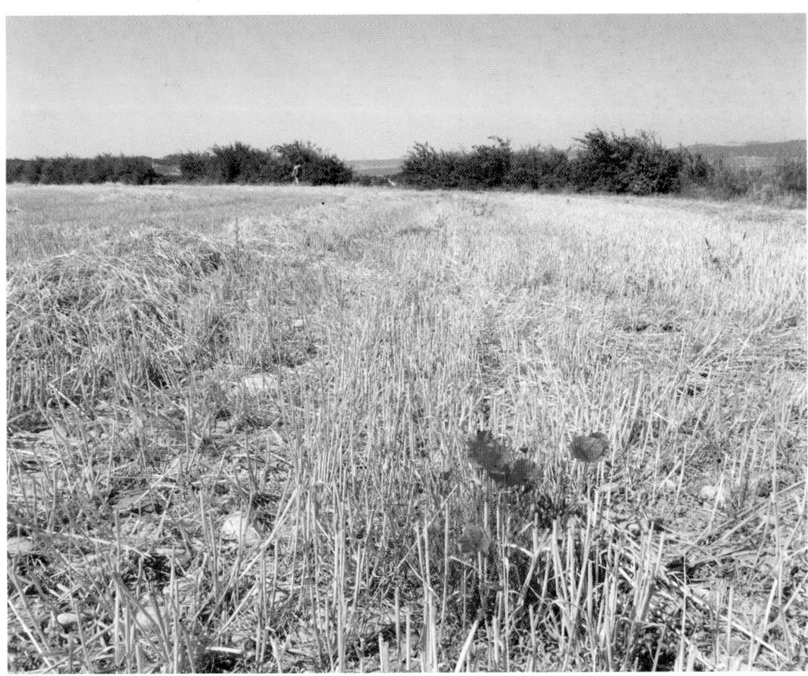

Poppies among the stubble.

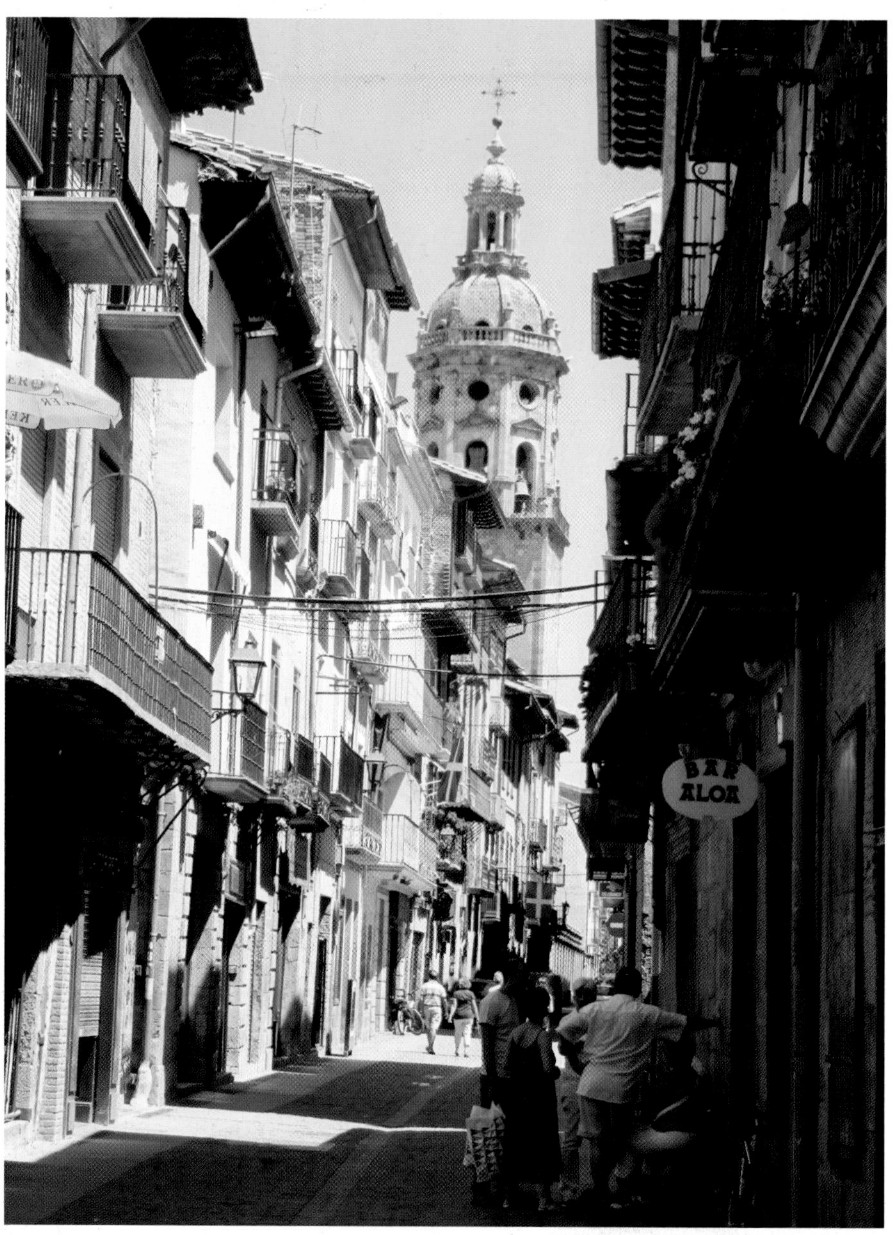

The bell-tower of the Iglesia de Santiago on the main street through Puente la Reina, which is also the Camino, towers over the town.

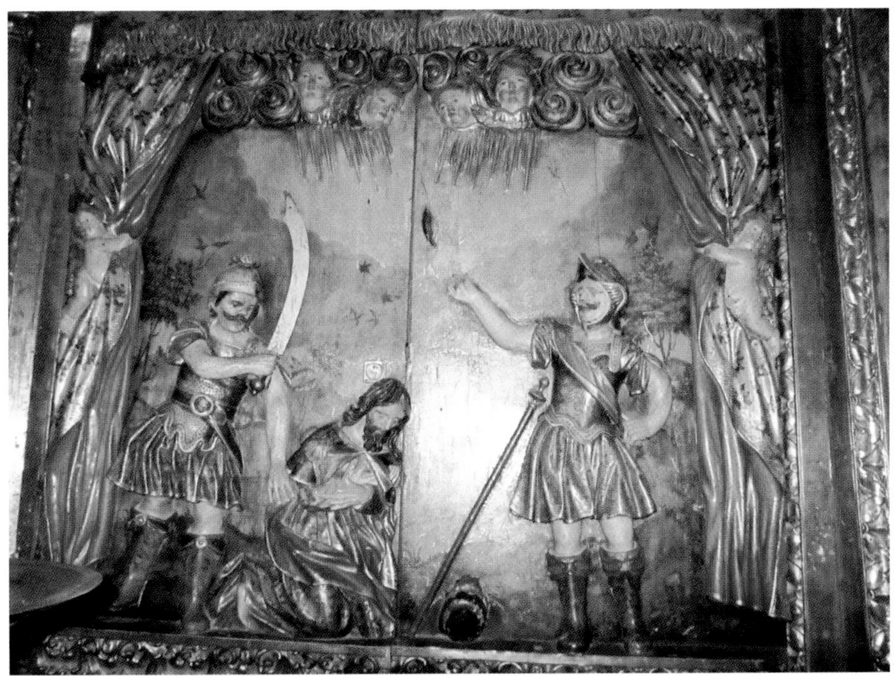

Church depictions of the beheading of James are often in naïve, almost Punch and Judy style, as in this *retablo*, or altarpiece.

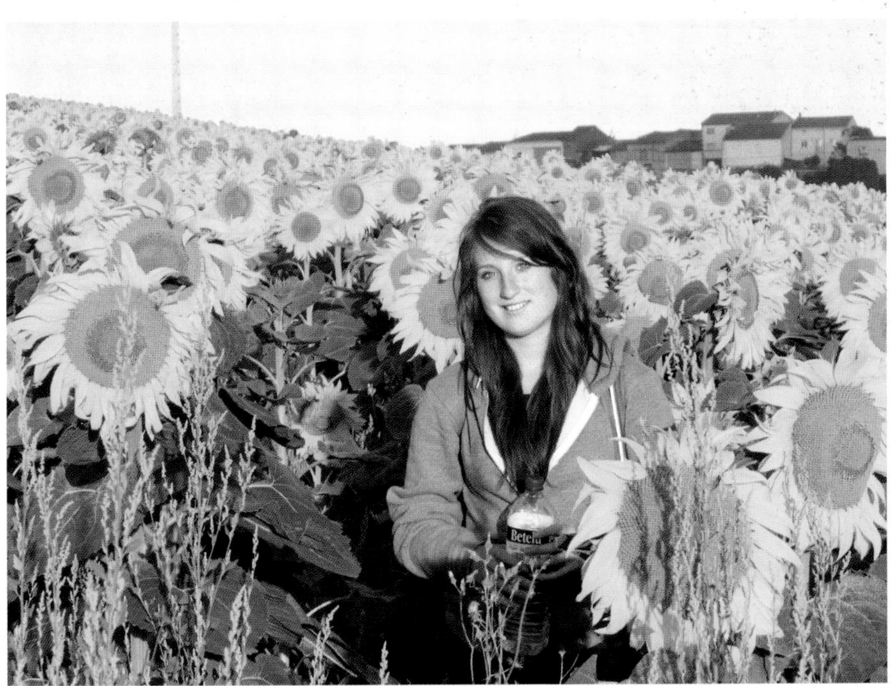

Among the sunflowers.

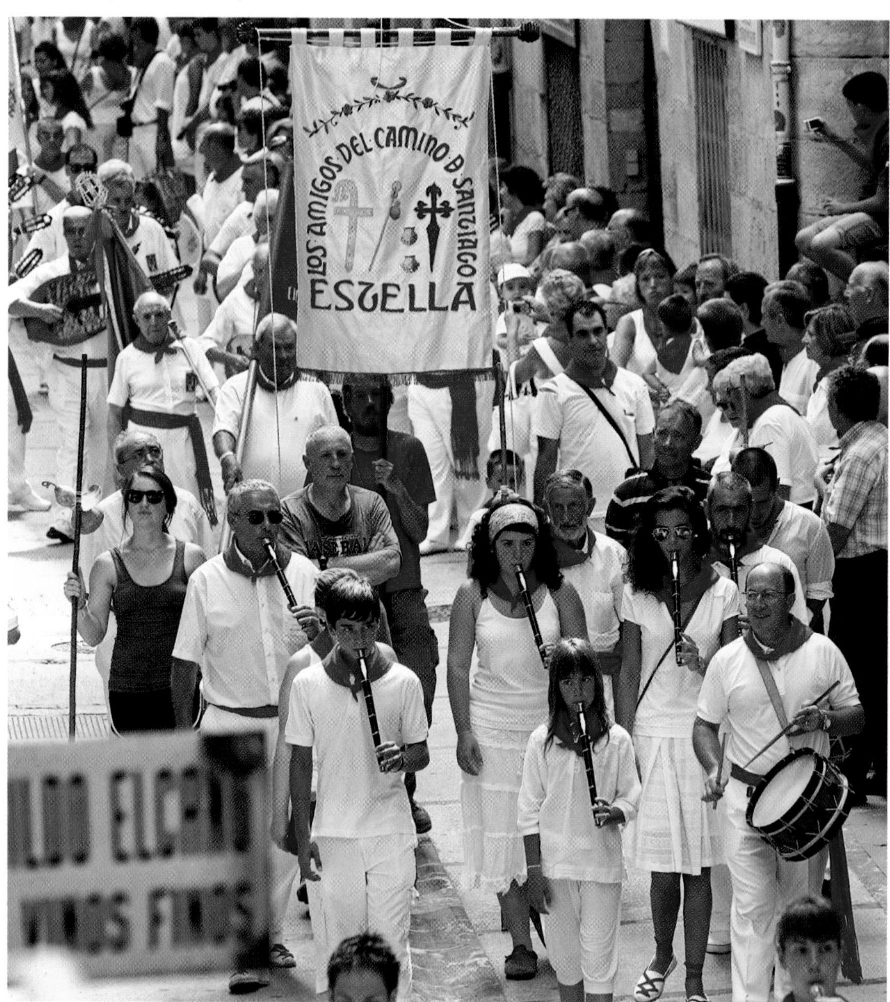

The Los Amigos contingent in the fiesta parade through Estella, as published by the local newspaper. The banner is carried by Oddball. (*Montxo/Diario de Navarra*)

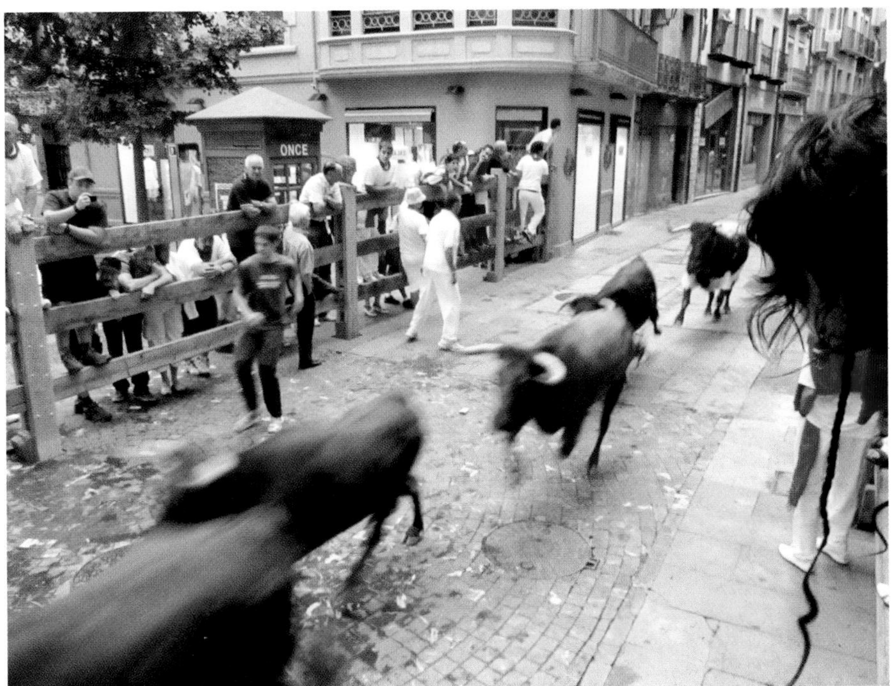

Estella's running of the bulls.

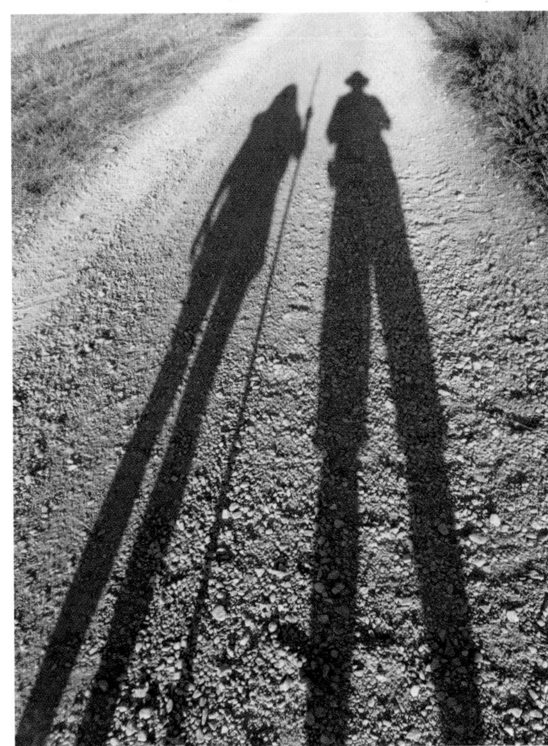

The early morning sun, always at one's back as the Camino heads west, makes long shadows of pilgrims.

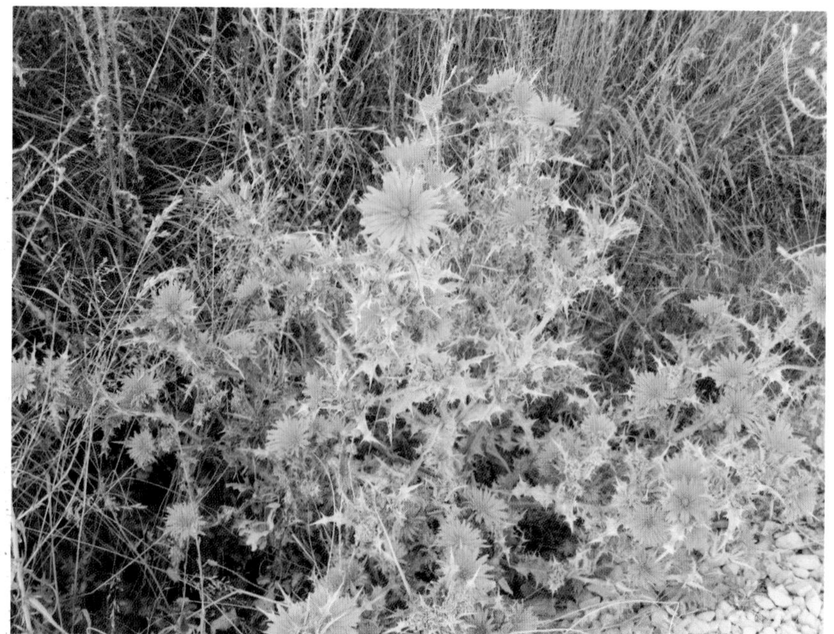

Wayside Camino flowers.

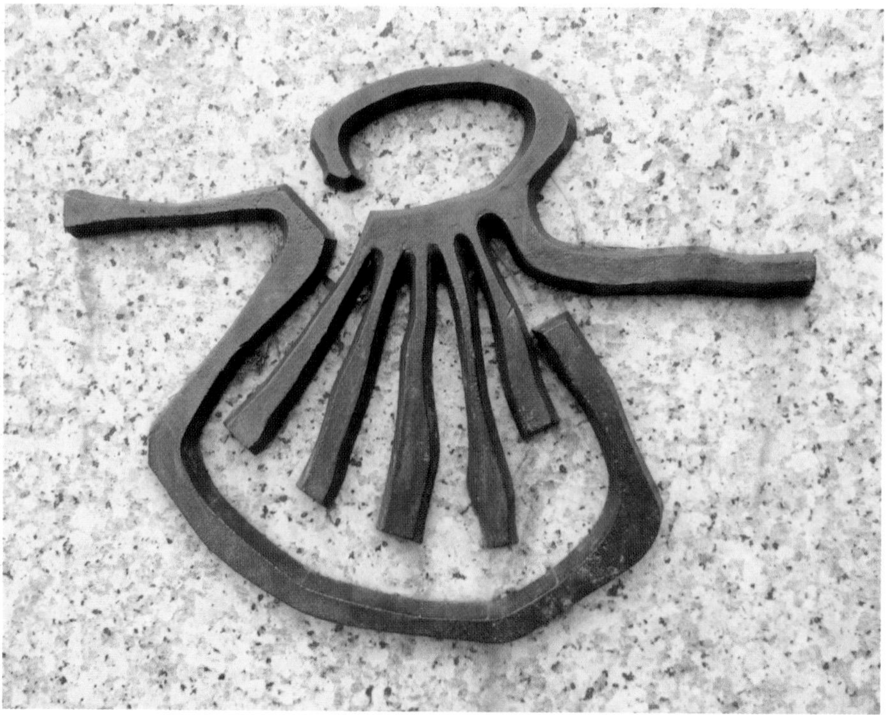

Logroño city's distinctive interpretation of the scallop shell Camino sign.

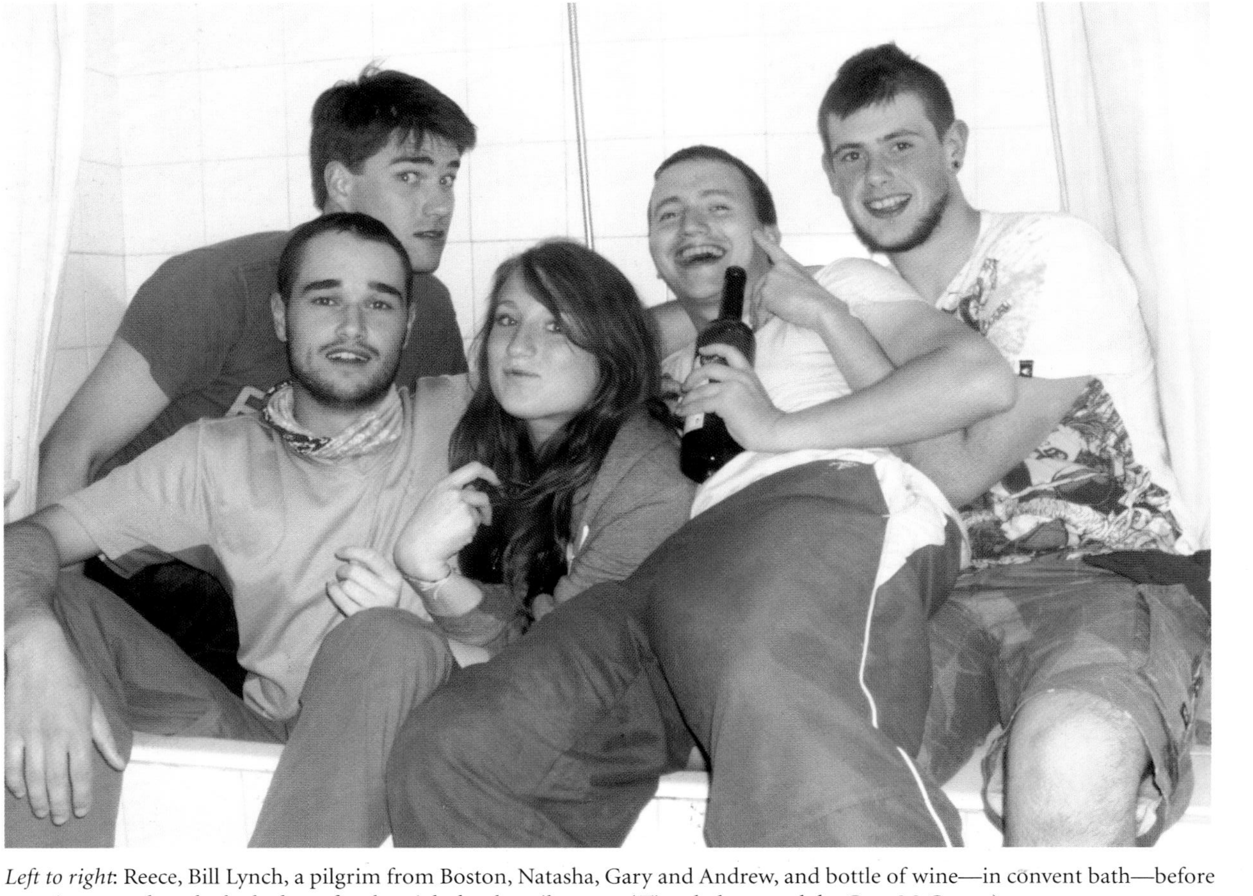

Left to right: Reece, Bill Lynch, a pilgrim from Boston, Natasha, Gary and Andrew, and bottle of wine—in convent bath—before escaping … only to be locked out for the night by the wily nuns. (*Timed photograph by Gary McCartan*)

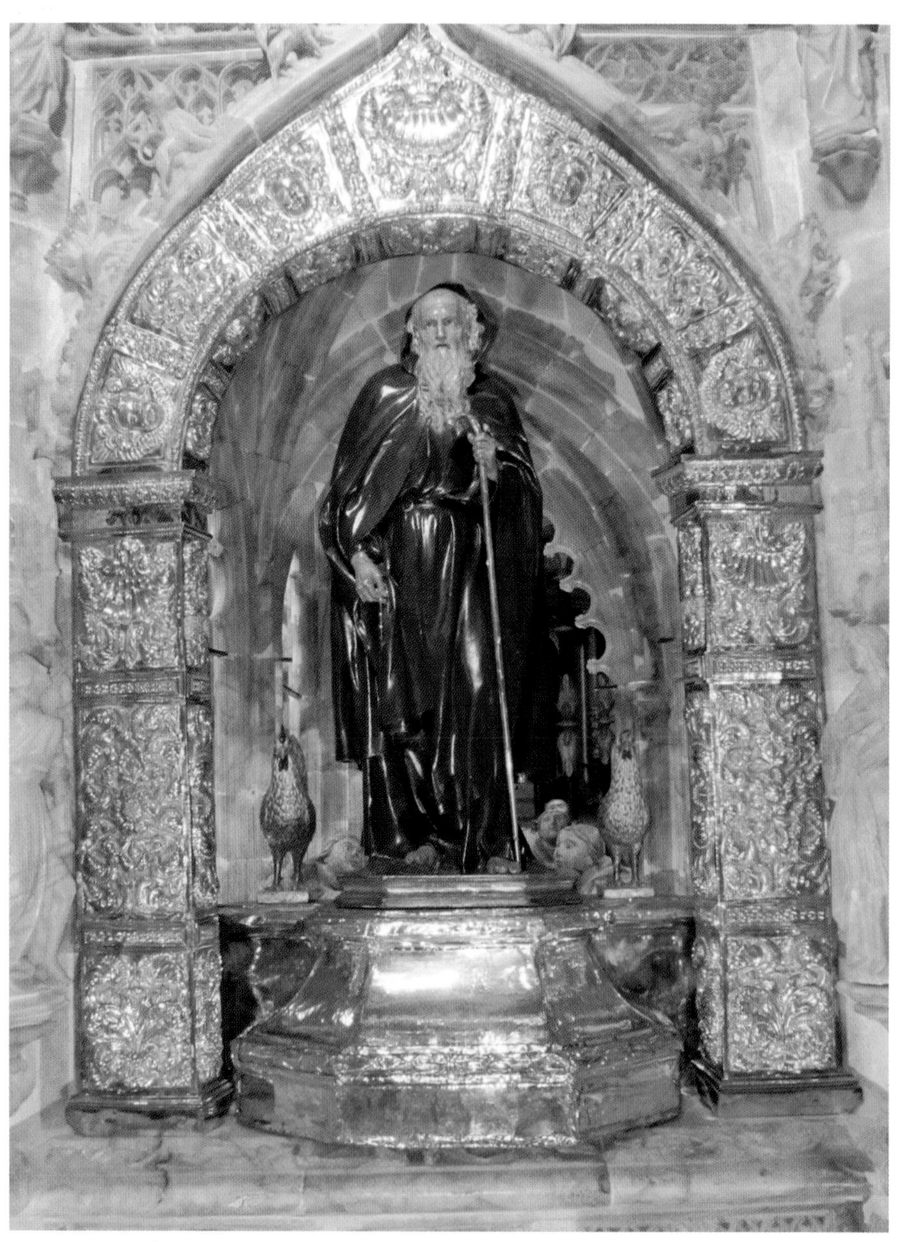

Statue of Santo Domingo in the cathedral named in his honour. Note the two chickens on either side of his feet.

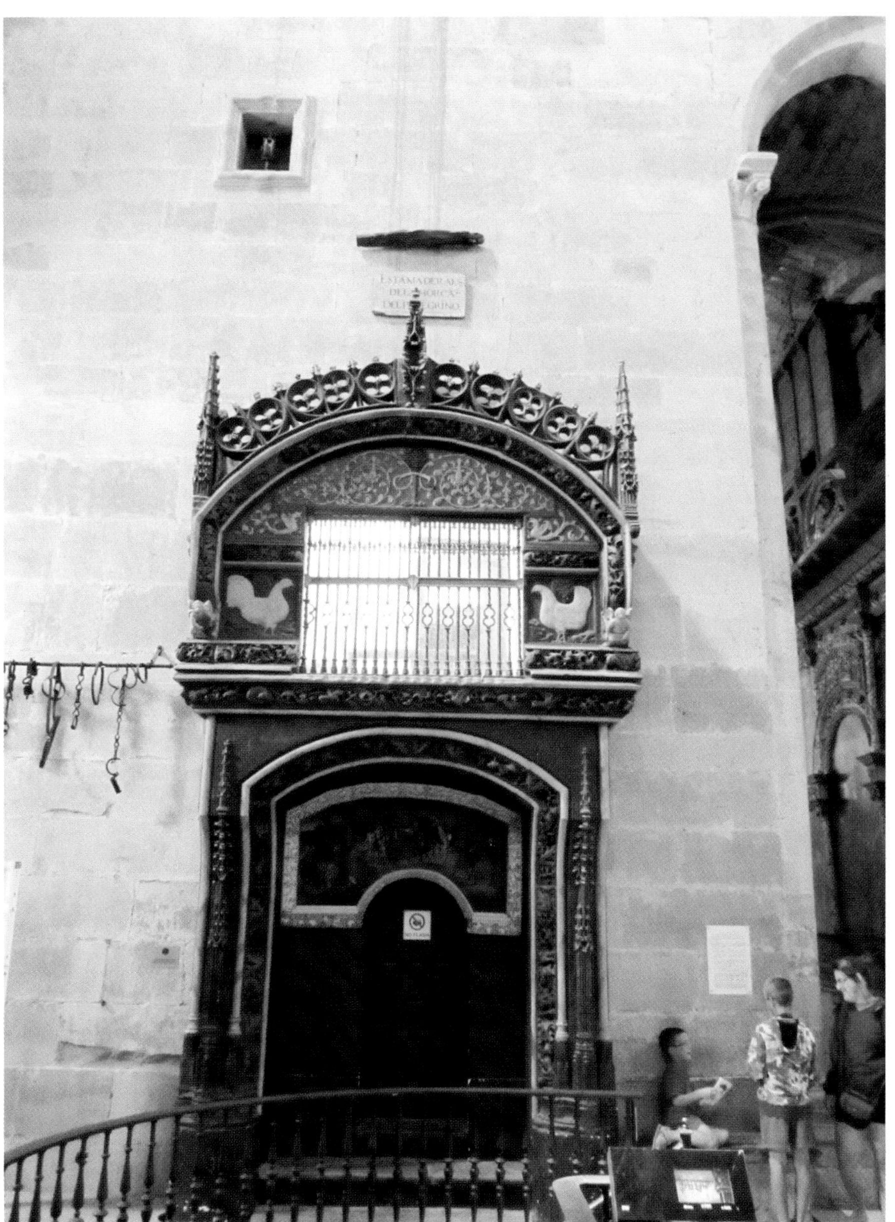

The 15th-century coop in Santo Domingo Cathedral, home to two live chickens, a cock and a hen, commemorates the 12th-century miracle involving the amorous barmaid and the wronged German pilgrim.

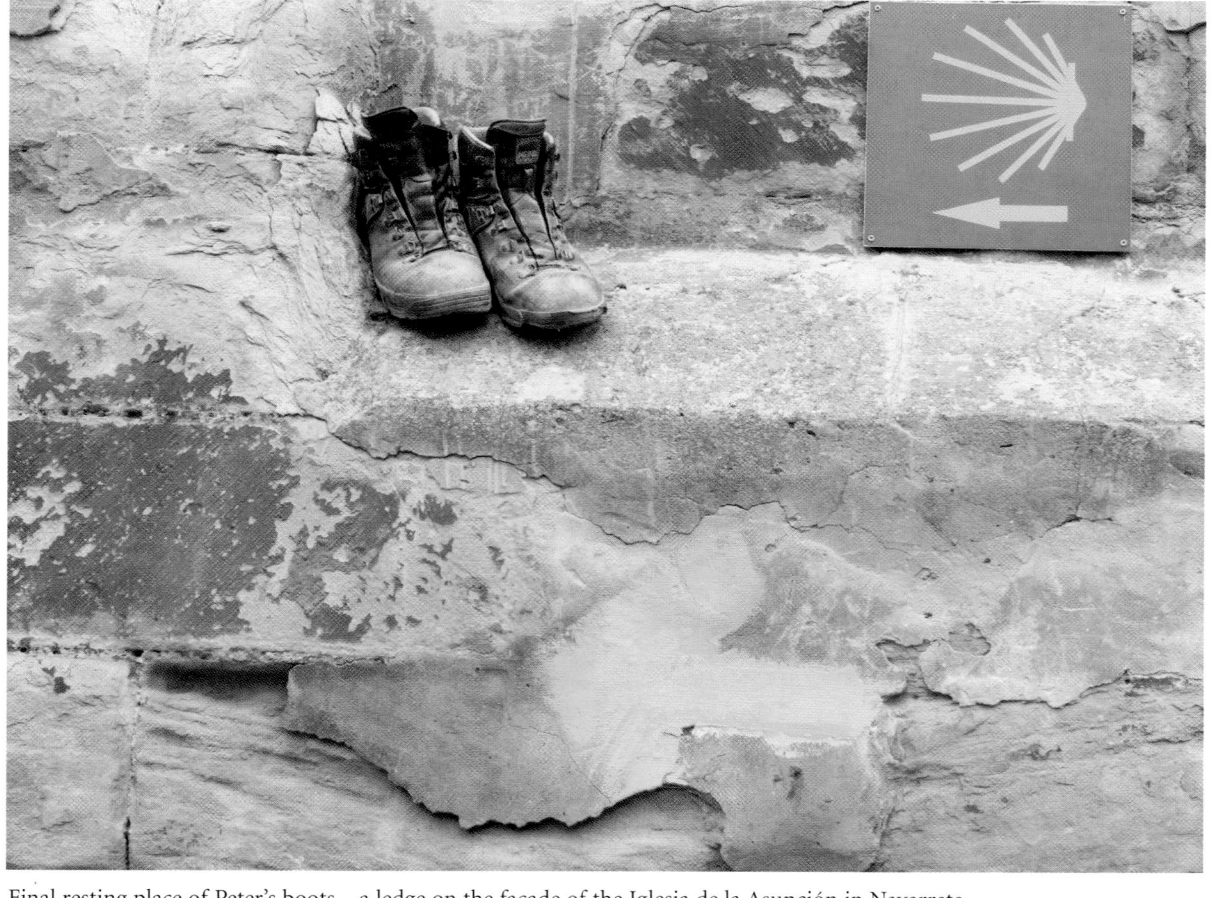

Final resting place of Peter's boots—a ledge on the façade of the Iglesia de la Asunción in Navarrete.

bulls: "Ha! So you thought this street was yours, torro; well, just you listen to my jolly tune. I'm not afraid of you!" And the young girls are everywhere, ogling the young studs who ran with the bulls, one of them grabbing a small one by the tail and almost dragging him to the ground.

And then the band disappears and the people melt away again and the wooden barriers are slid back into place.

NATASHA: 8.50 am and we were getting ourselves ready, turning to Andrew, who sat high up on the fence, for wise words on how to make it out alive. The locals and regular runners must have been laughing at the deal we were making out of something that was clearly like a run to the milk shop for them. Dad hopped down off the fence and agreed to join in too.

The bulls would be coming from the opposite direction this time, from down the town, up towards us and to the bull ring. We stood watching, waiting, feeling nervous and wondering at the madness of it all. BANG BANG! It was 9.00 am and they had been released. We waited.

Then we saw them. I was looking at Dad and Gary, who were closer to the bulls, to see when they started running. When the bulls were about 80 metres away, we started to run. They were synchronised in their running, and caught up with you very fast. I was getting nervous as I could hear them getting closer and closer.

PETER: As they rounded the bend and started towards us, I tried to take a picture, close the camera and then start running. Jazus! Where are all those little ones? These guys are HUH-YOU-AGE … Two blokes in front of me turn and start their run. If they're off, I'd better leg it. And so I ran and ran and ran like blazes, not looking back, just trying to make sure I didn't fall. "If you fall, Tash," I said to her before the run began, "roll to the side as fast as you can; don't let them trample you."

I'm fairly sure that's what her mother would advise as well.

So far, so good; done about 50 metres now. Pumping, pumping, not looking back. And then there's these two blokes, one on either side of the narrow street, holding a big, yellow, plastic, tarpaulin banner close to the ground as though they are about to lift it suddenly for us all to jump over. WTF!! Do not do that, lads; DO NOT DO THAT!!!!!! They read my mind and keep their banner on the ground and the whole herd—runners and bulls—trample over it. Then the bulls veer right into a large square and on up towards the ring; I carry on straight into a shopping arcade, scattering customers, slip onto my backside and lie there giddy with excitement.

Yes! Got away with it!

And then the thought: Where's Tash? A nanosecond of panic until she emerges, safe and in one piece and a massive grin on her face.

NATASHA: I pulled into a doorway, Dad pulled in a little further up, and then Gary. And on the bulls went, back to the ring. We were thrilled. Dad's wish to run with the bulls had finally come true. Hemingway would be proud!

PETER: Who? Hemingway? Nah, never heard of him but come here, did I ever tell you 'bout the time I ran with …

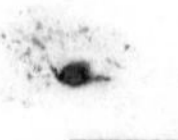

Estella to Los Arcos: 21 km in 5 hours

PETER: The Camino from Estella returns to countryside quickly. There are mountains in the distance: one, Monjardín, we will approach and then skirt around its shoulder but it's a climb nonetheless from a start of about 450 metres to about 650 metres. But the exhilarations of the bull run will carry us a long way. In the far distance, an escarpment, part of the mountains of Cantabria, signals the separation of Navarra and Rioja from the Basque lands.

NATASHA: I walked with Andrew and Gary almost the whole way. I was already happy that these boys were Irish, and that I didn't have to struggle with a language barrier talking to them. But I was even happier when I realised they were such nice boys. The nicest people I think I have come across yet. They were so nice because they were friendly and interesting and were both genuinely good people.

They worked in various hospitals around Belfast as part as their study. I asked them if they had ever had to deal with something difficult. Gary told me of this one man. He was in his early forties and was struggling with a lung disease from serious smoking. Gary explained that he was a very closed man and got angry when people tried to get to know him. But after a while of caring for him, Gary did become quite close to him, and the man opened up to him. Gary started to tell him about the Camino, and that he was going to do it over the summer. The man had heard about it and was very interested.

He had wanted to do it, but knew he would never be able to because of his condition.

A few days before leaving for the Camino, Gary's mentor contacted him to tell him that the man had passed away. The last thing the man said was, "Tell Gary to send me a postcard."

I was overwhelmed by the story and started to cry. It was like something you would read out of a Mitch Albom book. Gary should be proud of himself. I know that man would be.

PETER: We have begun our walk late—after 10.00 am—but thankfully the sky is cloudy; there will be no punishing sun today, perhaps even a little rain. Just before the Monastery of Irache we come to the vineyard of Irache. A sign announces that, just as Aymeric Picaud wrote in the *Liber Sancti Jacobi* all those years ago, the wines of Estella in Navarra are very good indeed. And just to reassure any doubters, the good people who run the Irache winery invite pilgrims to partake of their ... complimentary wine fountain. Well, bugger me, Oddball wasn't that whacky after all! It really is true: free wine, on tap. Okay not from monks but who cares? All of us—Tasha, Gary, Andrew and I—take a good draught, and water too. Gary reminds us why we are here. "You know," he announces to his assembled audience, "when St James passed this way, he said, and at this very spot I believe, 'Right lads, time for a piss up!' I believe this is what the fountain commemorates."

I think he read a different guidebook to mine but I love his cheeky, youthful, Northern Ireland humour.

At the tiny village of Azqueta a few kilometres further on, a café offers a welcome break, a real break for some coffee and juice. We sit there, the four of us, reliving the craic of the morning, when a small, slightly bent-over figure dressed all in white appears at the café door.

"Pablito! Buenos días!" I say with delight. He acknowledges with a big smile and comes to join us. His English does not stretch far beyond "Hello" but it matters little. We are with a friend. "Coffee?" "Sí, gracias." I get that morning's *Diario de Navarra* from my rucksack and open it on page 24. There he is: with me and Tash and Oddball holding the Los Amigos banner aloft. I try to tell him "Thank you for making our day exceptional," that he is a wonderful man and that his community of Amigos are special people. But I don't know if it got through; it is time we moved on—the Camino beckons.

But Pablito urges us to come, come this way. "Mi casa," he says and effects to stamp a non-existent document on the palm of his hand. Ah, he wants to put a stamp into our pilgrim passport. What a lovely souvenir; of course we'll come with him. And so he leads us slowly across the village street to his house, gently holding Natasha's arm. I try to ask him his age; my Spanish does not rise to the occasion and so I try French, writing down—57—for him to see. A little girl playing on a step hears me and understands. She repeats the question in Spanish, shouting in Pablito's direction. "Ah," he says and writes his down in my Moleskine. It is 76; the handwriting unsteady.

At his house, he opens the front door. Inside the hall there is some dark wood furniture, including a table-like desk on which Pablito has a rubber stamp and an ink pad. The image produced is of a Cross of Malta in a circle atop a plinth. Natasha asks him to sign his name also. We are both delighted with this little trophy. After all the fun and privilege of the procession, here is another special token. Pablito leads us out again and we are about to shake hands, embrace and leave. But no, there is more. He leads us gently around the side of his house to the garden. There, under a walnut tree with a child's swing, is the subject of the stamp carved in stone, the Cross of Malta on one side, the Cross of St James on the other, both hard to make out but there alright. I point to my age in my notebook, then his and then to the stone. Pablito understands and takes my pen; "800," he writes.

He takes Natasha's hand and leads her to a pile of gourds. He indicates she is to take one. Then he leads her further into the garden, to a stack of cut staves, each one about two metres long, beside a shed. He chooses one of the staves; not the first one to hand, he makes a careful selection. He bids Natasha to stand straight and takes the staff, measuring it against her height. He marks a spot about eight centimetres taller than her, rests it on a table and cuts it to size. He files the cut smooth. Then he shows Natasha how to hold it, where on the length of the pole to grasp it; one place for walking on the flat; another for climbing; and where forward to position the staff relative to one's stride.

I watch all this and am overcome with the moment. I turn away and look out over the landscape, cut wheat fields, some in stubble, some now ploughed and resting until next season's harrowing and sowing, vineyards and their harvest yet to come, groves of olive and walnut trees. Behind me, there is a gentle old man, lovingly passing on to a young girl with whom he cannot communicate in any conventional sense, something precious to him, which he hopes will be precious to her.

The gift made, we embrace and go our way, meeting up again with Gary and Andrew. I walk on ahead; I want to be alone; my eyes are filled with tears. This is what you cannot buy, what you cannot plan for. Long after I am dead, Natasha will remember Pablito and those precious moments when an old man in his garden made her a walking stick, gave it to her and taught her how to use it for no reason other than she should share in a ritual, the Camino de Santiago, to which he has devoted his declining years.

Dundrum Shopping Centre, Ugg boots, MTV and *The Hills* and all that other crap will never, ever top that. That's one of the reasons I'm on the Camino, because I know what it is giving Natasha.

Los Arcos to Logroño: 29.5 km in 6 hours

NATASHA: The journey to Logroño was longer than I expected. We woke up in Los Arcos early, and the sky was completely clear. Today's walk would be a long one, about a third more again than we had been averaging to date. Dad and I were sure we were going to have a difficult time because of the sun. We left our small, cosy *albergue* alone; we had been separated from the Irish boys because they stayed in the municipal *albergue* on the other side of the village. I was disappointed we wouldn't walk with them. They were good company.

PETER: Los Arcos has been settled since Roman times. It is strategically located on a raised part of the flood plain of the River Odron and was fought over by the kings of Navarra, Aragon and Castile throughout most of the Middle Ages. The land about it is very fertile and produces a wealth of grain, some grapes and vegetables.

We parked ourselves for the night in a privately-owned *albergue*, run by Austrians. It was a pleasing, higgledy-piggledy, hippyish sort of place and, for €8.50 a head, provided us with a good night's sleep.

NATASHA: Our first stop next morning was eight kilometres along the way. The sun was still very low in the sky and the air cool. At a café, we stopped for a drink and there, sitting at the bar, were Andrew, Gary and Reece. We shared tea and coffee with them and chatted for a while before moving off again on our own. I struck out and walked the whole way to Logroño alone. It was now 10.00 am and clouds had covered the sun, and there was a cool breeze. Thank God.

The scenery along the way stayed the same for a majority of the 28 kilometres. It was up and down small, bendy, dusty roads, passing through fields and crossing main roads. It was very pleasant, and the temperature made it comfortable. I passed a number of our friends along the way, having small conversations, and then going on alone. I didn't mind walking alone. I often found good conversation with myself.

For the last five kilometres of the journey, and the most exposed stretch, the sky decided to clear, and the blistering sun was hovering right above my naked face. I didn't now whether to stop and put on sun cream or just speed up and keep going. I decided to keep going and risk it.

I could feel my forehead sizzling. I tried lifting my hand to shelter my face, but my arm grew tired. Finally, after a very long five kilometres, I was protected by tall buildings. The *albergue* was only five minutes in from the outer city, and I found it quickly enough, and got there at 3.30 pm. Immediately when you walked in, there was an enclosed, paved rear garden. In the centre was a tiny, square pool, and sitting around the pool, with their blister-covered feet, were, of course, the Irish boys. I was far too sweaty and flustered to stop and make conversation. I had to get inside and shower.

Unfortunately, the boy behind the desk spoke English and was well up for a chat. With minimal words, I replied to the many of Diego's questions. He was delighted that I was Irish, as he had spent three months in Birr in Co. Offaly learning English. Diego showed me to my room, where I rested for 30 seconds, and then got straight into a freezing cold shower. When I had cooled down, and didn't smell of foot, I went out and joined the boys in the tootsie-pool. Seeing as I had lost a bet, I owed Gary a drink, so Andrew, Gary and I decided to go to the pub.

I love being with them. They are great fun. Conversation flows easily, and they are both really interesting. I love it when they talked about life in the hospital; it was like real life *Scrubs* episodes. We ended up having three beers each, and decided we should try a traditional Spanish drink. Gary told me to order three drinks. The barman's face alone let me know that what we were going to have was strong. He emptied an ice bucket and started pouring red wine into it, then came some orange liquor and about three types of vodka and two sliced limes. It was amazing. After that we hopped to another pub for a beer, just before heading back at 8.10 pm, to get Andrew's wallet, and come back out for more beers.

I met Dad briefly at the *albergue*, writing away. He didn't mind me going out again, as long as I didn't get 'jarred', and so he went off to dinner while we headed out to the pub. We had a couple more beers and I felt like I was at home in Dublin. We left at 9.15 pm to get back to the *albergue* as the doors closed at some time around then. Just as we were up in our room about to go to bed, Andrew went out for a cigarette and I went with him. He started talking about his best friend, Craig, as he was on the phone to him the night before. Andrew was missing him. He was telling me all about him, and how they became friends. I honestly don't think I've ever heard a boy speak about a friend as nicely as Andrew did. He really, really loved him. They haven't seen each other in a long time as Craig is in the army, and will then be going to Afghanistan to work. They seemed really close.

They reminded me of Andrea and me. I had told him all about her, and that it was Andrea's 18th birthday yesterday and that I was planning her present. Andrew and I made a promise to ourselves: one day we would meet each other's best friends. Then we were off to bed. Talking with Andrew made my homesickness go away.

Logroño to Nájera: 28.5 km in 6 hours

PETER: The morning was cold, dark and unwelcoming. The *refugio* opened directly onto the cobbled street that is the Camino passing through Logroño. Stepping outside, we were once more on our way—on his way. His church, the Iglesia de Santiago el Real (St James the King) is closed at 6.30 am. A great big lump of a building dominating a nest of narrow streets, it dates from the 15th and 16th centuries. Above the entrance door on the façade are two very substantial depictions of the saint: the lower one as a pilgrim, the upper one astride a horse, King Billy-style, sword raised and about to enter battle.

The Camino winds its way out of the old medieval city and into the modern city with its wide streets, empty offices and silent, empty shops. Logroño is a substantial provincial city, capital of the Rioja region. Like every decent-sized town we have visited, the historical centre is very well kept, its Camino heritage celebrated and preserved … and used to generate income for the community. As we walk in the cold early morning, we meet again the familiar dawn chorus of delivery vans, buses picking up and dropping off early morning workers, and other stragglers scuttling eagerly to their place of work or wearily making their way home. Shopping areas give way to modern apartment block suburbs, parks and, eventually, industrial zone wasteland grunge. Further on, a reservoir is home to many ducks (they look like female or young mallards), moor hens, coots and a lone grebe. Red squirrels scamper about furtively, gathering early morning food. Finally, the rural Rioja landscape unfolds before us with the rising sun: a patchwork of rolling fields and vineyards; all beautifully kept; most pruned now to push the hot summer growth into the fruits which seem today to be a long way off harvest.

Natasha is more than usually bright and perky this morning after her night out with the lads from Northern Ireland. They went to a couple of cafés and bars around the main square in the old town. She comments, not for the first time, how thoughtful and courteous are young men who are *not* from Dublin. Belfast 1–Dublin 0. Her face is glowing; I notice that for the first time since we started our Camino she is wearing eye make-up …

Thank Heavens for little girls
For little girls get bigger every day,
Thanks Heavens for little girls
They grow up in the most delightful way
Those little eyes
So helpless and appealing,
One day will flash and send you
Crashing through the ceiling
Thank Heavens for little girls …

Navarrete, the first settlement after Logroño, presents itself rather unexpectedly; even though it is 12 kilometres further along the Camino, we seem to come across it in no time at all. Just before arriving, my left boot disintegrates. This is quite upsetting. The boots and I have been companions for about 10 years; I know them and they me; we are both well worn and fit well together; we are a couple. The signs had been grim since Pamplona, it must be said. A cobbler there did his best, gluing everything back in place while not promising things would last to Santiago. As it was, I got another 100+ kilometres out of them. But I didn't come on the Camino to *lose* my soul; rather the opposite if that's possible. Still, a pair of hideous, cheap trainers from the nearest market will have to suffice for now. The boots I left, with a certain solemnity, on a wall of Navarrete's Iglesia de la Asunción, beside a Camino scallop sign and a yellow arrow showing the way to go. A more suitable resting place for boots that had earned their rest I could not imagine.

Inside the church there is one of the most extraordinary and loud Baroque *retablos* to be seen anywhere. It rises from the floor behind the altar and the side aisles right up to the ceiling and then into the half dome above the altar. The entire structure is covered in gold leaf and twinkles and glistens even in the half light of the church's otherwise gloomy, unlit interior. The solomonic (that is, twisted) pillars of the central tableau are extravagantly decorated by climbing vines with bunches of grapes; the pillars of the parts that face the side aisles are festooned with the faces of cherubs. The panels themselves tell the story of the Virgin's assumption into Heaven and carry one's eyes gradually upward as they tell their story. At the top, on the curve of the dome, is God himself looking down benignly on all His works below. The structure is magnificent and I am glad for stopping and obeying my guidebook's entreaties not to pass this place without seeing the spectacle. As I sit there in awe, a lone voice behind me, that of a middle-aged woman, the only other person in the church, recites the rosary under her breath. Outside, two pilgrims are taking a photo of my boots. I feel I should tell them that the real show is inside. But I don't.

As Navarrete yields to the countryside once more, I fall into conversation with a woman I have noticed—watched—over the past several days. I saw her sitting near the foot pool at the *albergue* in Logroño; and several times along the way as well. She has been reading a book that Natasha first showed me and we have both read: *Tuesdays with Morrie* by Mitch Albom. I know the appeal of this book. The woman is slight but broad shouldered; she has short-cut, fair hair and walks with firm, confident strides. But it is her face that catches my eye: her face is strong, really strong and filled with character. Her voice is slightly gravelly; she's a smoker. I'm turning away from photographing a Romanesque gateway to a modern cemetery and taking notes, as one does, when there she is, walking along the side of the road out of

Navarrete. There's a moment of mutual recognition and we begin walking together as the Camino veers into vineyards once again.

"You are writing," she says. It's a question, not a statement.

"Yes," I reply.

"You are a writer?"

"Well, not really. I am a journalist but I am writing a book with my daughter."

"Yes. I have seen you together with her. You are writing together? This is very special. What is it about?"

I agree it is very special, that Natasha is a very special girl to her Dad and I explain what I hope the book will be about. "Why are you doing the Camino?" I ask. This is her answer.

The woman I am with is named Gloria and she is 37 years old. She comes from Barcelona but speaks flawless English, a legacy of seven years in Edinburgh where she studied the European Union and communication. Now she teaches English in Barcelona. "I went travelling but then, you know …" There was someone else? I ask knowingly. "There's always someone else," she replies, smiling. So, come on, why are you doing the Camino?

"Well, something happened recently in my life and I needed time, time to get away and process things; time to think. In January my mother, how do you say? [She indicated to her head; had a stroke? I say.] Yes, had a stroke. And it was terrible. For four months, I went to her each day in hospital and held her hand and talked to her. Work during the day, work hard, and then in to see her in hospital that way she was. Horrible. But I loved her and we had time, I had time, to say things that now I am glad I was able to say.

"At the same time, my relationship broke up and my partner's father died. It was a really bad time and I just needed time away from all that. And so here I am."

Gloria's mother lived in a coma for months and then, mercifully, slipped away.

"It was very hard. You know, we moved her to a special hospital, a hospital that deals with the head only. She was examined and some doctors said 'She is going to die and there is nothing we can do,' but others said 'No, we think she will live.' And all the time, we do not know and I am there holding her hand. She was crying all the time—yes, crying—while she lay there for four whole months. You know they say this is what happens to some of them [coma/stroke patients]. My mother just cried. She was religious, spiritual, and she did not want to have an end like this."

When Gloria's mother died, Gloria was already dealing emotionally with the death of her relationship after seven years and with it, the possibilities of children and life-long partnership. As her mother lay dying, suppressed family history rose to the surface. When Gloria was three and she went to her first school, the school asked (as was apparently the norm) for her to bring with her the 'family book'. This is the book in which the family keeps its own story, the story of births, birthdays and special family occasions which, when read by an outsider, tells the story of the family itself. Gloria brought her family book and the teacher went through it with the little girl, page by page, learning for herself who this new little charge in her care was.

"After the last page, there was another page that I didn't know about," said Gloria.

This was the page recording the life of Gloria's dead three-year-old sister about whom no one had said anything to her. The sister, it transpired, had become ill as a baby. The family believe that a diseased cat somehow transmitted something to the little girl that made her sickly and eventually she died.

"And you know we never talked about it. Never. I was shocked to learn about this."

"How old were you at the time?" I asked.

"About three. I asked my mother what this page was about and she got so angry, so angry. And we never spoke about it again. My mother and my father never spoke about it. And you know, after this baby died, their relationship was not the same. They never spoke about it and they grew apart, and when I was 15 they divorced. When my mother was dying and I was holding her hand and talking to her I told her how angry I was about this, angry she never told me, angry we never talked about this, angry she and my father never talked and then went apart. And you know she leaned over and she kissed me."

We talk about religion and spirituality. "They're really the same thing," says Gloria. I don't know, I said. I am not religious; I am spiritual, emotional; I'm not Roman Catholic; I don't like the institutional church—what it has done to women, what it continues to do to gay people; I don't like its conservatism, its authoritarianism.

I lose Gloria at Ventosa, a place so utterly unremarkable it merits a single line in my guidebook ("The parish church is dedicated at San Cernin," it tells helpfully!). We fall into company again a while later and share some fruit, sitting in the shade under a tree, marvelling at the beauty of the Rioja. "Like the wine?" I ask. "Hmmmm, yes!" she says. "Me too!"

And dwelling on Gloria's story, I realise the time is coming when I should write about my mother.

NATASHA: I arrived in Nájera just after 2.00 pm. I judged the municipal *albergue* on the first look. It looked dirty, uncared for and very small. But it turned out to be very nice, and the people working there were constantly asking if you were okay, and every 15 minutes you would get a refill of red wine. There were about 60 beds, all in the one room. Everybody we had met along the way was there.

I was queuing to book in when a man I had seen before along the way came up to me.

"Do you speak English?" he asked.

"Yes, I'm from Ireland though," I said.

"Did you start today?" He seemed confused.

"No, I started in St-Jean."

"Oh, it is strange because I have never seen you before. I don't recognise you."

He was Spanish and very smiley and friendly and he was playing with me.

Later on, after dinner and when Dad had gone for a walk, I sat down outside to write. The same man came over to me again.

"I'm sorry; my friends just told me you are doing this with your Dad. This is very special, no?"

"Yes, it is very special, for both of us," I told him.

"You must have a very good relationship with him. If I was to walk 800 kilometres with my Dad, I would end up killing him. You are a very lucky girl."

He smiled and left me to write.

I thought about what he had said to me. I had always known that doing the Camino with Dad was special, and more meaningful than doing it with just a bunch of friends. But I had never thought of myself to be lucky, lucky that I could do something that not many could do. I began to appreciate this particular part. I thought about it, and realised that not many of my friends would get to do this, because they wouldn't have the relationship with their Dad that I do with mine.

The further we walk, the better things get. I make more friends. I get stronger, more capable. And Dad and I get closer. Nearly everybody we have met has told me Dad's great. He makes people laugh and is always offering food and help to others. He talks to anyone and is always happy. Dad told me yesterday, when we arrived to Nájera, about the lady he had walked with, Gloria. She was a lovely woman who had had bad luck. It didn't show, however, as she was always smiling and showing a strong personality. At dinner I was looking at her talking with all the people around her dinner table. She was an example of a person whose personality comes through and makes them beautiful. Her story about her dying mother made me think about Dad and Granddad. I often think that when Dad and I are walking separately he is thinking of Granddad. I think about him. Granddad was the grandparent I was most close to. He lived with us for five or six years after Granny died, so I saw him almost every day. Granddad's last year had been difficult, as that's when he started to become really sick and had to go in and out of an old people's home, where there was 24-hour care for him.

When he lived with us and I would go down to the little cottage in our garden where he was, our small conversations were often about the same things—the family, school, writing, piano, tennis, jewellery making, friends and the many things that irritated Granddad. He always loved that I played tennis, because Granny had. He always loved that I made jewellery, because he had been a jeweller. He always loved that I played the piano, because he lived for Lyric FM and was in St Patrick's Cathedral choir when he was younger. And he always loved that I wanted to be a writer, because that's what his little boy had become. Granddad was funny like that. He loved to see his streaks develop in family members.

When Granddad moved into the nursing home towards the end of 2009, we all kind of knew he was going to pass away soon. Dad was often a little fragile after seeing him. I began to cycle down to the nursing home when I could, to pay him a visit. He was always happy and surprised. I would trot into his room welcomed by a: "Oh, who's that? Who's there?"

"Granddad, it's me, Natasha." His blindness had taken away the emotion of his eyes, but you could always see it in his face. I would only spend 15 or 20 minutes with him, as he got very tired. I remember going to see him the day before Christmas Eve. I went with Dad. It was the worst I had seen him look, and it was very hard to talk to him. I was really upset. So was Dad. Dad left the room to get something and I sat leaning on the edge of the bed right beside Granddad. I told him I loved him. I had never said it to him before. He replied slowly: "That's all I care about."

It was one of those things I'll be happy I said for the rest of my life. The last time I saw him was New Year's Eve.

—

MUM

PETER: One of my earliest memories of my mother is of being with her in Courtown in Co. Wexford. We went there occasionally as a family when I was growing up. We stayed in Mrs Grace's farm; Seafield House it was called, a big country home with a gong in the hall that called guests to meals. Sometimes, maybe after a walk on Courtown beach, Mum would take me to a café overlooking the harbour. I was probably about eight years old then. I remember there was a big sailor figure on the roof whose arms would turn in the breeze. There was a juke box inside and I'd badger Mum to play a song, *Hello Mary Lou.* Even now, walking the Camino, I can hear Ricky Nelson …

You passed me by one sunny day
Flashed those big brown eyes my way
And oo I wanted you forever more
Now I'm not one that gets around
I swear my feet stuck to the ground
And though I never did meet you before
I said 'Hello Mary Lou
Goodbye heart
Sweet Mary Lou
I'm so in love with you
I knew Mary Lou
We'd never part

So Hello Mary Lou
Goodbye heart'
I saw your lips I heard your voice
Believe me I just had no choice
Wild horses couldn't make me stay away
I thought about a moonlit night
My arms about you good an' tight
That's all I had to see for me to say
I said 'Hello Mary Lou
Goodbye heart
Sweet Mary Lou
I'm so in love with you
I knew Mary Lou
We'd never part
So Hello Mary Lou
Goodbye heart'

I think of her all the time on the Camino; she is with me through my little silver box which used to belong to Dad. As I walk with it in my pocket, it bounces off my thigh, making its presence felt. I think of Mum and see her during various replays of my life. There was the woman who did weekly shopping with £5 in a local grocery store near Rathfarnham in Dublin where we lived. There was the woman who adored the scenery of the Dublin mountains, who could get enough inner satisfaction from sitting in the sun on the Featherbed with her back against a granite boulder to carry her through the next week. There was the woman who would lovingly pick a yellow rose and place it in Dad's button hole as he went off to work where his style and dash would be admired, to his great satisfaction, not least by other women. There was Mum who nursed me through illness, who fed me steamed fish and sautéed tomatoes when I had yellow jaundice aged 11. There was the woman who I made cry as a teenager by demanding too much when she could ill-afford it and was thinking first of food and not of some stupid fashion thing I wanted. There was the woman who had a great sense of style, of composure, who could look a million dollars with effort that seemed effortless but that I now know required talent and taste. She was beautiful was my Mum. There was the woman who took deep pleasure and satisfaction from simple things and taught me how to do the same.

She wasn't religious in any obvious way. Sure, we were sent to Sunday School and church afterwards every Sunday and Dad participated in the parish by serving on the select vestry and being church warden several times. But their religiosity was, as I think for many Church of Ireland people of their generation in the Ireland of the 1940s, 1950s and 1960s, a quiet affair that was intimately connected to self preservation and the preservation, for their children in the main, of a set of values that they saw under attack but which, in my view, their country came largely to embrace in due course. Mum went to church for much of her life and prayed and sang hymns and participated in the weekly ritual but I still don't know if she believed in God in the conventional sense. Rather, she was deeply spiritual. I think she saw God in nature—in flowers, in birds, in breathtaking landscape, in the purple headed mountain, in the birth of a child. She is with me as I walk the Camino and look at the plants and animals that abound and I hear in my head one of her favourite hymns, the Irish hymn *All Things Bright And Beautiful.*

All things bright and beautiful,
All creatures great and small,
All things wise and wonderful:
The Lord God made them all.
Each little flower that opens,
Each little bird that sings,
He made their glowing colours,
He made their tiny wings.
The purple headed mountains,
The river running by,
The sunset and the morning
That brightens up the sky.
The cold wind in the winter,
The pleasant summer sun,
The ripe fruits in the garden,
He made them every one.
The tall trees in the greenwood,
The meadows where we play,
The rushes by the water,
To gather every day.

He gave us eyes to see them,
And lips that we might tell
How great is God Almighty,
Who has made all things well.

I don't think she could look at an Irish mountain with its cloak of heather and not think of that phrase 'the purple headed mountains' and see a Paul Henry painting in it. When I was about 13 years old and was going to Austria on a camping holiday with the Boy Scouts (at a time when she had never been outside England or Ireland), she said to me, "Take it all in! I want to hear all about it when you come back." I sometimes think that all my writing, all my reporting ever since, has been for her.

Mum was of that generation that was short changed by circumstance. She grew to see the world change in a way that allowed women have infinitely more opportunity than was afforded her, but she grew also to see her children and grandchildren given those opportunities and take them. The sadness was that in seeing this, she saw also what she had been denied. It wasn't that anyone consciously ordained it thus; it was just that was the way things were. She left school at 16, I think, and went to work in the office in Newell's, a department store long gone but then on the corner of Chatham Street and Grafton Street, at the other end of which worked her future husband. She probably would not have gone very far had she stayed in employment; she didn't have the sort of drive, or qualifications, that are necessary. But she had an iron will and determination and was competitive. She was a club and provincial tennis champion and in her later years was a better than average amateur painter. She loved doing landscapes in oil and her children now all treasure examples of her work. She brought us up to understand frugality, perhaps because her own upbringing had its testing times and rough edges.

Her father, John de Lacy, was a Roman Catholic seminarian who dropped out before becoming a priest. More than that, he then eloped with a 16-year-old Protestant girl, Annie Jane White, when he was nearly 40 and converted to her faith. It is family lore with us that her family never spoke to her again, but I recall visiting a great aunt, Sue, in Harold's Cross in Dublin, so some connection was maintained. John and Annie Jane went to live in Limerick, hardly a bastion of liberality in late 19th-century/early 20th-century Ireland. They lived in Barrington Street and took in paying guests, PGs as Mum called them. They had eight children, five girls (Mum, Olive Clare de Lacy, being the youngest) and three boys, two of whom achieved the distinction of playing rugby and hockey for their country. John de Lacy had various jobs, including a stint in the Royal Irish Constabulary, but the PGs were necessary to supplement his income. It appears that he was born a straightforward Lacy but added the 'de', possibly in an attempt to 'Protestantise' himself, as it were, or distance himself and his children from his original family. I have a sepia picture of the pair of them, John in a double-breasted jacket, looking formal and grandfatherly, and Annie Jane appearing to be not a lot younger. Standing in front of them is a tiny, cheeky little girl, Mum, winking at the camera. She looks about eight years old, the same age from which I can trace one of my earliest memories of her.

Very little of this mixed marriage background was known to us—me, my brother, Nigel, and sister, Jane—until I was in my late 20s or perhaps early 30s. I think it was one of Mum's sisters, Auntie Muriel, who let the cat out of the bag by telling me the story of John and Annie Jane. Mum was private to the point of paranoia about this hugely interesting aspect of her past. When my sister and her husband went to live in Limerick and remarked casually that she would now have an opportunity to look at the parish records and trace the family, Mum was on the train from Dublin to Limerick almost immediately, telling her to let sleeping dogs lie. I don't think it was a matter of any sense of shame or embarrassment (and why should it be?); I just think she had some memories she wanted to leave tucked away in the bottom drawer of her mind. One of them may well have been of her Dad dying in Limerick. According to Muriel, when a family member went to see how John was doing, there was a Catholic priest at his bedside imploring him to reconvert on his deathbed. It seems hard to credit the story; it sounds more like an Irish Protestant urban myth and yet I can't think that my aunt would have made it up and no one in the family ever denied it to me. Sometime after John's death, Annie Jane moved to Dublin and Mum spent the rest of her childhood in Ranelagh.

Mum fell ill in June 2002 when she was 79, an age she did not look. She was fantastically fit through walking and exercise classes, and should have had another five years at least. She knew something was wrong inside her abdomen but it took the doctors a while to pinpoint the problem. The delay wasn't their fault; pancreatic cancer is not always easy to detect, but by the end of the summer an ultra sound showed what was described as 'a shadow'. The doctors were wonderful: thoughtful, gentle, patient, inclusive. Nothing was said bluntly; a small amount of information was given, and if Mum asked a question it was answered. She didn't ask too many; she didn't have to. She knew. A course of mild chemotherapy was prescribed, not, I'm fairly certain, with any great belief of a positive outcome; it might slow things down; it would certainly give her something to hold onto, something to focus on …

She came to our house for a few days' rest after the diagnosis and a sort of serenity descended on her. She and my wife Moira had a number of intimate conversations about life and death. On the day Moira's own mother died in England, Mum asked to see her, to comfort her. Moira was distraught, naturally. She asked Mum how she was coping when we all knew she was frightened of death. Mum said, "Something just happens; I don't know what it is, something just happens and you are able to cope."

I went into her bedroom one morning and she put her arms around me and said, "I don't want to leave you all." And then she added, "I don't think I ever told you that I love you. I don't think I ever said the words. I love you and I want you to know that." I was devastated. I was so upset that she could think I didn't know she loved me. Everything she ever did for me was done with love and I knew it.

The doctors said she could live for between two and six months. In the event, she lived for nine. When the end was approaching, she and Dad moved from their house, a cottage near us, into a granny flat mews in our house. That way he was settled before she was gone, the trauma for him minimised, to whatever extent that was possible. He was in denial; we'd try to explain as gently and specifically as we could but the information just didn't go in, didn't register. One day in May 2003 when she and we could no longer cope alone, Jane and I drove Mum to the hospice in Harold's Cross. We didn't say where we were taking her; we could not bring ourselves to do that—her generation remembered such places as Rest Homes for the Dying. We couldn't do that to her. But the hospice was wonderful; the staff exceptional. For 10 days she had a room that opened onto a patio and a flowerbed; Cashel, a Labrador dog, would amble into her every now and again and they'd have a chat and share a Marietta biscuit. One of my last memories of her is of her sitting in a chair, withered and shrunken to almost nothing, wrapped in a blue dressing gown, looking contentedly through the open patio doors watching birds feeding from a table. She was at peace at that moment. After she slipped into a coma and I was sitting with her one morning, a Catholic priest tip-toed into the room and asked me if I would like him to pray beside her. He knew, he said, that my mother was Church of Ireland but he would be very happy to pray for her, if I wanted it. I said I would like that very much. He recited *The Lord is My Shepherd*, slowly, softly, and then blessed Mum before leaving the room. In a beautiful way, I felt a circle had been closed on what happened in Limerick all those years ago and that she would have approved, very, very much.

She died on 4 June 2003. She simply curled up and stopped breathing—shallower and shallower and shallower ... and then no more. The nurse who was present pronounced the formality. "I am sorry to have to tell you that your mother is dead." The finality, the enormity of it, cut us to the quick. Dad was holding her hand. The nurse offered to take off her ring. "No," said Dad through tears, "I put it on 56 years ago and I'll take it off now."

Next morning I woke with a start. There was a single, crystal-clear, instant thought in my head: this was the first, the very first, morning of my life when my mother was not alive to share it with me. I loved and missed her so much on that morning and I have loved and missed her so much every morning since.

You passed me by one sunny day
Flashed those big brown eyes my way
And oo I wanted you forever more
Now I'm not one that gets around
I swear my feet stuck to the ground
And though I never did meet you before
I said 'Hello Mary Lou
Goodbye heart
Sweet Mary Lou
I'm so in love with you ...'

Nájera to Santo Domingo: 21 km in 5 hours

PETER: A kilometre or three outside Nájera, as one approaches from the east, there is a place named Poyo de Roldán—a place 'where an enormous treasure is said to be hidden buried', according to a tourist information poster there. Roldán is the Spanish name for Roland, he of Charlemagne and Roncesvalles fame. The sign is interesting as, once more, it provides evidence of the great soup of truth, half truths, legend and myth surrounding both the Camino and medieval history.

Roland and Charlemagne were knocking around Navarra in the latter half of the 8th century. The seminal Battle of Roncesvalles in which Roland died took place on 15 August 778. But a huge amount of 10th, 11th and 12th-century myth-making related to the intertwined French and Spanish imperatives of, firstly, ridding Spain of the Moors and replacing the Saracen with Iberian regimes friendly to France; and, secondly, asserting French Catholic influence along the Camino. We know that the 'discovery' of the remains of St James in Galicia did not occur until around 814. According to the version of events at Poyo de Roldán, Roland was on his way to Santiago several decades *before* the saint's remains were allegedly found, thereby creating the shrine to which Roland could not possibly at that time have been going. No matter; as all propagandists know, it is the essence of the message that matters, rather than the facts.

Poyo de Roldán is the location of a legendary battle between a Syrian giant named Ferragut, said to have been seven metres tall and to have had an enormously wide nose and the strength of 40 men. He was, according to the legend, from the race that gave us Goliath. The emir of Babylonia sent Ferragut and 20,000 Turks to rebuff Charlemagne's incursion into Spain. They met outside Nájera, the story goes, Ferragut challenging the best of the French to come and get him. The French sent their best, one by one, and, one by one, the giant made mince meat of them. Roland, ever the hero, demanded to be given his chance. After hours of battle, Ferragut offered Roland a truce but the knight rejected this and battle was joined again for 'two days with its nights', as the sign puts it. Over the two days, they had occasional breaks and seemingly amiable chats, arguing the pluses and minuses of their respective religions. And just like the wily lad of many a legend, Roland did not miss the key bit of information that Ferragut let slip: like Achilles and his heel, Ferragut had just one weak spot—his navel. And so when battle resumed and Ferragut got Roland on the ground and was sitting on him, squashing him to death, the knight whipped out a dagger and stabbed the giant in his navel, killing him. Or, as the sign puts it, 'he arduously unsheathed his dagger and plugged [*sic*] it into him killing him'. Roland thus liberated Nájera from the heathen Moors and released imprisoned Christians. Or, as a graffiti 'artist' has added to the tourist notice: 'Then he [Roland] went and burned Pamplona, despite his promising not to. And the Basques ambushed Roland at Roncesvalles and killed him. Moral: You can kick giant ass but don't mess with the Vascos [Basques].'

All of these stories were central to underpinning popular support for the Reconquest of Spain from the Moors (which took several hundred years more) and in portraying that battle as one of good Christian against evil Moor, proselytising support for the Camino and the push to establish the French Cluniac model right across northern Spain.

Nájera is in a lovely setting. The word Nájera comes from Arabic and means 'between cliffs'. The town is indeed located, or the old part of it anyway, tucked onto a tongue of land beneath red sandstone cliffs and hemmed in by the wide but very shallow Najerilla River. The town authorities keep the river banks beautifully manicured and the water is home to a great variety of reeds and rushes, including a forest of bulrushes in full bloom. It is popular with local fly fishermen trying for trout. Like many other of the settlements along the Camino, Nájera was developed on a Roman settlement base, held a strategically important place for east–west traffic and stood sentinel over fertile plains to the town's north. The town's importance was cemented when members of the Navarran royal family were buried at the Monastery of Santa Maria, founded in the 11th century.

The *albergue*, run by the town's Los Amigos, didn't look great but in fact turns out to be one of the best so far. It has a great atmosphere, exceptionally pleasant staff … and better than average wine for an irresistible €1.50 a bottle. When Gloria and I were eating fruit under the tree just before reaching Nájera, a walker went past us at a rate of knots. A tall, slender man looking well into his 60s and with an impressive moustache, the ends of which were twirled and pointed, he walked like he was in a race of life and death. He held walking poles in both hands and jabbed them into the ground as he went. The tap-tap, tap-tap, tap-tap, tap-tap, tap-tap sound they made was matched by his small but urgent steps. He must have been moving at about eight kilometres an hour and there was something beyond urgent in his walking method; it was almost violent. It was like he was punishing himself.

Gloria and I looked at him bemused. "God, that was like a steam train," she quipped as he disappeared down the track.

Getting up in the Nájera *albergue* next morning, there he was again, seconds after the lights went on—out of bed in a flash, down onto the floor for a series of rapid-fire press ups. Up-down, up-down, up-down, up-down, up-down with such force and determination it was as though he was trying to hurt himself, pushing himself to some limit, waiting for his system to crack. I carried on into the shower, and when I came out he was just finishing. He stood up, ram-rod erect, chest glistening with perspiration and stuck it out as though he had something to show everyone. His pectoral muscles were enormous and his seeming 60-whatever-year-old torso sported a six pack of which Brian O'Driscoll would be proud. With his moustache twirled and pointed, he looked like the weightlifter in an Edwardian circus. I felt like telling him to chill out, relax, have a coffee; talk to Gloria …

I got dressed, had a coffee and went online for five minutes. And no sooner than that but your man was off. "Bonjour!" he announced to all and sundry as he rattled through the dining room and out the door like a TGV …

Walking out in the early half light a little later, the Camino rises through a pass in the sandstone cliffs and up onto a vast plateau given over almost entirely to vines. And for the first time we experience rain; a light, penetrating drizzle which seems to irritate other pilgrims, but after so much sun and heat it doesn't bother me that much at all.

After a brisk five-hour walk, the town of Santo Domingo presents itself to the pilgrim. The first *albergue* we come to is in a 17th-century Cistercian monastery. A rickety door opens from the street into a cobble-stoned courtyard, the left into a small reception area and a glass box in which sits a rather severe-looking, middle-aged lady. It's all rather reminiscent of an Intourist hotel in Omsk, c.1985. There's a little warren of rooms, all badly in need of modernisation and a lot of TLC; very old linoleum predominates; there are ancient, ill-fitting doors everywhere. But it is genuine; the dining room is wonderfully ancient and an elderly and kindly nun pads about the place welcoming us. There is no charge; a donation of €5 is suggested.

Santo Domingo has a wonderful story to tell. In the early 11th century when devotion to St James was really taking off and the Camino attracting a steadily growing volume of pilgrims, the location of today's Santo Domingo was little more than a swampy mess interspersed by forests that were infested by rogues and thieves who preyed on travellers. Domingo Garcia was born in 1019 in nearby Viloria de Rioja, and in due course he received a vocation to serve God. So he gave up sheep herding and tried to become a monk. But the monasteries at both Valvanera and San Millán found him so thick when it came to studying that they effectively threw him out. Undeterred, he went off into the forest determined to be a hermit and build a hermitage in honour of Mary, mother of Jesus. In this role, he noted the stream of pilgrims travelling to Santiago and their determination to press on, regardless of the obstacles in their way that made the journey such an ordeal in the Middle Ages. Domingo Garcia resolved to try to make their passage through the area a little more bearable. He built a bridge over the River Oja and he began chopping a 37-kilometre path through the woods with sickle. When he stopped to rest, angels picked up his sickle and the clearing continued. Finally, the king (Garcia III Sanchez) told him he could rehabilitate a ruined fort as a pilgrim hospital. Through the efforts of Domingo Garcia, the area around present-day Santo Domingo de la Calzada became among the safest for pilgrims travelling to Santiago.

A place in history well earned, one might say. But what happened next raised Santo Domingo to superstar status.

In the early 12th century, a German husband and wife, together with their son, were going as pilgrims to Santiago when they stopped at the town that had grown up. An amorous innkeeper's daughter took a shine to the lad but he, being a pilgrim, was not about to allow himself to be distracted by matters of the flesh. Angry at being rebuffed, the innkeeper's daughter stole a goblet from the church, hid it in the boy's belongings and promptly informed the authorities of the dastardly theft. A search was mounted, and when the church silver was discovered the young man was convicted of theft and hanged.

In those days it was common practice to leave a criminal corpse on a gibbet for days, if not weeks, the flesh rotting, the mortal remains becoming food for birds and other scavengers—a frightful sight intended to be a deterrent to other would-be thieves. The young man's heartbroken parents continued their pilgrimage despite the appalling tragedy that had befallen them. On their way home they approached the town of their grief with trepidation, but when they came to the gibbet a voice told them that their son was alive, that Santo Domingo had saved him! Delighted, they rushed to the home of the judge who had passed the death sentence to inform him. He was roasting chickens at the time. He was having none of it and poo-pooed their silly claim. "Your son is as alive as these chickens I am going to eat."

And at that very moment, the chickens, a cock and a hen, leapt from the spit, crowing: "*Santo Domingo de la Calzada / que canto la gallina después de asada*" (Santo Domingo de la Calzada / where the chicken crows after being roasted). And to this very day, two chickens, a cock and a hen, always white, are kept in a display case high on a wall of a transept in the cathedral of the town that bears the name of Santo Domingo. The ornate black and gold wooden case, with a window through which the cock and hen may gaze down at worshippers in the cathedral, was made in 1445. The cock and hen are changed every month and it is said that today's pair are bred from descendants of the very two that leapt from the roasting spit all those years ago.

The chickens are in fine fettle the day I visit them. The cock is a-doodling to his heart's content, his crowing echoing all around the cathedral. It is bizarre, ridiculous and utterly enchanting. The cathedral is a wonderful, well-lit building full of interesting medieval art and, of course, a mausoleum and crypt for the great man himself, Santo Domingo, the idiot hermit in whose name a 1,000-year-old tradition endures and delights tourists and pilgrims alike.

Santo Domingo to Belorado: 23 km in 4.5 hours

PETER: Things were a shade, shall we say, fraught before setting off for Belorado.

I had gone to bed as usual at about 11.00 pm; Natasha had stayed downstairs with her Belfast Musketeers, which was fine ... except by 1.30 am her bed remained unoccupied. I lay there debating whether to go downstairs and tell her, in no uncertain terms, to get to bed pronto. Except there was no sound coming from downstairs. Maybe she was asleep down there, or maybe in another bed. Either way, the implications of rooting about the multiple-bedroom *albergue* disturbing all the other pilgrims (and maybe also waking the nuns), were not attractive. By 2.00 am, I gave into parental instinct and went down. There was no sign of her; no sign of anyone. The rear door from the dining room, where just hours before eight of us had enjoyed a fine communal meal and a variety of Rioja wine, from the basic to the not half bad, was wide open. In the tiny garden a single chair was against the wall in such a way as to suggest an escape …

Oh fuck.

Think. Think, think, think.

They're not nice blokes from the North; they're lunatics. They're not gentlemen; they're having their evil way with my little girl. They all collapsed paralytic drunk on the pavement and are being pumped out in the nearest hospital as medics mutter about the plague of young foreigners coming to Spain and acting like eejits. They got in a fight after shouting in the bar in the main square that the Spanish team were, actually, like, crap, know what I mean, really crap?; the Dutch were robbed; if it weren't for the ref etc etc etc … Hang on; what's likely to be the case? She's in Sancho Fritzl's basement already! Pull yourself together. This is a small town; there's no big river of which you know. There's been no clatter of police or ambulance sirens. Oh yes there was and you were asleep and you didn't hear, you feckless git, and now you're in REAL BIG TROUBLE. What sort of a feckin' father are you?

Hang on, hang on, hang on. Isn't it far more likely that they got locked out? Or maybe met some others after doing their bunk and are still, well, having a good time like young people do all the time (eh, like you did)? Hmmmm, doesn't make it any easier. But yes, like I did and, yes, that's more likely.

And so back to bed and lie there rigid, wide awake looking at the ceiling and reacting to every tiny sound to see if it's her tip-toeing to bed … And then someone's mobile phone alarm goes off (one of those really silly tunes) and suddenly it's 5.40 am and a couple are rousing for their day's walking. I'm out of bed in 1.75 seconds, dressed in 1.85, and down at the *albergue* door in 1.95. There's someone knocking.

"Tash?"

"Yeah."

"That you?"

"Yeah," voice sounding a tad sheepish.

"Are you okay?"

"Yeah. I'm real sorry, Dad. We got locked out; we were just minutes late getting back."

Not entirely true, young lady.

"Well, you'll just have to wait there a while longer. They'll open up at 6 and you can get in then."

Relieved voice: "Thanks, Dad."

"And then it will be time to pack and start our walk."

"Okay, Dad." Voice slightly more relaxed at evident absence of volcano on other side of door.

I guess when you are 18 and 21, the old chair-against-the-wall wheeze seems fiendishly clever, original probably. But the wily old nuns have seen it all before; the chair on the outside, the one in the adjoining yard that made the re-entry possible, had been removed and they were stuck. In a kind of weird way, it reminded me of a book that was hanging around our house when I was a child, a 1949 book about a nun who escaped from a convent after having a change of mind about her vocation but when it was too late and she was just going to have to stay inside for the rest of her life. It was entitled *I Leap Over the Wall* and was written by Monica Baldwin. It was the sort of volume Protestants read as affirmation of all they assumed about the Catholic Church!

Tasha's leap over the wall got her to a little local festival in the village square, and then a hotel lobby that didn't want to know about a couple of clots that got themselves locked out of the *albergue*, then a couple of street benches, and finally a bus shelter. But the important thing, I guess, is that she and her Musketeer stayed calm, stayed together and looked after each other.

Oddly enough, I walked much better than Tash today …

The mix of vines and grain gave way, as we left Rioja, to grain and sunflower fields. Dozens of fields and millions of bright yellow flower heads facing east as the sun rose and began to pound on our backs.

NATASHA: So, now my side of the story.

We had just had an amazing dinner, all eight of us; American Bill and his parents, the three Irish boys, Dad and I. A feast was prepared. One course included Gary's family recipe chicken and vegetable soup, and wine was drunk in large quantities, mostly by us as it was Bill's last night with us and we planned on staying up past the oldies.

By 11.00 pm all seven bottles of wine, six cans of beer and one carton of white wine were empty, and Dad announced bed time. Quickly, before closing time, I ran to the nearest pub and bought a bottle of wine for us, and a sneaky beer for myself. Now we had to make a plan.

The plan was 'to go to bed', along with Bill's parents and Dad, and then in 20 minutes we would meet again and have the bottle of wine between us. A very excited Gary reminded us every five minutes that we were to meet in 20 minutes. I got into my pyjamas so that I could hop right into bed when we came back up.

We took the bottle of wine and went to the tiny bathroom where there was a bath. Bill and I sat in the bath, while the other three huddled around. The wine took about 15 minutes to open as our cork screw wasn't very good at all; eventually it was opened by Andrew's teeth. As classy as we Irish are, we began to pass the bottle around and we quickly became noisy. To sort the noise levels out, we decided to be responsible young adults: use a toilet paper roll as 'the conch' and one could only speak when they had 'the conch'. Of course this didn't work out too well.

When the bottle was drunk we wanted more. We decided we were going to take our adventure to the outside world. We were going to fool the nuns, and escape. We snuck downstairs and out the back door. We put a chair against the wall, and then one on the outside for our return. The wall was high enough and it would have been difficult to climb back over without it. We thought we were geniuses. What could go wrong?

One by one we hopped over and walked towards the centre. There we found a huge square packed with people and *Mambo Number Five* was being blasted out. Of course we had a dance, and then onto the nearest pub.

Beers were being bought right, left and centre. I lost track of how many went down, but it was enough for me to forget I was wearing my pyjamas. We were keeping up the Irish reputation. We played drinking games and talked to strangers like they were our best friends. We were having such a good night.

At 1.30 am we decided to head back. This is when things got complicated and our plan was shattered. Somehow, Andrew and I fell behind the others. But as far as we were concerned, it was only 5 minutes. I would kill for a picture of our faces, when Andrew and I walked down the street where the *albergue* was, and saw no chair, no Gary, no Bill and no Reece. Shit. We were stuck outside. This was when

I noticed the cold for the first time, and it only got colder. Damn nuns caught onto our plan, we thought. We also thought that the others just hadn't got to the *albergue* yet, and that they would come trotting around the corner any minute. They never came. We waited. They never came. So 2.00 am came, but they didn't. We began knocking on the door and ringing the bell. No one was coming. The whole city was silent. There wasn't a soul in sight.

The only light we could see was a hotel. A really fancy one. In stroll Andrew and I, looking rather rough. "Can you help us get into the monastery, please?" All we got was a laugh. "It closes at 10 am. You can't get back in." We left, found a bus shelter and slept there until just before 6 am, when we slowly walked back to the *albergue.*

"Fuck, fuck, fuck, fuck, Dad's gonna kill me," I said.

"Fuck, fuck, fuck, your Dad's gonna kill ME!" said Andrew.

I told him he wouldn't, but in my head I sort of thought Dad might blame Andrew, or else praise him for looking after his little girl.

There was the shuffling of keys and the mumbling of a nun on the other side of the door when we got there. That's when I heard Dad's voice. It wasn't as furious sounding as I had prepared for, and he didn't call me Natasha, so this was a good sign. As soon as I got into the room I had to grab my things and come downstairs to begin our walk. Dad thanked Andrew for looking after me; he knew I was safe with him. After a few scowls from him, he began asking me about the night and he turned out to enjoy our antics in Santo Domingo. I later got a few giggles out of Gary's sleeping position which Dad described to me. I believe it was like a turtle on its back, legs in the air, almost struggling.

PETER: Your version, eh? So, just which bit did I get wrong in mine?

Belorado to San Juan de Ortega: 24.5 km in 5.5 hours

PETER: We are later than is sensible leaving our Belorado *albergue.* A certain person is more tired than might be expected had that certain person not slept in a bus shelter the night before ... And so now we are setting off in full sunlight and the day ahead promises to be hot. The Camino rises from about 800 metres to around 1,150 and then falls again to around 1,000 before reaching our destination. I just hope we don't fry. Belorado seems, on an admittedly scanty viewing, to be a fairly unremarkable place. However, near the Church of Santa Maria is the

El Corro district, now a UNESCO world heritage site. In 1116, Alfonso I—Alfonso The Fighter, as he was known—granted the district special privileges to hold a market (the special bit usually meant that Alfonso and his ilk got a slice of the financial action thus generated, let it be said). The market quickly became one of the most successful in Spain and claims to be the country's oldest. One side-effect of the resultant boom was the growth of a Jewish quarter at the foot of the nearby castle, now in ruins.[7] Behind the church, carved into what look like sandstone cliffs, are caves that used to be home to saintly hermits.

The Camino graduates into open countryside once again and for the first time the bulk of the grain being grown is barley, yet to be harvested. Pretty much as far as the eye can see, the land is given over to grain—wheat and barley. It is not the most interesting countryside, mostly rolling fields of stubble. At the second village en route, Villambistia, a lovely, tiny hamlet of perhaps half a dozen houses and a large, 17th-century church, I see the first memorial connected to the Spanish Civil War, fought between 1936 and 1939, between government, or republican, forces and usurpers of that power who were a conservative, essentially fascist political movement known as the Falange, and some army officers led by a general, Francisco Franco. A tablet over the entrance door lists seven men under the statement: *Caídos Por Dios y Por España*—They Fell for God and Spain. Memorials are erected mainly by victors and the word 'caídos' would not be accepted by the republican, losing side because it implies sacrifice in a noble cause.

7. Jews played a significant role in communities across northern Spain in the Middle Ages. Major urban centres in Navarra and Castile all had vibrant Jewish quarters in settlements along the Camino. There were significant Jewish communities in Pamplona, Estella, Burgos and León. For the most part, Jews, Christians and Muslims lived in peace, but not always, and Jews were usually the victims. In 1196 the Christian armies of Aragon and Castile attacked León and took hostage an entire Jewish population living on a hill just outside the city. In 1276 there were Christian-inspired anti-Semitic riots in Pamplona; and there were anti-Semitic riots across Spain generally in 1391. On both occasions many Jews were murdered, and in the 1490s the Jews were expelled from Spain altogether.

After Villambistia, the Camino rises steeply into a national park in the Montes de Oca which is afforested with sessile oak and Scots pine. The path is lined by several varieties of heather, from light to deep purple, and broom, which is sadly out of season. In spring the riot of yellow and new season green must be spectacular.

At the top of the hill there is a memorial to the losing (i.e. government) side in the Civil War. Some of the worst atrocities were committed by the rebel falange forces in and around Burgos in the summer and early autumn of 1936. People with known or presumed republican sympathies were rounded up, often in pre-dawn raids on their homes, and bundled away, either never to be seen again or only as a bloodied corpse dumped on a street corner some days later. A concrete obelisk at a high point in the Montes de Oca commemorates something altogether greater in scale. Under the date 1936, the obelisk says this: *No fue inútil su muerte, fue inútil su fusilamiento.* My fellow pilgrim, Jesús (pronounced 'hay-zeus') Sanz Castro, an architect from Madrid, translates this as "It was not unuseful their death, it was unuseful their execution." The obelisk is a memorial to some 400 men, presumed republican sympathisers, who were 'disappeared' from Burgos, murdered and buried *en masse* at that spot. Jesús says that across the other side of the Camino the bodies of their women are buried. Even today, the obelisk can arouse passion as is evident by several layers of paint under the words. I assumed it was covering graffiti, but Jesús explains that the people behind the monument had the flag of the 1936 government painted onto the obelisk though it was repeatedly painted over with the post-1939 (i.e. Francoist) Spanish national flag. Recently, everyone gave up and now there is just white paint and no flag.

The Camino runs through the forest for what seams like an eternity. The sun is high in the sky; our shadows stretch less than a metre from our bodies and even my hat is dripping with sweat.

NATASHA: For the first time, today my feet are sore and I feel them as never before; I feel they are beginning to tire. The first stretch of the walk was boring and unexciting. We walked out of the village, which seemed to all be under renovation. Nearly all the buildings looked like they hadn't been touched for 200 years, some had been knocked down, and some were being done up. When we came out of the village we passed over some main roads, a falling-apart petrol station, and then finally we were in the Camino world of the countryside. Here, we were protected. Clean from dust coming off speeding cars going by, and covered from the sound of the tyres beating over the hot tarmac. We were surrounded by different noises and peaceful imagery. It was like every insect in the ditches on either side of us was trying to wish us a good journey.

We stopped off at around 9.00 am at a café in a passing town. Every time Dad and I decide to stop in a particular café and have some breakfast, I always find it funny that almost every other pilgrim chooses the same café, and you soon find yourself surrounded by your friends once again. It's a Camino thing, I guess.

We get talking to a Spanish man I have seen around before. He spoke to me briefly in Nájera, but we never caught names. He has a very good-looking face and a beautiful smile. His name is Jesús, and he is 35. He's an architect from Madrid, but is originally from Pamplona. He was very interested in Dad. They had an interest in history in common and conversation flew with them. He found Dad very knowledgeable and reminded me of this later on, when I spoke to him again.

Unusually, we stopped off a second time, because there wasn't another village after that one for 12 kilometres. We had a drink and some nuts in a nice beer garden attached to a hotel. That was the last time we stopped. The journey to San Juan de Ortega was mostly on dusty field paths, winding along the countryside and disappearing over the horizon. I hadn't noticed the sun that much yet, although I could feel it on my shoulders. I had plenty of sun cream on, so I wasn't worried about getting burnt.

The walk was quiet; it was just Dad and I for a majority of the walk. Andrew and Reece had decided they were incapable of walking any further, and were in fear of damaging their feet more, and so they got the bus to Burgos. They would stay there for two days recovering, and we would see them when we arrived on foot. I wasn't envious because they are now going to hell as this is cheating the 'Camino spirit'. A real pilgrim would have cut his feet off to deal with blisters, bandage the stumps of their legs and just crawled on. Simple.

The moment where the heat became noticeable was when we veered off the roads and onto a wide, red, stony forest path. The width of the path meant the tree shadows didn't reach you, and you were totally exposed to the sun, directly above. The noise of the forest, however, was incredible. It was even louder than walking through the fields. I came to the idea that it was the forest creatures' equivalent of the running of the bulls' festival, because there seemed to be a synchronised chanting coming from beneath the tall trees.

The forest path was endless. Looking down towards the end made it worse as it only disappeared into the horizon, suggesting no end. Every corner we turned I was expecting to see a little village, or at least an end to the forest. I had the idea we were 20 minutes away from our destination.

It was here that my feet suddenly began to pain me. I could feel blisters sprouting like new potatoes in a crop field, all over my heels. The only way it didn't hurt was walking like a horse, on the balls of my feet. After a while this hurt my calf muscles. I was slowing down rapidly, and prolonging my time in the sun. I tightened the straps on my bag and gradually began to jog. Then I sped up and it turned into a run. There was no pain. This was great. I passed Dad. "Tasha, why are you running?" he shouted after me.

"It's the only way it doesn't hurt," I replied, my voice being left behind.

I passed single pilgrims. Odd looks came my way. I even passed out a chubby cyclist. Before I knew it, I was running into the shade of forest trees, on a narrower path. It was slightly downhill, making it even easier for me to run. I passed a man and his son who were with an Australian woman I had talked to before. "That girl," the man exclaimed, "she is running." "Aye, she's Irish," the Australian replied.

I ran out of the forest shade and into an open area where the town became visible. I was so relieved. The trail ahead was dotted with clusters of pilgrims. I didn't know whether to start walking of not. When I slowed down the pain came back, so I ran. As I ran past fellow pilgrims they clapped and cheered me on. They told me later I was crazy.

When I arrived into San Juan after about 2 kilometres of running, I saw Gary sitting under an umbrella. There is a small trail of pilgrims' rucksacks outside the closed *albergue.* I sat my bag down in the queue. As red as a poppy, I came over and enjoyed a well-earned Coke with him. Twenty five minutes later, Dad arrived.

PETER: San Juan is most welcome. It is little more than a very large church and *albergue* and a café/bar all in one row—a substantial terrace of cut-stone buildings. There are a few village houses around the corner but as one arrives after a very long and hot walk, there isn't anything else that one can see to San Juan. However, the café provides me with fantastically welcome draughts of Tinto de Verano (essentially a red wine spritzer) that refresh instantly. And then, as pilgrims lounge about on the grass outside the café trying to cool down and catch their breaths, around the corner from the direction of Burgos come two men on horseback. They are in full military uniform—hats, trousers tucked inside impressive black boots—and sporting shiny, polished cavalry sabres. The horses are white and fine looking. The men progress with a certain stately indifference towards the crowd of sweaty pilgrims. Could they be latter-day Francoist forces re-enacting something, perhaps? Probably not as, on closer inspection, they appear to be dressed in mid-19th-century hussar-style uniforms of the sort common in many central and eastern European countries.

Lieutenant-Colonel Barnabás Ádám, aged 44, and Second Lieutenant Pál Mike Bugnics are in fact cavalry officers with the Hungarian Army on a 3,500-kilometre trek from Lisbon to Budapest. When I try talking to them by saying, "Peregrinos?"—the Spanish for pilgrim—Barnábas replies in accented but perfect English, "No understand. You speak English?"

"Great!" I say. "This is going to be easier than I thought. Why are you doing this?" I ask.

"Why not!" says Barnabás with a big grin as he and Pál dismount for a break. We all sit on the grass and they tell me their story.

There are just two of them riding and two support colleagues up ahead making sure there are supplies and somewhere suitable to stay each night. The route is well planned and what they are doing is official, not some retro jolly by a couple of soldiers having a lark on their own time. On 15 July they left a NATO facility in Lisbon, the JALLC (Joint Analysis and Lessons Learnt Centre)—armies the world over cannot function without expressing themselves in acronyms—and aim to cover an average of about 50 kilometres a day. The penultimate highpoint of their extraordinary journey will be on 6 October at Pákozd, a place between Budapest and Lake Balaton where, in 1849, the Russian Army of the Tsar executed 13 generals of the Hungarian Army, five of them hussars, having intervened, at the request of Austria, in the Austro-Hungarian war, in which Hungary was seeking its independence. In between, they are visiting a network of places including Tarbes in France and from there following the old Napoleon route into Italy (to

Maranyo, Lodi, Castiglione and Solferino), Slovenia (Gorjansko) and into Hungary via Lenti and on to Pákozd and Budapest.

The horses were bought in Portugal and are named Pretty Girl, a half Arabian, half Luzitano; and Mimo, a half Arabian, half Garucho. They are eight and nine years old and seem perfectly content munching away and drinking water as Barnabás and Pál slice a side of what purports to be bacon but looks like 95% fat, slap it onto bread, offering me a sandwich sitting on the grass in the welcome shade of a small sycamore tree. "The main aim [of our trip] is to explore the links between Nato countries' light cavalry units and also visit some places particularly associated with Hungarian history," says Barnabás. He and Pál have small rosettes in their national colours pinned on their chests but not a lot else evident to me declaring their nationality. We talk about Hungary and how it has changed since the end of communism and joining the European Union; and about NATO and the Irish Defence Forces and Kosovo and Chad. Both men are well up to speed on Ireland's position on neutrality and NATO and Partnership for Peace and EU battle groups.

A middle-aged man with a dog strolls over and chats to the men. He's evidently also Hungarian; a bit of a coincidence, I think. As he talks to Barnabás and Pál, they stand, straighten up and become a little more formal. A woman, a small woman with a Camino hat, shorts, walking boots and a warm smile, also strolls over and introduces herself. There are big smiles all around. Barnabás and Pál take the woman's left hand in turn and kiss it in the old-fashioned, rather formal style. In a moment, Barnabás turns to me and says, "May I introduce the Hungarian ambassador to Spain?" The woman turns to me, we smile and shake hands, in contemporary style.

This can't be true, surely? I remark. But it is true, confirms Edit Busci-Szabo, Ambassador of the Government of Hungary to Spain—and Camino pilgrim! Weird! Did she know to meet them here, today? I ask.

"Yes, of course I knew they were doing this. The embassy is told of these things routinely," said Edit, "but I did not know they would be here today. Miklos [her husband] and I are walking from Belorado to somewhere beyond Burgos. When I saw [Barnabás and Pál] and their uniform, I wondered, and then of course I saw their rosettes with our national colours and I knew who they must be. Seeing them is just a coincidence but a nice one."

And so we all stand there in the shade of the little tree chatting about Hungary, the hussars, the Camino, and the EU, Edit's speciality as a diplomat on her third term in Spain, the first time as ambassador. Whisky the dog ("I prefer the Scotch variety to the Irish," says Miklos explaining the name spelling. "Sorry!") is altogether sniffy of Pál's offer of a thick slice of the pig blubber. Must have been reared on Ferrero Rocher, I suppose …

NATASHA: When the *albergue* opened at 1.00 pm, we brought our bags to our beds and relaxed for a while. At 6.30 pm every night, this *albergue* upholds a tradition: they serve all pilgrims staying with them a bowl of garlic soup in their dining hall. It was a hard day's walking—and running—and was just what we pilgrims needed. It was lovely soup, and we were surrounded with lovely people, having lovely conversations. I guess it's another Camino thing.

San Juan de Ortega to Burgos: 26 km in 6 hours

NATASHA: As we left San Juan at 5.00 am, we arrived in Burgos at an impressive 11.00 am. I was hobbling. My feet were in a bad way, and for the first time I was worried about the next day's walk. Dad said we could take a rest day in Burgos to let them heal. But I didn't want to fall behind and lose everyone, again. I had developed five blisters. They were small, but in very awkward places.

Tim and Louise are an Australian couple we met on our way to Nájera. They have been travelling the world for nearly three years, and are finishing it with the Camino, before heading back to Melbourne. They are reluctant to go home, but say it's time to get married and eventually have a family. "Pop a few kangaroos," in their case.

They are really lovely people and I like them very much.

PETER: Tim is a radiologist and Louise a physiotherapist. They have been paying for their long trip through Europe by using their skills in temporary employment wherever they can. They spent several months in Scotland and hoped to get work in Ireland but found it impossible. Nonetheless, they visited and liked the country.

Louise has a natural, seemingly effortless prettiness. Her hair is cut short, she has freckles, glistening eyes and is always smiling. She wears pearl stud earrings. She's the sort of girl who could throw on a skirt, her boyfriend's shirt and a pair of sandals and look a million dollars. The people who make the ads for Gant clothing and Tommy Hilfiger should look her up.

Tim is also a handsome man and has that slight laidback drawl that many women seem to find attractive. When we meet again in Burgos, he and I fall into conversation. For some reason we both mention TGV man and his extraordinary walking speed.

"You know, he's got a tombstone tattoo on his leg," says Tim in that Aussie way of inflecting the sentence at the end so it sounds like a question.

"Go way," I said. "I hadn't noticed that. I must look out for it."

NATASHA: As soon as we arrive outside the municipal *albergue* in Burgos waiting for it to open at 12 noon, Louise sees that I'm in pain and immediately rummages through her little sanitary bag, squeaking in a worry in her little Australian accent. She tells me exactly how to treat them and gives me a needle and thread so I can burst the blisters later. And she tells me the name of the medicine to buy to dab on them so they won't become infected. She was caring and kind, and I felt like I was back at home, with Mum nursing me over a little tummy ache. Then they are off, for a night of luxury treatment. We filthy pilgrims with our smelly feet watch as they disappear around the corner. It's Tim's 32nd birthday and so they are staying in a hotel—with actual duvets, room service, air conditioning and other wishes a pilgrim longs for after nearly 300 kilometres.

Andrew and Reece had come from a café where they had been relaxing for the morning, after their sinful bus journey to Burgos the morning before. Their feet were all cared for, clean and on the way to mend. Reece was looking extremely pleased with himself.

After getting through the outskirts of Burgos, which is industrialised, covered in petrol stations and a huge airport, we were in the heart of the city, filled with sandy-orange cobble stones, little boutiques and cute cheese and meat shops. Burgos was alive with people on their morning missions. Small elderly women, with their little slipper shoes, would tootle by with fresh bread for lunch, and men would occupy the small cafés, reading the paper, with an espresso and a cigarette. Pilgrims were scarce at this hour as many wouldn't arrive until later.

The most famous thing about Burgos is of course the cathedral. It's the largest in Spain and is known for its extravagance and burly essence. Sitting outside the *albergue* on the bench, I could see the peeks of the towers breaking through the skyline. I decided to have a quick look.

As I walked around the corner, the enormous beast sat, threateningly, like a spider on the edge of its web, in the centre of the square. No words can describe the gothic cathedral in a way that one will understand. The towers were smothered with creatures hunched over, looking down on the people of the city, and appear like claws, or bat wings, closed over. The guardian angels of the parapet stand, protectively, over the flying buttresses. It looked like something out of *War of the Worlds* that had risen from the earth and was going to start destroying the city at any moment. Later I looked inside at the cost of a small fee. The inside too was like no other cathedral I have seen. To me, it looked like every detail of every statue and carving had been created with the idea to intimidate and terrorise. I do have to say I was more impressed with the outside.

PETER: The Cathedral of Burgos reflects the city's status as a regional capital and the most important city in Castile before the rise of Madrid. Burgos developed on a hill overlooking the Arlanzón River that was fortified by the Romans. Later, the Visigoths and Muslims didn't pay the area much attention, concentrating instead on the kingdoms of Navarra, León and Aragon, and on the emirates around Córdoba and Granada in al-Andalus to the south. It wasn't until the 11th century, when Sancho el Mayor of Navarra took possession of the area, and Fernando I el Magno became the first Christian ruler of the medieval era to preside over a semi-unified northern Spain, that Burgos began to develop its position. Its wealth was based largely on trade, part of which related to its being more or less in the middle of the east–west Camino de Santiago, and part because there were good connecting routes between Burgos and north coast ports such as Laredo, Santander and Castro Urdiales. The Meseta Alta, the vast upland Castile plateau that is Burgos' hinterland and was then a wool-producing area, was thus linked via the city and the ports to the textile-developing nations of England and Flanders. Successive monarchs pump-primed the Burgos economy by decreeing tax incentives, such as the abolition of duty on goods imported to the city. As trade led to more trade and a growing economy produced wealth, the city developed a metropolitan character together with all the varied bureaucracy of government.

The first cathedral, built in honour of Saint Mary, was Romanesque and dated from 1075. But what one sees today has its origins in the 13th century with Mauricio, Bishop of Burgos. This man had studied in Paris and travelled in Germany, and as a result of what he saw there he determined that Burgos should have a great gothic cathedral. The Romanesque one was knocked down and, on 20 July 1221, work on the new cathedral began. It was to be in the characteristic Latin cruciform, measuring 84 by 59 metres and made of pale limestone. But building went on throughout the 13th and 14th centuries ... and the 15th, 16th, 17th and 18th.

Inside the cathedral, separate individual chapels are two a'penny—17 of them in all. The building is filled to capacity by religious art, medieval and Renaissance, and religious sculpture, *retablos* and other carvings and statuary. The cathedral museum's collection of gold, silver and gilded goblets and crosses, and heavily embroidered vestments going back centuries, must be among the finest, possibly the most concentrated, anywhere in Europe. The square choir located in the centre of the aisle is breathtaking—two rows of walnut stalls, 44 on the lower level, 59 on the upper, face each other across a recumbent effigy of Mauricio, who died in 1238. The bishops' stalls are at right angles to the choir stalls and face forward, looking up the remainder of the nave to the altar. Above the stalls is a carved frieze of panels that tell the story of Genesis; the back of each stall tells an individual biblical story. The cathedral is littered with alabaster sarcophagi of the great and good (and not so great and good) of Spanish history, temporal and religious.

If there is a single masterpiece in the entire building (and it is near to impossible to select one), it is the crossing—the ceiling of the tower and what lies beneath. In 1539 the original gothic ceiling collapsed and what one sees today was built between 1540 and 1573. The tower is held up by four heavily ornamented and sculptured pillars. The ceiling is a geometric, star pattern that, from the floor gazing up, looks like delicate filigree, light streaming through the openings onto all that lies below. In between the top of the pillars and the ceiling, there are two tiers of windows and, between them, reliefs that tell the story of the assumption of Mary and of several Old Testament characters, including Daniel, David and Moses.

And beneath all this? Under the floor of the crossing, the literal pivotal point of the entire building, is the tomb of El Cid and his wife,

Doña Jimena. El Cid, Rodrigo Diaz de Vivar, is one of the heroes of Spain's long battle to rid Iberia of the Moor.

Burgos Cathedral does not do subtlety.

NATASHA: When the *albergue* opened Dad and I were in first. It was very nice. Modern, massive and equipped with everything one needed. All the rooms were big, white, bright and open planned. There were big glass windows and large, wooden sliding doors everywhere. The downstairs had a kitchen and dining area full of big tables and benches.

After I had gone to the pharmacy and bought iodine and plasters, I showered, and prepared to pop my blisters with a needle and thread. I then took a nap. Dad went to Mass in the cathedral. I dined on my own later on, as I finally found a café that could tame my craving for calamari, and I just couldn't wait for Dad. I bought a couple of bottles of white wine for later for whoever wanted it.

PETER: 2.00 pm Mass was held in St Thecla's Chapel inside the cathedral. It was Sunday, after all, and I felt strongly that after two whole weeks of pilgrimage and walking almost 300 kilometres, I wanted to participate in a religious service, if only to praise God for giving me sturdy feet. Where better than in perhaps the most extraordinary cathedral in Spain?

The Chapel of St Thecla is probably as large as at least half the churches in Ireland and yet it is merely one chapel of 17 that are housed within the cathedral itself. It is rectangular and dominates the left-hand side of the south entrance to the cathedral proper, the Santa Maria doorway into the main aisle. One side of the chapel looks out onto the aisle through four huge, arched openings that are glazed and have iron grills. Each of these arches corresponds to the entrances to four small medieval chapels that occupied, until 1731, the space that is now St Thecla's. Behind the medieval chapels stood the parish church of St James the Fountain. So in all, no less than five smaller churches were demolished to create St Thecla's. I labour the point only to give an idea of the enormity of everything associated with Burgos Cathedral.

St Thecla's has two rows of 14 pews, each capable of seating 15 or more worshippers, on either side of its aisle. At 1.45 pm, it is lovely to just sit there soaking in the peace and calm and take in the religious art and, most of all, the spectacular *retablo* behind the altar. The Rococo ceiling is a sight to behold. There is a main dome covering most, but not quite all, of the chapel interior. It is heavily decorated with geometric patterns that remind me of nothing more than one of Indigo Jones's 18th-century garden designs. One could be looking at the plan for a series of interlocking rose garden flowerbeds in a stately home. The colour of the plasterwork is pleasing as well: deep greens and blues, red, gold and white—nothing vulgar, nothing garish. For that, one must turn to the *retablo*.

It is dedicated to St Thecla, a saint of the early Christian church and a follower of Paul of Tarsus. She was saved from martyrdom—burning at the stake—by the onset of a storm. Overall, the *retablo*, which is Baroque and was made between 1730 and 1736, is typically ornate, gold and extravagant in design and execution. Four pillars separate the main vertical panels from the two side panels. It is perhaps 20 metres tall and maybe seven metres wide. The lower part of the central panel is dominated by Thecla, in a beautiful, flowing red and gold dress, looking a little nervously into the middle distance. Hardly surprising as she is standing on a mound of logs, the pyre of her would-be martyrdom, being added to eagerly by two very obviously Muslim-looking characters. Immediately above Thecla are three much smaller statuettes—the Boy Jesus of Prague, St Ignatius Loyola and St Francis Xavier. On Thecla's right we meet again Santo Domingo, reading his bible, two white chickens clucking about his feet, and, on her left, a very severe, disapproving looking St Anthony. What has him so grumpy is not entirely obvious.

Above all this, we have the top panel, the crowning glory of the whole edifice: St James himself, on that horse again looking very King Billy-ish, sword raised, hat festooned with scallop shells, smiting his enemies. And who might they be? Two Moors, looking very Moorish in their turbans and flowing Arabic clothing, being trampled upon by James's horse. And all made in the 1730s—some 600 years after the Moors were expelled from Spain, with no verified help from St James!

On the other wall, the one facing the glass panels looking out onto the cathedral aisle, there are four wall-mounted reredoses (essentially, much smaller *retablos*). One is dedicated to Santa Lucia, which seems appropriate as she is patron saint of the blind. With me I have my little silver box, one of my father's prized collection of snuff boxes. He being blind for the last eight years or so of his life, I think this would amuse him.

There are about 45 people present at 2.00 pm when Father Victor Ochotorena walks from the sacristy to the altar to say Mass. It is a perfectly ordinary Mass from what I can tell because it is, of course, in Spanish. But as always, I find the Mass a little impersonal because I am used to something different, something by definition more familiar and which always seems to be more involving of the congregation, especially because of hymn singing which the Church of Ireland does quite well. In time, Fr Ochotorena calls the faithful forward to take the body of Christ. I queue with the others; it seems wrong not to, not to acknowledge and participate in the observances of others when I am their guest. After the Mass, I chat a little to Fr Ochotorena. He is a very nice, warm, friendly man, a little bemused, I think, at this pilgrim seeking his name.

As I leave the now empty church, there is a middle-aged Spanish women sitting in the rear pew weeping quietly to herself. I'd like to give her a hug but don't; I'm fragile enough myself with my little silver box rubbing my thigh through my pocket as I walk.

NATASHA: At around 7.00 pm, Andrew, Reece, Gary and I had a few drinks down in the kitchen area. Somewhere in between a bottle of wine Reece disappeared with his phone. He returned to the table looking very happy. He had been talking to home, which included a little hello from Eddie, his Jack Russell dog and mountain walking partner.

Reece and Andrew hadn't eaten anything but a croissant from earlier that morning. I often forgot they didn't have a Dad to take them out every night. So when Dad arrived with bread, salami, olives, crisps and more wine, their faces were priceless. It was a good night, and later, Jesús joined me, and we had a glass of wine before heading to bed.

Burgos to Hornillos del Camino: 20 km in 4.5 hours

PETER: The municipal *albergue* in Burgos must rate as being in the five-star category of *albergue*. It is right by the cathedral, and in a small courtyard by the entrance there is an appropriate bronze statue of a pilgrim anxiously examining his toes for blisters. Inside the *albergue*, there are ultra-modern sleeping, washing and eating facilities. Each bunk bed has its own light and plug, and permanent screens afford a large measure of privacy.

Getting ready for the off at 6.00 am, TGV man (who is obviously delighted with his nickname after I tell him) is limbering up, imitating a train. I get down on my hands and knees to examine his calf muscle. "What is it?" I ask, looking closely at the tombstone. He projects his calf muscle towards me and I see that it is a milestone tattoo. And then he shows me the corresponding spot on the calf muscle of his other leg and there is a tattoo of the cross of St James. "Ah oui," he says proudly, smiling and putting his arm around me.

"You know my name is Pardon," he says, "Yes! Pardon!"

"Pardon?"

"Yes, Pardon. Unusual, non?"

"Yes. And what's your other name?" I ask.

"Alain. So I am Monsieur Alain Pardon. And you know what?"

"What?"

"I really was a TGV driver."

"Go way!"

"Non. It's true. I drive TGV until I retire about five years ago. Yes. Really!"

"How old are you?"

"56."

Good grief, he's a year younger than me.

"And after, I, eh, how you say, I go …"

"Went?"

"Oui, I went to Asia to teach TGV there. But now I am retired and I run in marathon. Yes. In Paris and many other places. Okay, now I go. See you later!"

And he's off; out the door, tap-tap-tap-tap-tap with his walking poles, passing all before him.

I fear the walk today. Today we take our first steps up onto the Meseta Alta, the rolling plateau on which much of central and north-west Spain sits. It is a vast, largely flat region that stretches from north of Madrid right up to the Cantabrian and Picos de Europa mountains in the north, and lies between Burgos on its eastern flank, right across to just beyond León in the west. The northern meseta is Spain's breadbasket—a huge area where grain is grown en masse, and not a lot else. The meseta is the sun's anvil and there's no way around it—the pilgrim must walk through the meseta to reach his goal.

The start of the walk from Burgos takes us through the usual grungy outer city areas and then before us we see a great escarpment a couple of hundred metres high—the way up to the meseta. But happily today the sun is not breaking through the early morning cloud cover and we make haste up and along the flat plateau. There are some early morning farmers about and rows of wind turbines but the walk otherwise is dull. Coming down a steep incline to the village of Hornillos, the leg muscle just above my right Achilles developed a deep, dull pain that I could not seem to alleviate in any way. It was clear immediately that it would be foolish to go on. It's funny how after two weeks on the Camino, 20 kilometres seems a short walk and something of a lost day.

NATASHA: I was worried about the walk we had ahead of us as we left Burgos. Firstly, I was anxious to get out of bed and step on my feet for the first time since treating my blisters. To my surprise I could feel nothing. I was relieved. They were only tender, but no liquid had gathered overnight in the punctured blisters and they were only dead skin now. Secondly, Dad had kept mentioning the hot, flat meseta and all I could think of was Alexander the Great, and his men, travelling along the Georgian desert, which I studied for my Leaving Certificate exam. I'm terrible in heat, and get burnt very easily. Being pale, and having red hair, I fear the sun deeply, and must apply serious protection before starting the walk as, once I get warm, it doesn't stay on as well.

Thankfully, the sun hardly ever came out. Dad and I keep thanking our blessings, as we have been ridiculously lucky with the weather so far. We haven't really had any horrific days of sunshine.

The walk out of Burgos was quick. Being a large city, I thought it would take longer to get out. We walk the familiar yellow dusty Camino path straight into the expected barley and wheat fields. The colour of the blue, red and yellow ditch flowers is stolen by the white dust from the road. The leaves look like silver, spray-painted Christmas decorations.

On the horizon sits a sausage-shaped bulge of land. Dad fears that once we reach the top of the hill, the meseta will be the only thing our eye can see.

As we get closer we find ourselves walking parallel to the motorway, and once we cross over the bridge that's the last of 'the other world' we see.

The roaring of the lorries and vans disappears behind us, and we are soon enveloped in the quietness of the Camino. Dad and I walked alone for the whole journey today. Depending on my blisters, we had planned to walk the usual 25–28 kilometres. My blisters were absolutely fine, and so that was the plan. We were heading for a town called Hontanas, where everyone else would be going. Finally, after miles and miles of nothing, a small town became visible in the distance, as we slid down a rocky path. I was relieved we would have a break.

Dad had been having a little trouble with his ankle, but said it was fine and wasn't giving him any bother. When we had got down the slope, we began on a straight road into the village of Hornillos del Camino. Along the last kilometre, we passed a number of our friends, including Gloria and her Italian fan club—three fellows she has fallen in with and who seem to like her a lot. About 300 metres from the entrance to the village, Dad bent down quickly and grabbed his calf. His faced showed he was in pain. Slowly, he hobbled into the village. The first bar had a squad of cyclists outside it, so it seemed many were stopping here for a break. Dad said he wanted to book in for the night. I presumed that others would too, then. We went to the *albergue*, Dad in pain, and put our bags outside, ready to book in at 12.00 pm.

The village was based around one tiny main street of houses, two bars and one shop. It wasn't the best town we had stayed in. I walked towards the shop to buy a drink. Sitting outside on the bench was Jesús, Gerry, an Englishman, and a few others. I asked them if they were staying here. They said no. They were walking another 10 kilometres to Hontanas, with everyone else. I was really disappointed; 10 kilometres could separate us from the others for the rest of the journey to Santiago. I told him Dad had hurt his calf muscle badly and that we were going to stay here. I headed back through the village towards the *albergue*. Dad had taken our bags, and was booking us in. I sat outside in the sun on the steps of the Church, looking onto the main street, where other pilgrims were passing, on their way to Hontanas.

My ankle had formed a cut, where my boot had been rubbing; it wasn't sore, but looked bad. I clipped my heel on the step I was sitting on, and within seconds my foot was sitting in a large pool of blood. It looked horrific. In my disappointed, bad mood, I did nothing. I just sat there and let it bleed; I would clean it when I was bothered. People passing were pointing and whispering at my dying foot. A bunch of women bent down beside me and started speaking Spanish. With all the energy I had, I told them I don't speak Spanish, and that I was okay. They shook their heads and walked on.

Then a man, around 60, walked past me. He saw the pool of blood, and had the same reaction as the women. He disappeared and came back five minutes later with a little toilet bag. He was Spanish and didn't speak one word of English. Yapping away to himself, he lifted my foot and started to clean it and plaster it up. As he was cleaning my cut, he pointed at the sun, and then on his legs. He had psoriasis and his whole body was covered in skin that was purple, tight and very scabby. It looked extremely painful. I felt sorry for him.

This was a moment that summed up for me the kindness and care you find along the Camino. This man didn't know a thing about me. He could have happily carried on walking past me, down to the bar, to enjoy a nice cold beer, after his walking. Instead, without hesitation, and in the most natural way, he went back to his room to aid my cut, that I was too lazy to clean myself. Without any understanding of each other's language, we spent 15 minutes with each other, communicating by gestures.

As I sat with my leg on his knee, Jesús, Andrew, Reece and Gary passed, saw me, and walked over. Again, the concern expressed by them was touching. They were all asking after Dad, as Jesús had informed everyone of his injury, and then asked how I was. I felt guilty, as I was in no pain; it just looked bad. Their departure onto the next village was sad. None of us was sure if we would walk together again, yet we all said, "See you tomorrow."

I wasn't going to make Dad push on. Permanently injuring his calf muscle would be much worse and could ruin our whole trip. Instead of sulking about it, we had an early dinner, an early bed, and a promised 5.00 am start, to catch the others.

Hornillos del Camino to Frómista: 46 km in 10/11 hours

NATASHA: As promised, we got up at 5.00 am, and were out the door, walking, at 5.15 am. I was determined to catch up with the others, who were 10 kilometres ahead of us, having spent the night in the next town, Hontanas. It would take us about two hours to reach them. Andrew had told me they were going to leave at 7.00 am, so I was hoping we would arrive there just as they were leaving and we could carry on with them.

It was completely pitch black outside, and the sky was unbelievable. It looked like a sheet of black velvet, with white diamonds scattered across it, the Milky Way sliding through the other stars dexterously. Our path was flat, open and straight for the whole 10 kilometres.

Nearly every time I go to the gym back home in Greystones, I see this man. He's about 28, very athletic, and good looking. When I'm with my best friend, Andrea, which is usually every day, and we're wandering around the town, I see this man regularly. And every time I do, I say, "There's the guy that's always in the gym!" And every time, she replies, "Where!? Where!? Oh yea!" And then we move on. These are the kind of things Andrea and I get excited about, along with really good doppelgangers.

When we were on our way from Hornillos in the dark, I got a text from Andrea telling me she was on the night link bus, on her way home after being out in Dublin, and that the guy who's always in the gym was on the bus as well. I started laughing. I replied, telling her that's brilliant. She was shocked to see that I was out walking, and she was just getting into bed, from a night out.

We got into Hontanas just after 7.00 am. We met Gerry, the Englishman, just as he was leaving his *albergue*. The others were a little further ahead but Dad and I stopped for coffee. Dad's ankle muscle wasn't giving him any bother and he seemed up for a good day's walking. I was relieved. A lot of the walk was alongside a quiet road, with large trees on either side, creating a sort of avenue look. Walking along the overgrown ditches, you could hear rustling noises. If you stopped for a moment and followed the noise, you would find a little mouse, or a shrew, standing completely still with fright, with their little black, beady eyes staring at you. After another 10 kilometres, we came to a large town named Castrojeriz. We stopped again, for coffee. We met a few of the others here. After coffee, Dad slowed down at a church. But the clouds were clearing, time was ticking, so I kept going. I was really reluctant to get caught in the midday heat, as I was wearing tight black clothes, and no sun cream. But once again, thankfully, a thin cloud sheet blocked the sun's full potential rays and heat. I didn't see Dad for the rest of the walk after Castrojeriz. I walked alone, and quickly.

We had mentioned trying to make it to wherever everyone else was heading. We had done 21 kilometres when we reached Castrojeriz, and both agreed it didn't feel at all like it. I don't think either of us realised how far we would be walking to keep up with the others. The nine kilometres to the next town, Boadilla, was along the meseta, and I was praying the skies didn't clear. And they didn't. In the distance, I could see a little picnic area beside a water tap, and a man was selling fruit here. I also found Andrew and Gary here. They were impressed at how far and fast I had come. They mentioned making it to Frómista, another 14 kilometres after Boadilla, which was just a kilometre away. I had already done 32 kilometres and wasn't sure if I was capable of another three hours walking. I was also worried about Dad, who was far behind. I left Andrew and Gary at the picnic area, and carried on so as not to allow my legs get stiff.

When I reached Boadilla, I found Reece, Steve the Australian and Jesús, having a drink. They couldn't believe how far we had come. I didn't want to think about it, so bought a Coke, and just kept walking. They told me they were aiming for Frómista too. I badly wanted to make it there. The walk from Boadilla to the next town, which was eight kilometres away, was horribly difficult. I struggled the most here. The skies had cleared of all cloud and I was completely exposed to the sun; the temperature was around 35 degrees—really hot. I slapped on some cream while walking. Reece, Jesús and Steve were always on the horizon ahead.

I got a text from Dad then, asking where I was. Surprisingly, he suggested we keep going to Frómista. It sounded very unlike him, and I thought he might have miscalculated just how far that was for us to go. However, when I got to the last town before Frómista, I kept walking, as agreed. I had severe Bambi legs at this point, and was finding it very hard to walk. It was the last six kilometres, and after now, that's nothing.

Walking in front of me as I left the town was a lady. I had noticed her before along the way, staying in the same *albergue*s and that, but I had never spoken to her. She turned around and saw me, and like we were best friends, she called me over, shouting "Hola! Hola!" Looking behind me, I saw no one, and so ran up to her.

"Italiano?" she asked.

"Eh no, Irish. I speak English," I replied, looking at the flustered, tiny lady. She was about 53, much smaller than me, very tanned, and walking with difficulty. She had the most ridiculously large rucksack on, that looked like it had a child in it.

"Oh. No English. Only Italiano," she said stubbornly, waving her arms about. However, she began making small conversation in English, every fourth sentence being a groan and a complaint about the heat.

"My name is Angela, Angie," she said.

"My name is Natasha."

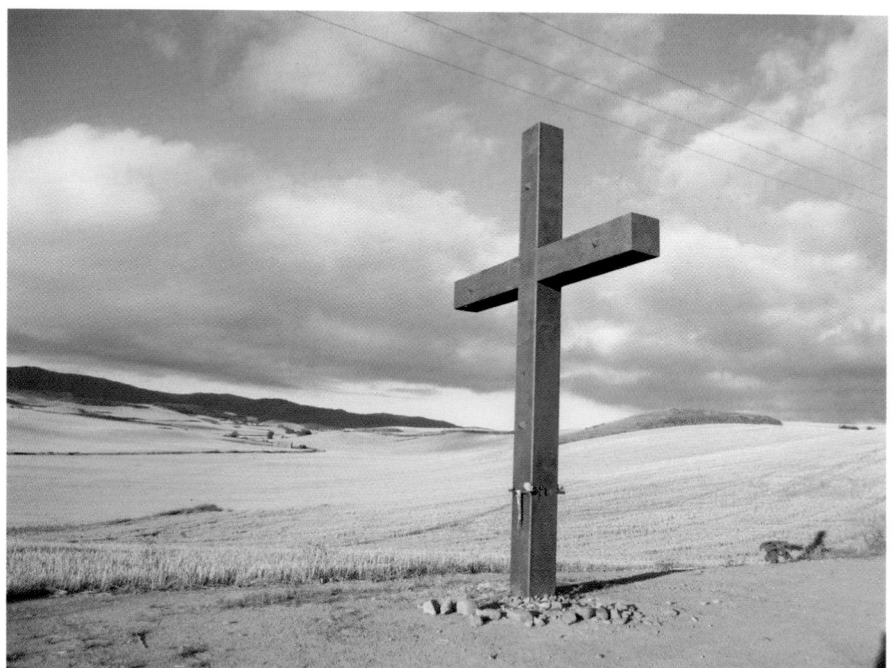

Crosses are commonplace along the Camino. Many are medieval but this one, not far from Belorado, is modern. (*Spanish pilgrim, Antonio Cebrián*)

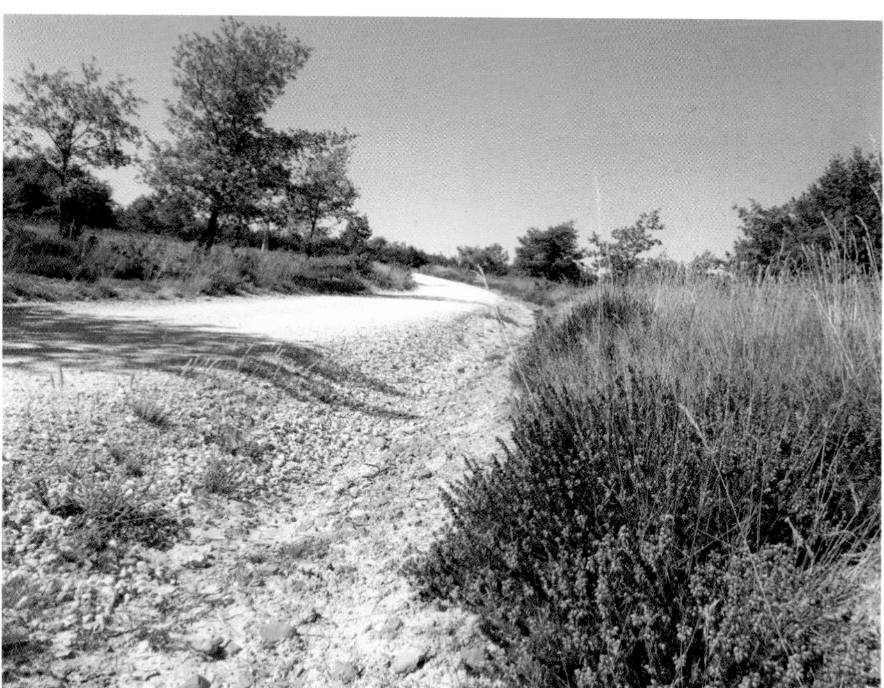

Purple-flowered heather.

Lt-Col Ádám in full dress uniform on his return to Hungary. (*Hungarian Ministry of Defence*)

Hungarian hussars: Lt-Col Ádám Barnabás (*left*) and Pál Mike Bugnics.

Plump, ripe sloes.

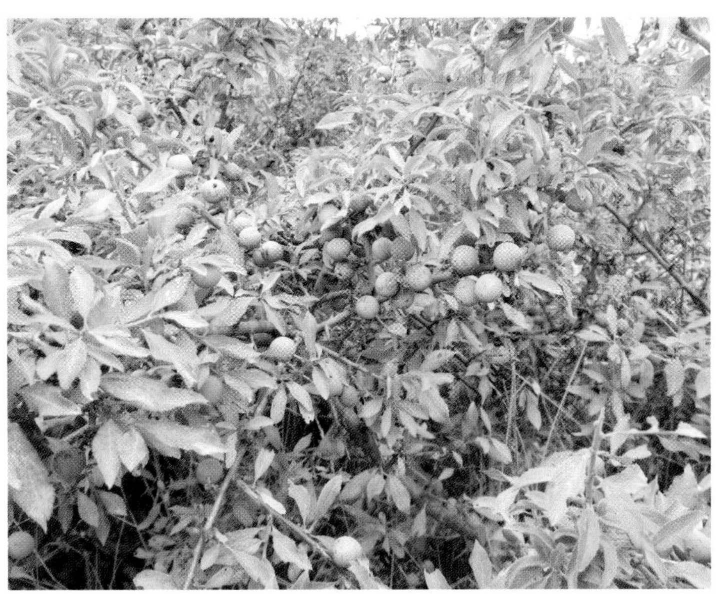

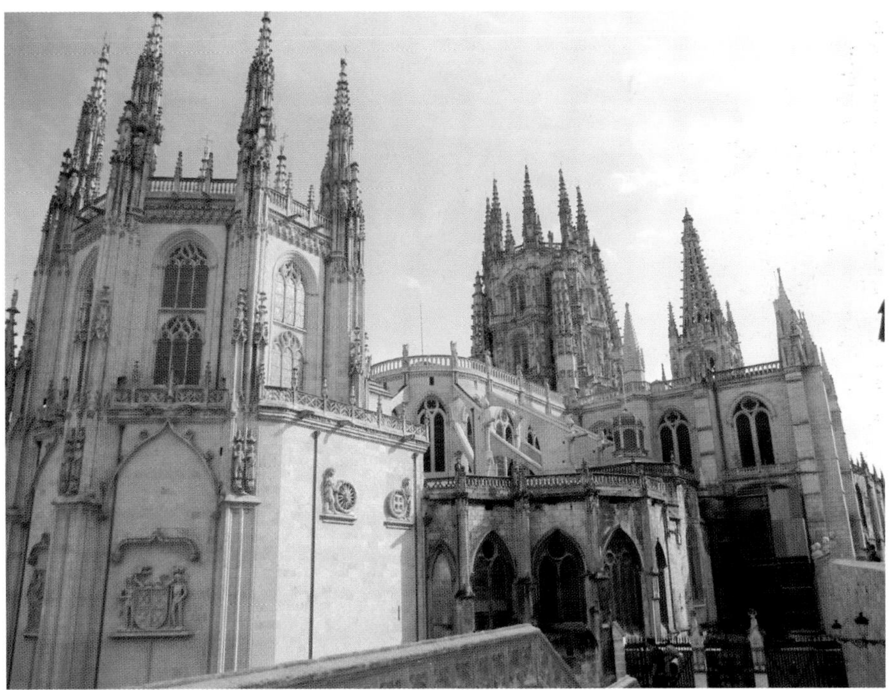

Like something from outer space, Burgos Cathedral. (*Sascha Thieme*)

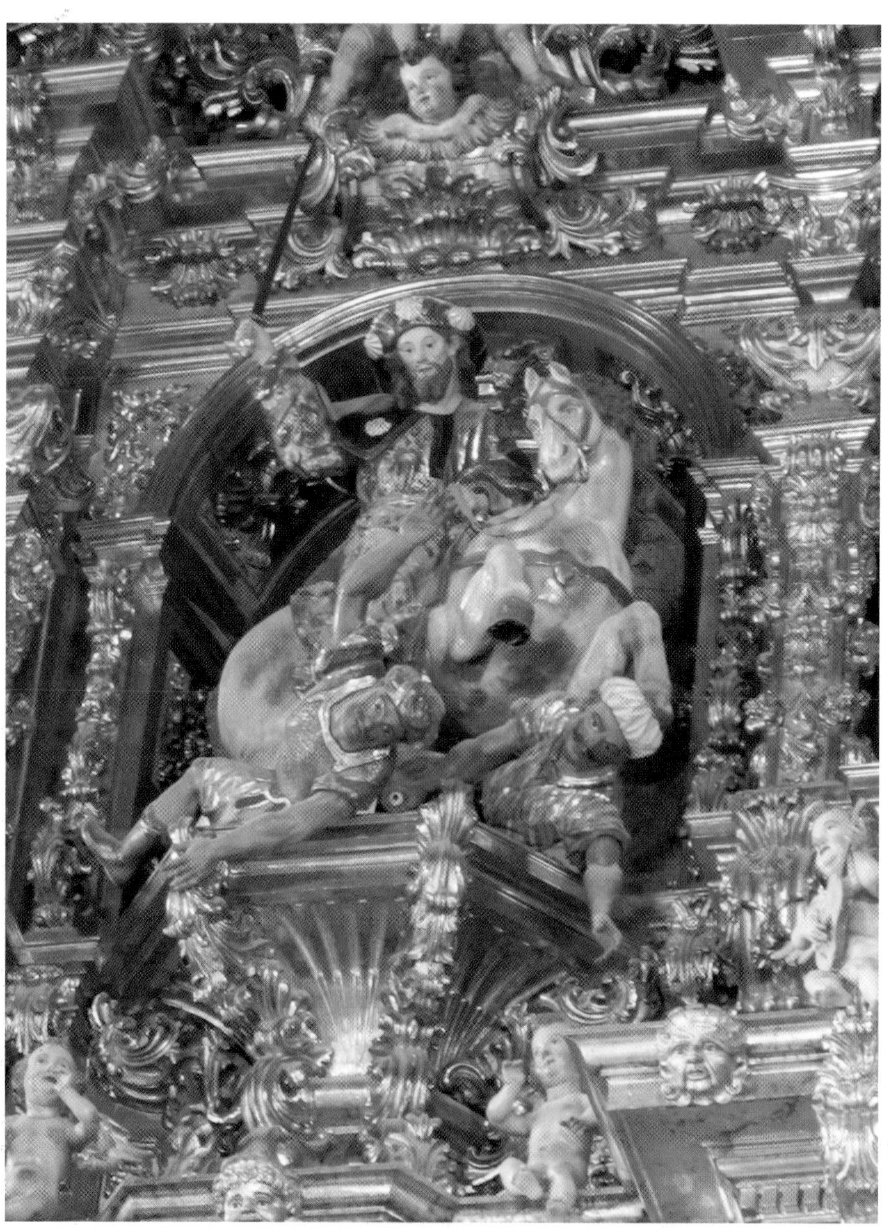

Santiago Metamoros—Santiago the Moor slayer—from the *retablo* in St Thecla's chapel in Burgos Cathedral. Note the two figures being trampled on.

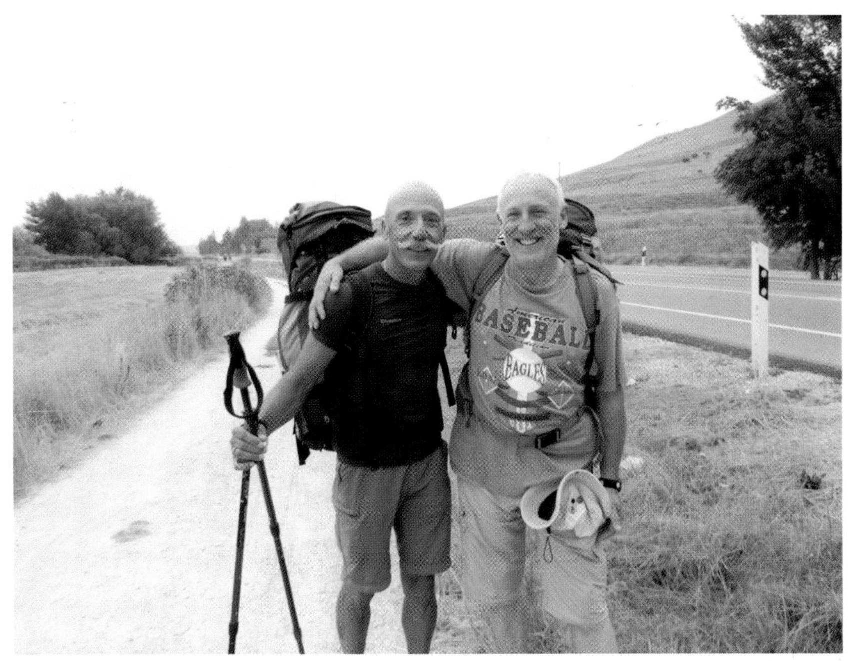

TGV man, Alain Pardon (*left*), with Peter.

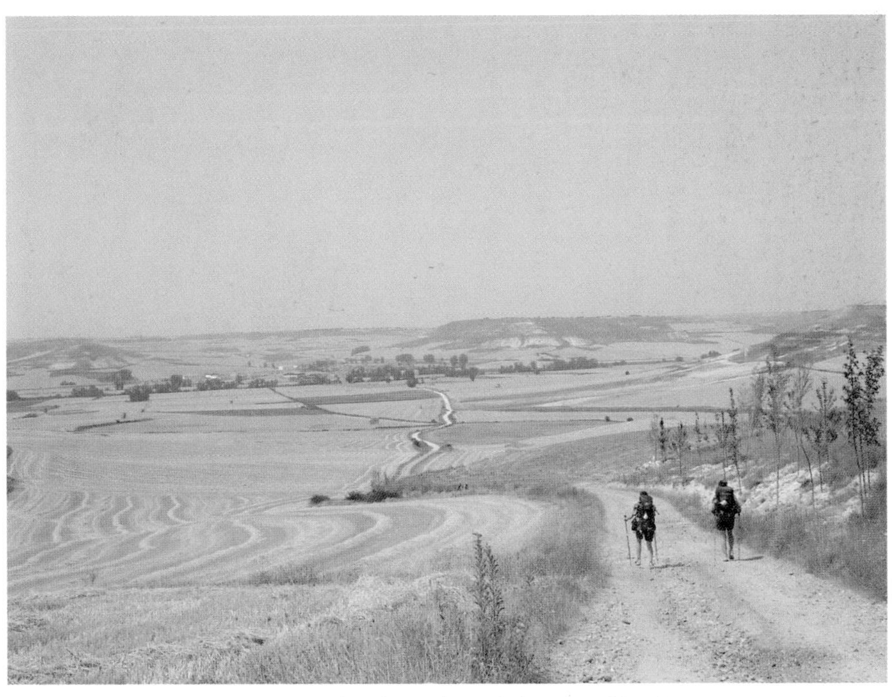

The Camino traverses the Meseta Alta, the sun's anvil. (*Sascha Thieme*)

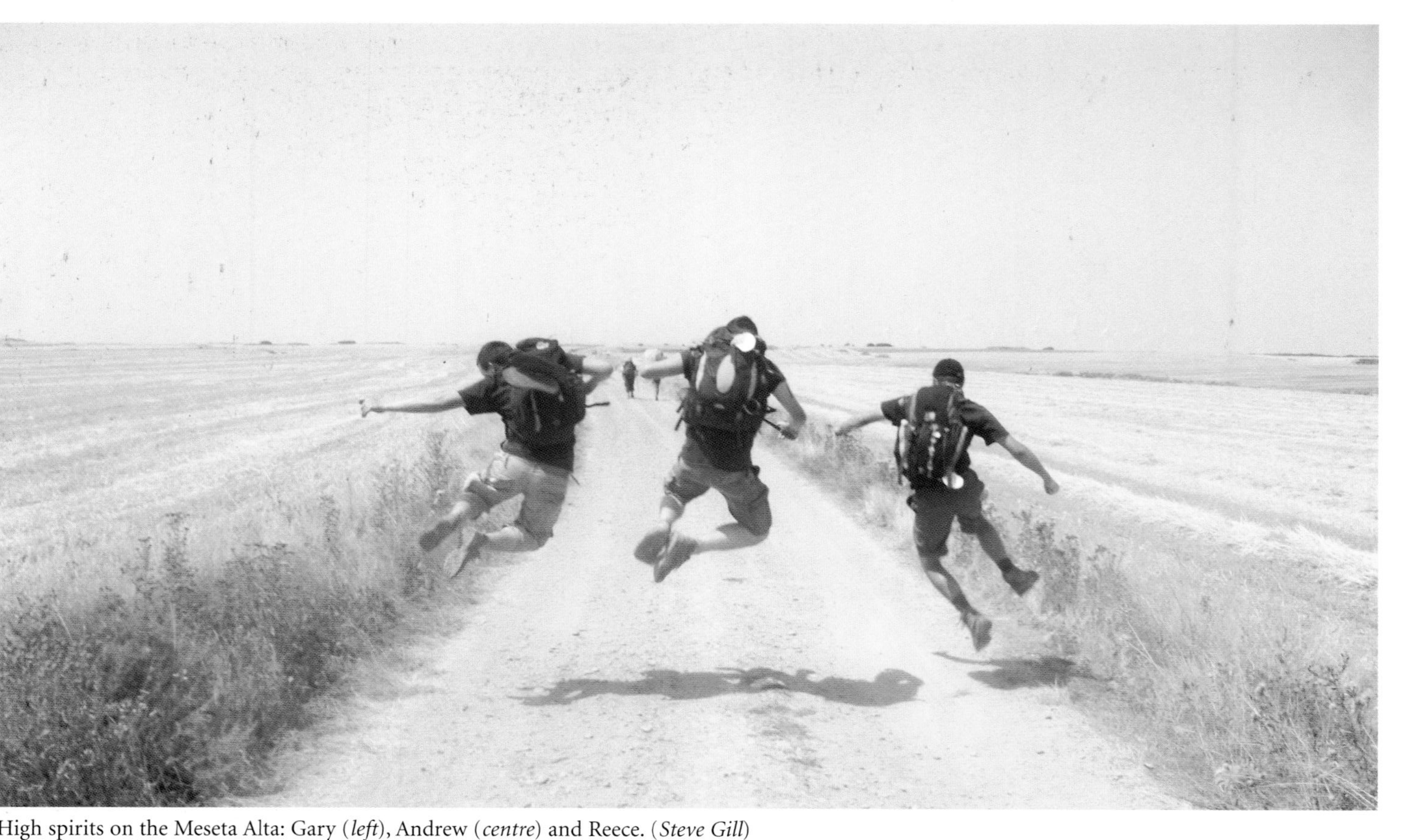

High spirits on the Meseta Alta: Gary (*left*), Andrew (*centre*) and Reece. (*Steve Gill*)

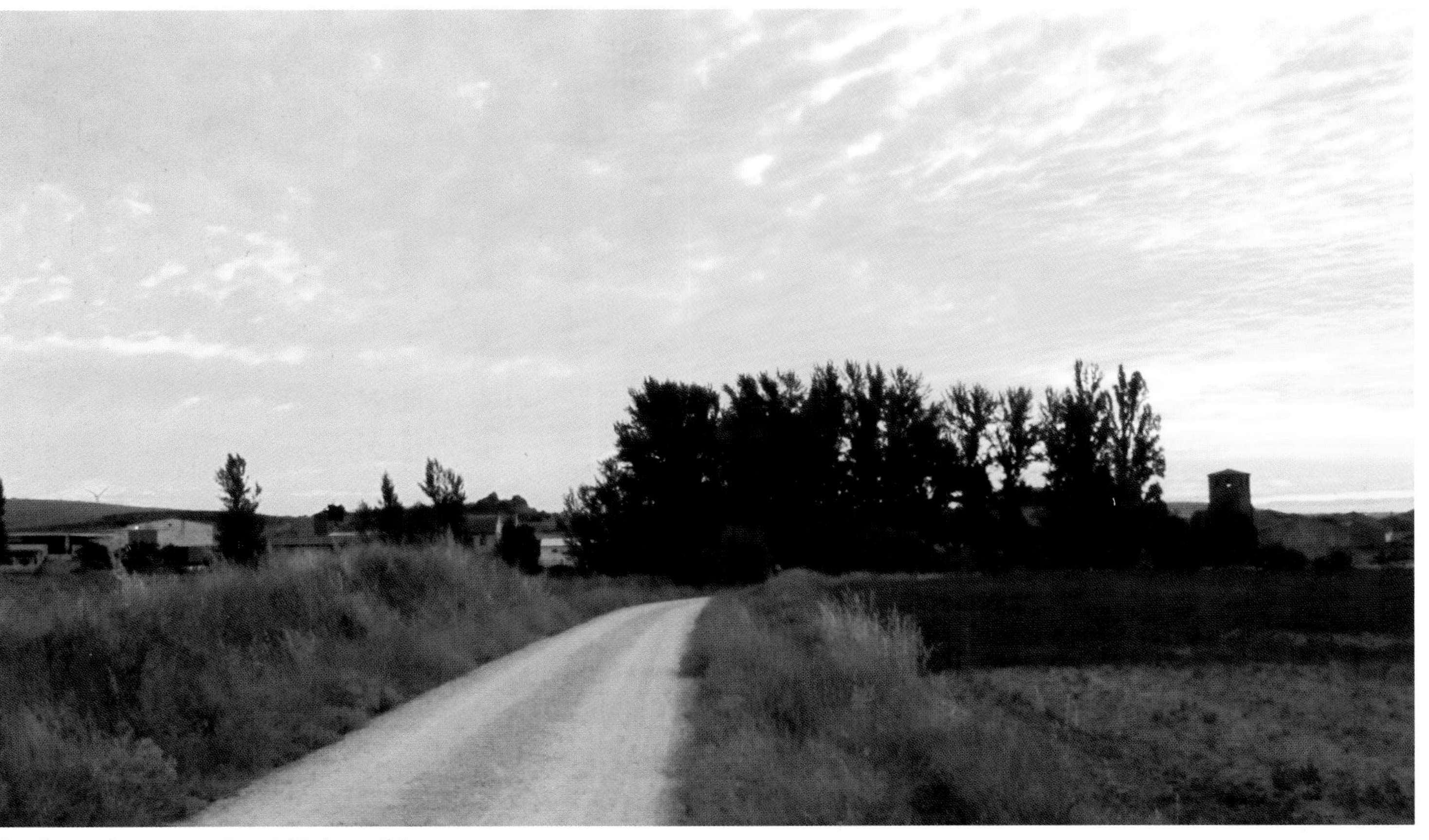

Sunrise on the meseta—invariably beautiful.

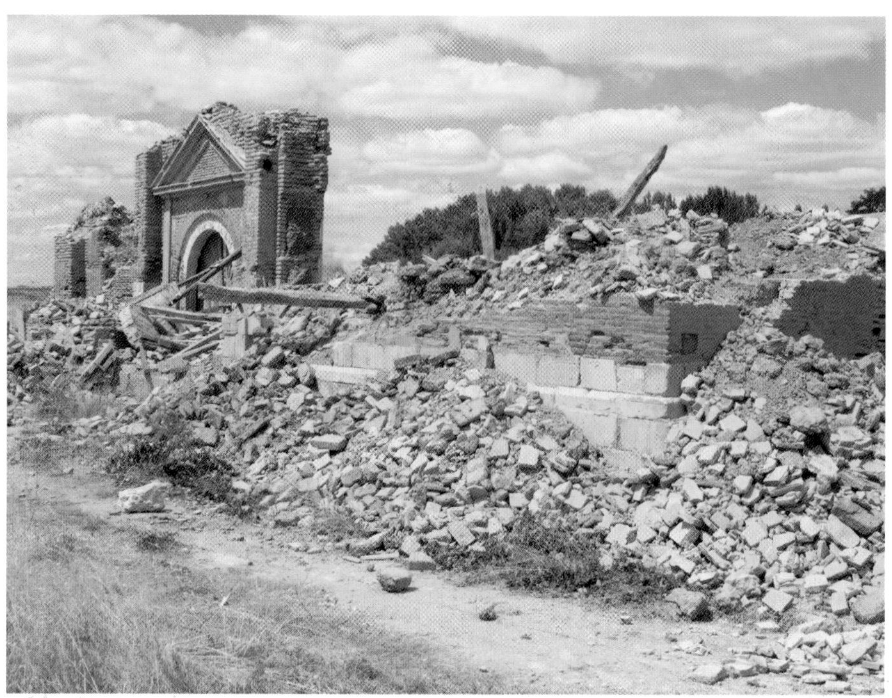

Bercianos: all that remains of the church of El Salvador, emblematic of the whole village.

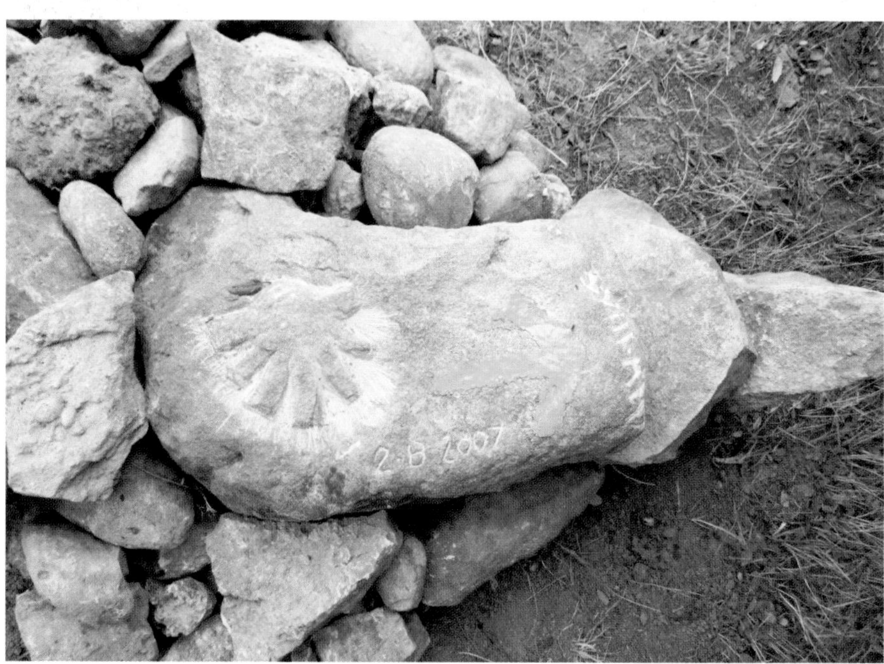

Camino direction sign carved into a wayside stone.

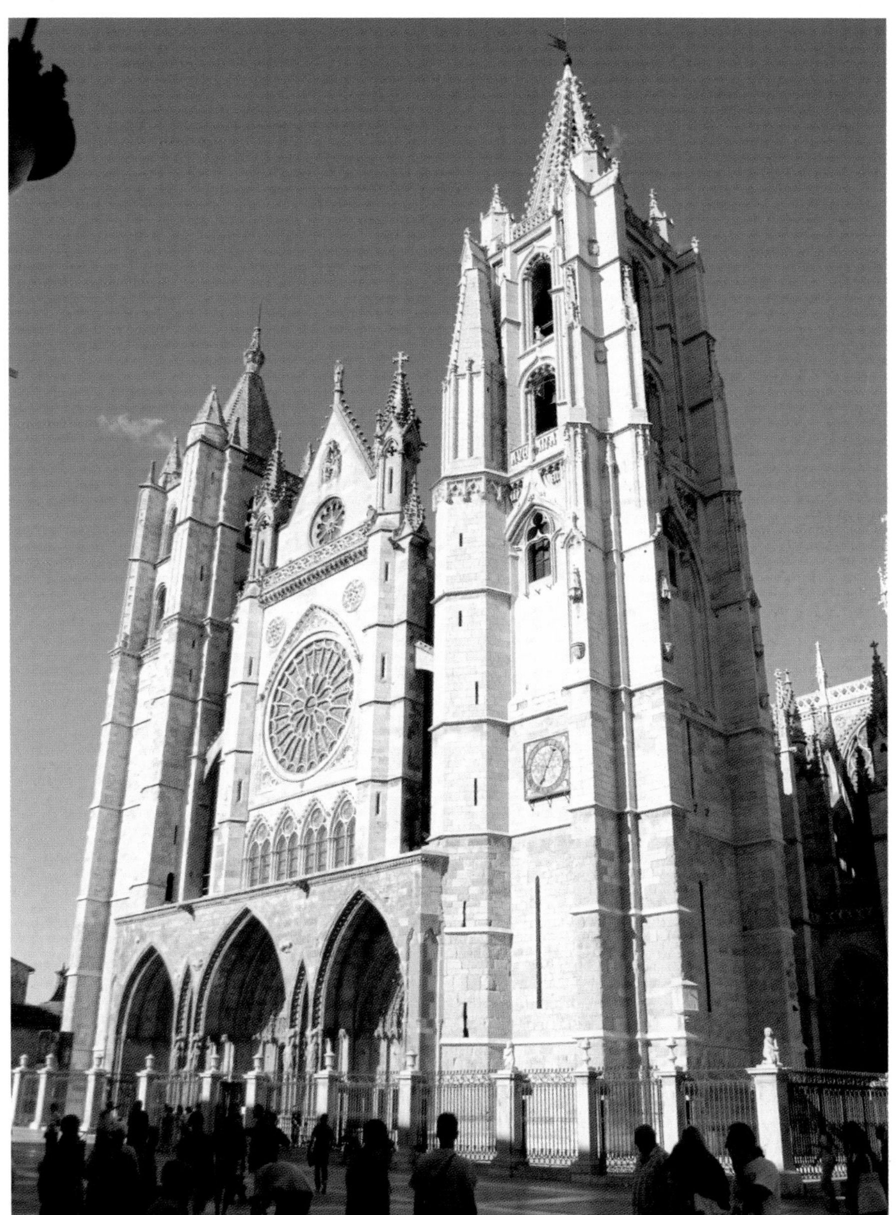

León Cathedral—a gothic beauty: majesty without vulgarity.

León Cathedral's *retablo* and, above it, some of the amazing 1,800 square metres of stained glass that floods the interior in coloured light and defines the whole building.

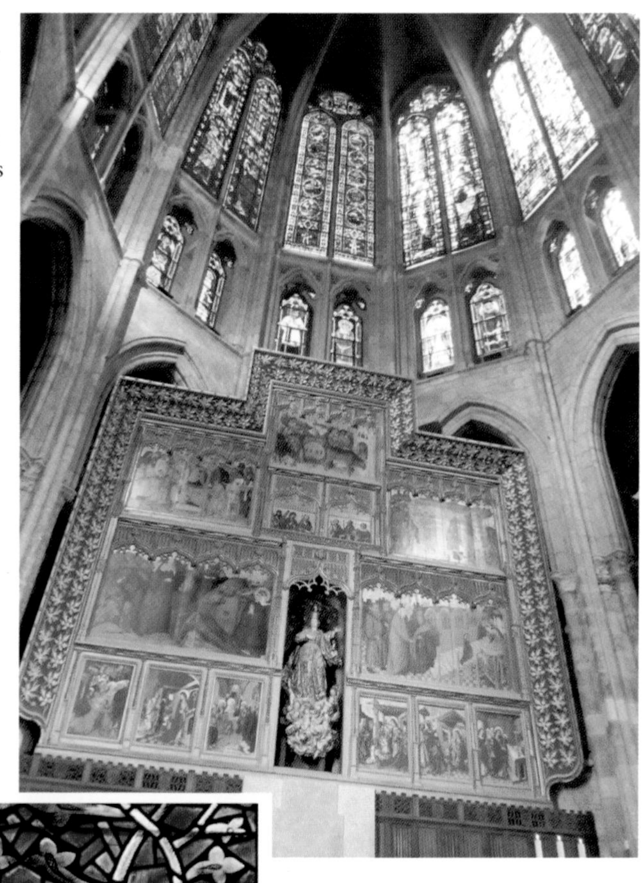

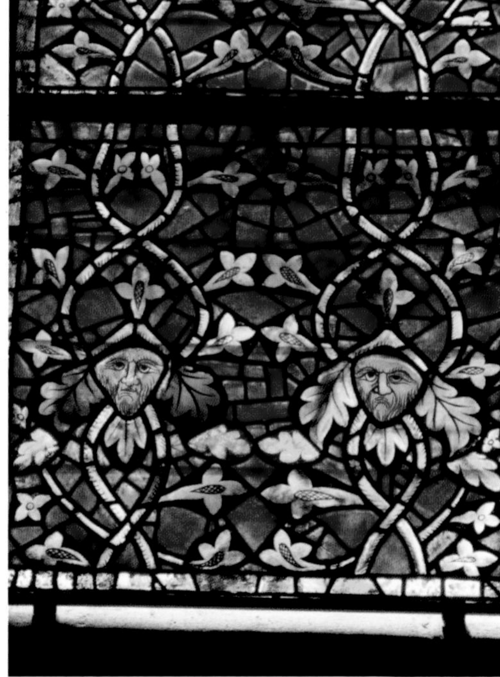

León Cathedral stained-glass detail.

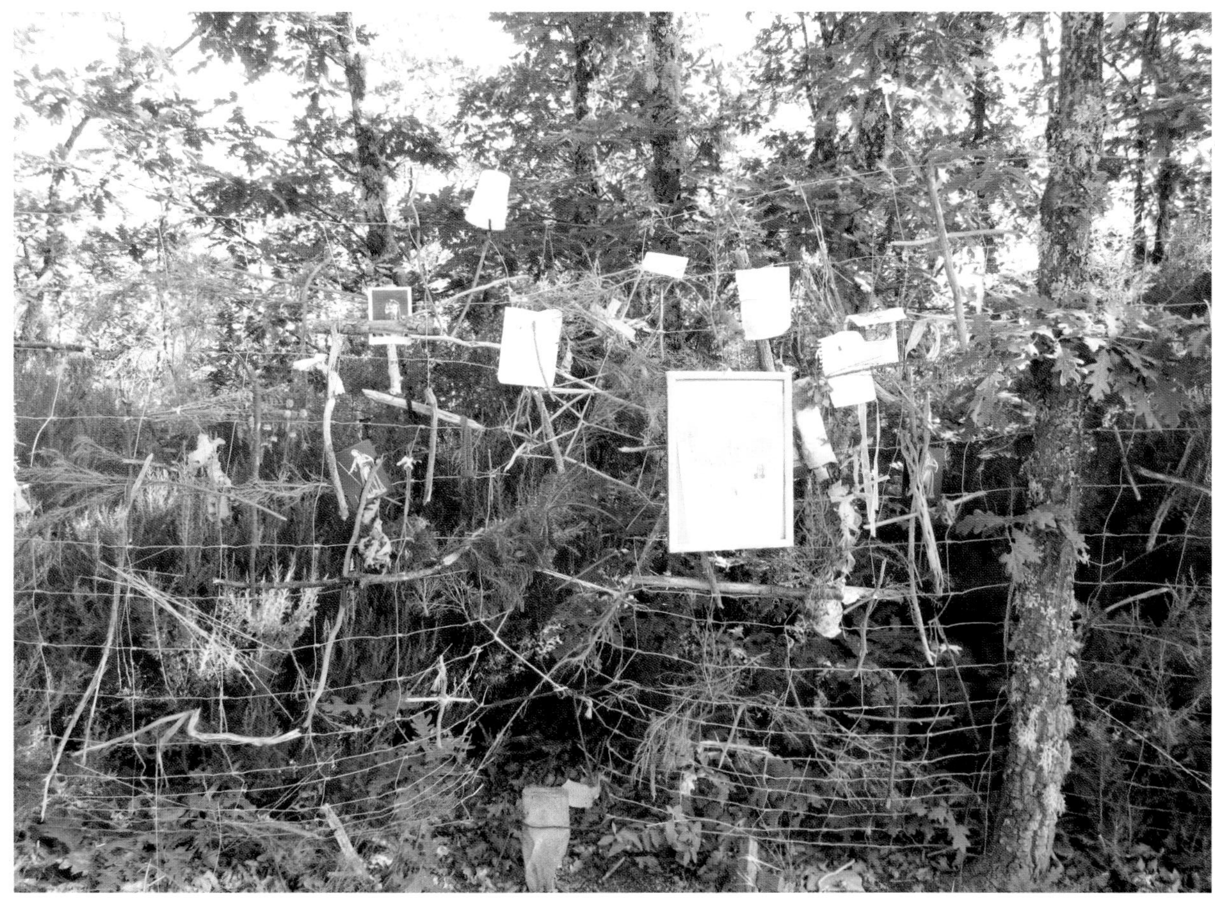

Pilgrims frequently lace crosses and other messages into wire fencing along the Camino.

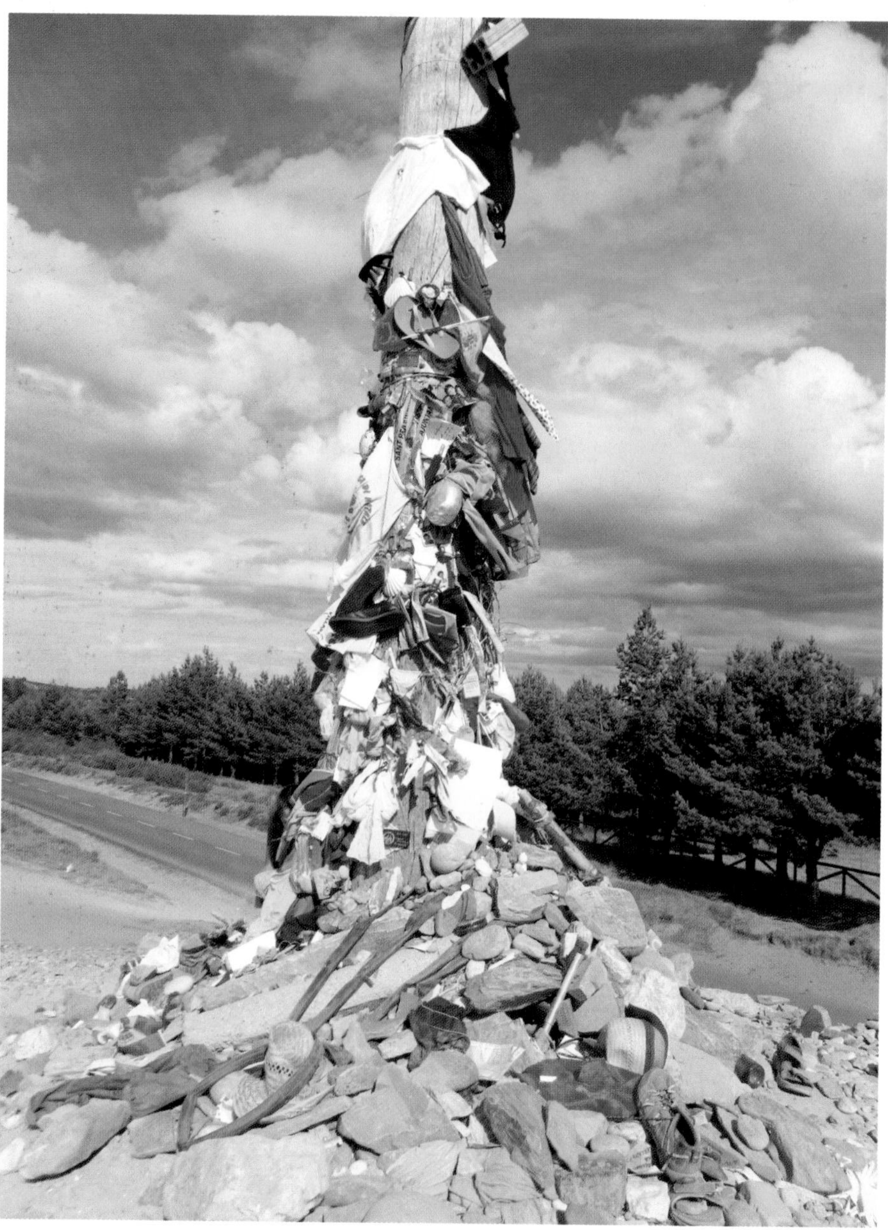

The Cruz de Ferro, highest point on the Camino at 1,504 metres above sea level; a focal point of pagan, Roman and finally Christian ritual.

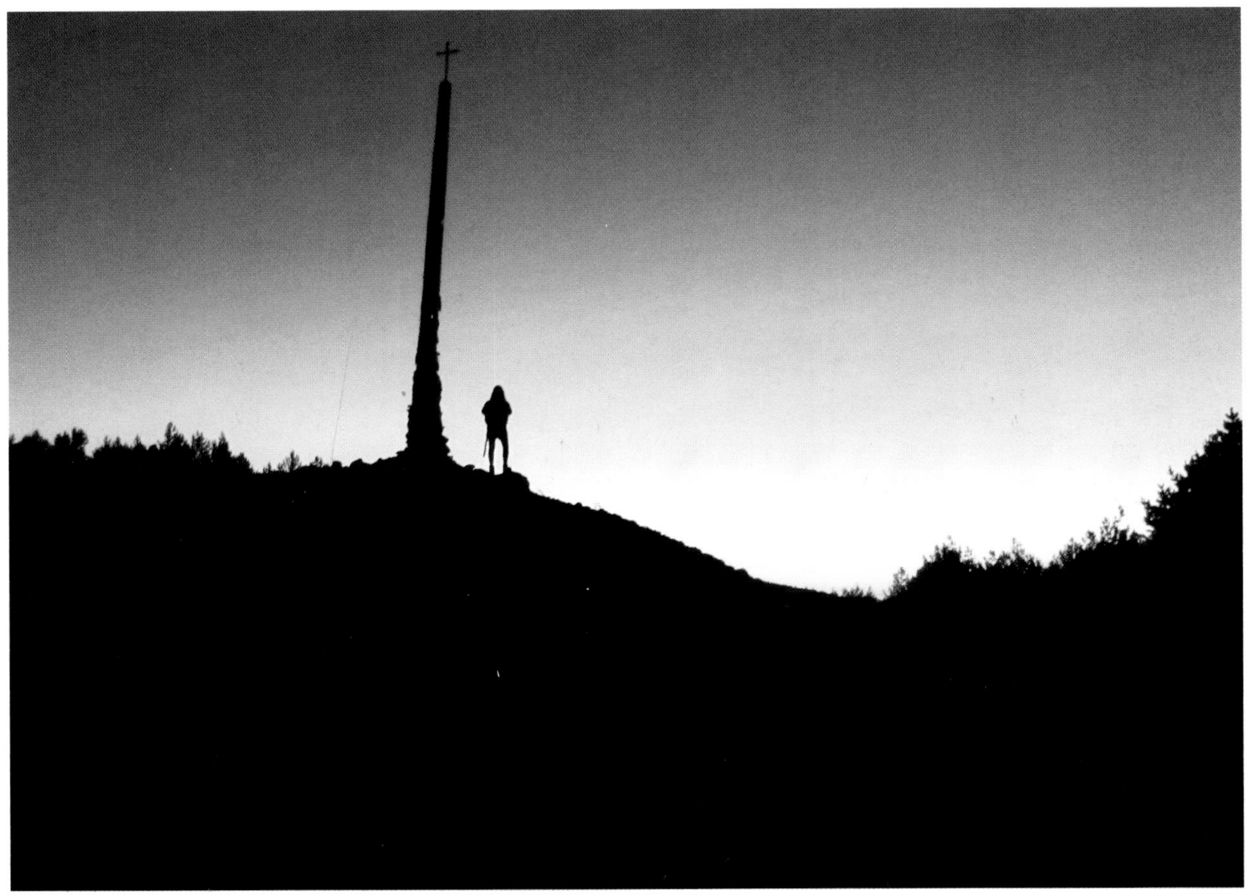

Natasha at the Cruz at dawn.

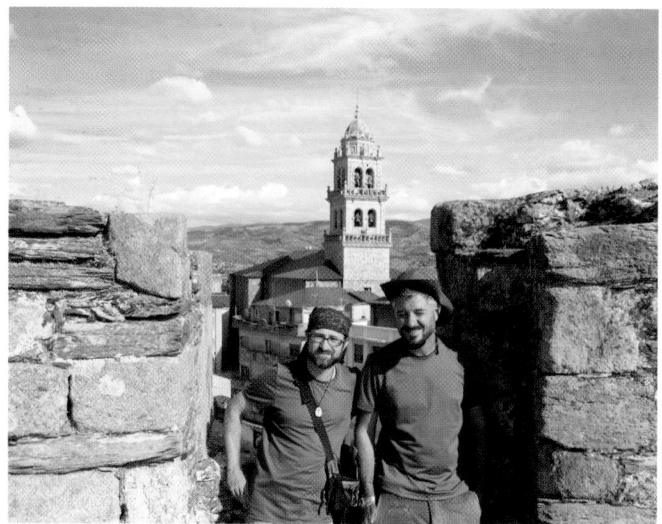

Antonio Cebrián (*left*) and Jesús Sanz Castro on the walls of Ponferrada castle. (*Photographer unknown*)

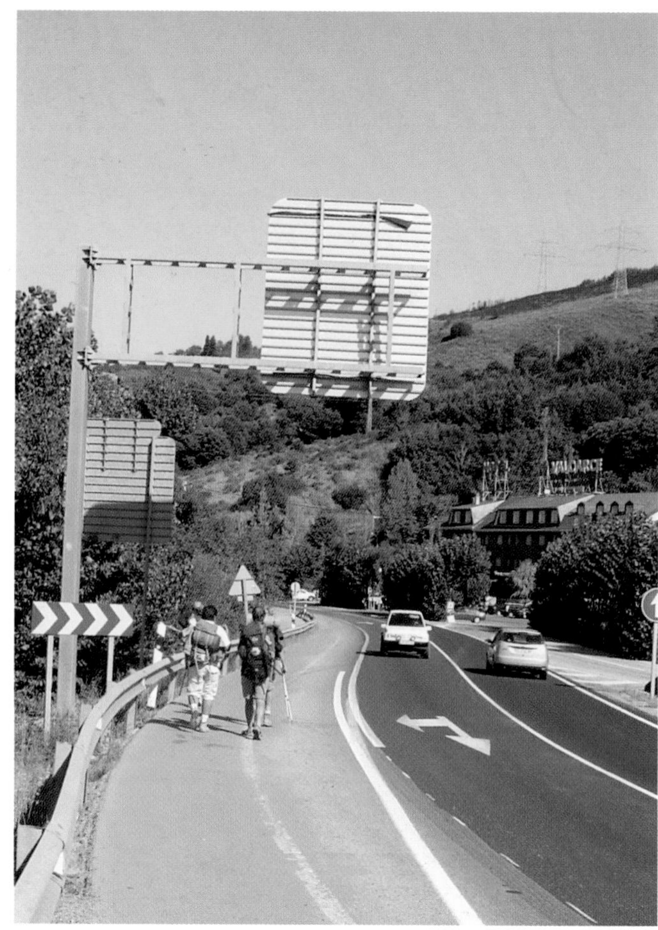

At times the quiet, slow-paced world of the Camino and the modern world of speed and technology come uncomfortably close to one another, such as here in the Río Valcarce valley. (*Sascha Thieme*)

Walking shoes and staves resting in an *albergue*.

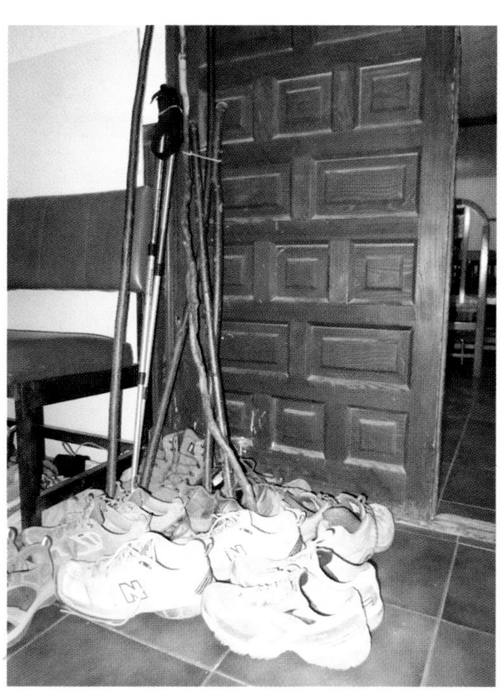

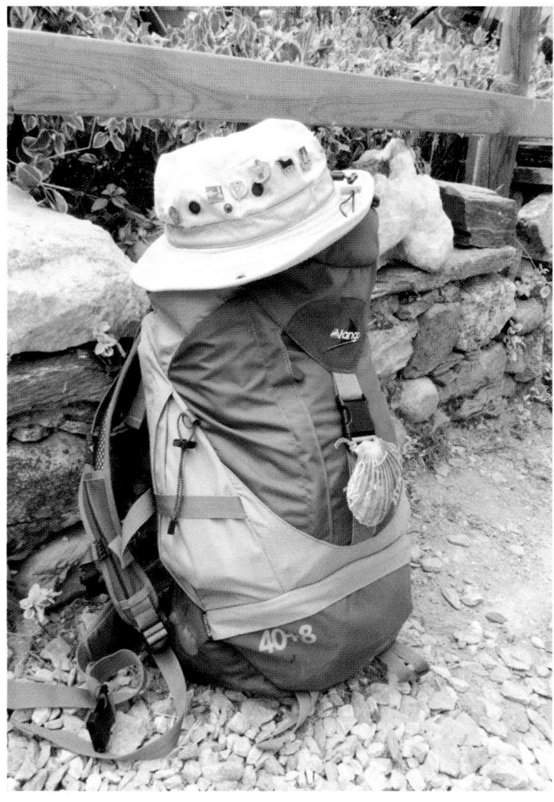

What you bring, you carry …

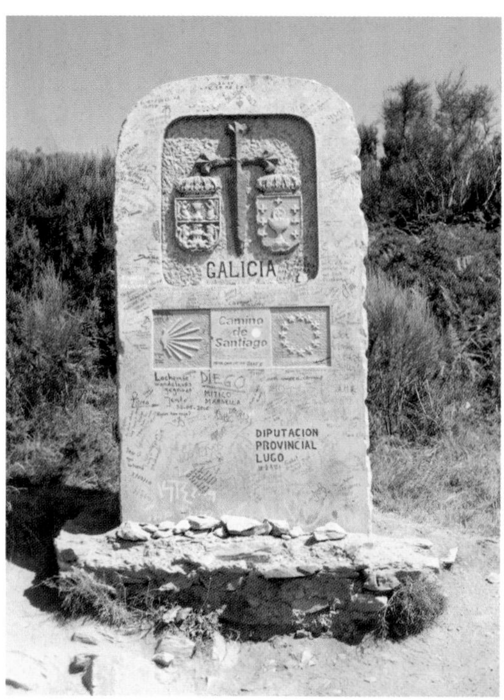

Boundary stone near O Cebreiro marking where the Camino leaves the province of León y Castile and enters Galicia. Note the dagger-like red cross of St James.

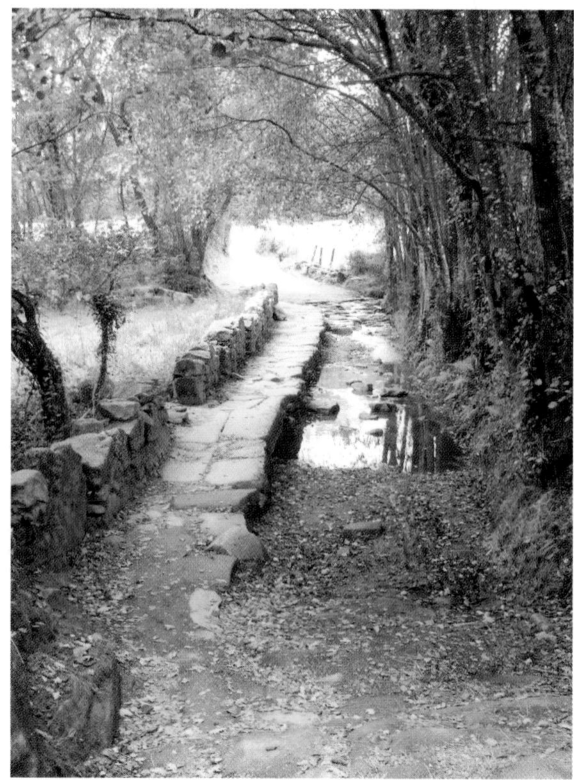

The mixed woods of Galicia are a delight. The bridge over this stream is designed like the Clapper Bridge at Killeen, near Louisburgh in Co. Mayo. (*Sascha Thieme*)

She grunted.

"Atención! Atención!" she grabbed my arm dramatically, and pulled me to the side of the rather large road, to allow one cyclist to get by. With his passing, she shook her head and grunted. This would happen every time a cyclist passed. There were lots of cyclists, resulting in an even angrier Angie. She appeared to be someone who harboured a lot of anger. With that thought, my phone started to ring. This bothered angry Angie. "No answer! Silencio! No answer." She waved her arms around. I saw it was Dad calling, and presumed he had just realised how far it was he had told me to walk. Very quietly, as to not disturb Angie, I answered.

"Hello."

"Natasha. Where are you?" blunt and angry Dad asked.

"Eh, about four kilometres away from Frómista," I replied.

"For God's sake. I'm not going any further, Natasha. I'm staying here. I'm not going any further."

"Well, do you want me to turn back?" I asked.

He huffed and grunted.

"Let me think about it." And then he hung up. About 20 minutes later I got a text from him: "I come." I always knew he was a marshmallow.

After that, I was shooed on by Angie. Clearly I was too loud on the phone. She reminded me of a gerbil I used to have. His name was Sid Vicious. He appeared harmless and cute, yet held a lot of anger. Angie is from Lombardy in Italy. Dad calls her Lombardy Lady.

I crossed over a lovely little canal and into Frómista, after nearly 11 hours of walking, and covering 46 kilometres. I have never been so exhausted and drained. I didn't have any specific pains anywhere on my feet or body, just general tiredness. I met Reece and Steve at the reception. I booked Dad and me in. The lady was shocked at the distance I had covered as she looked at my pilgrim passport and saw the town I had come from, 46 kilometres away.

Jesús, angry Angie and Dad arrived later. Dad wasn't angry any more, and rested. I got a text from Andrew saying he and Gary had booked into an *albergue* six kilometres back, thinking it was the one everyone was going to. They caught up the next morning. Later, we all went to the pool and had a beer, rather deservingly, particularly for Dad and me.

PETER: A day after having to stop because of a leg muscle problem, I can't quite believe we walked 46 kilometres. The little minx just wouldn't slow down, her eagerness compounded by my misreading where I was and making her think I was much closer to Frómista than I was. At one stage I thought the town just eight kilometres ahead was Frómista when in fact it was Boadilla; Frómista was in reality 22 kilometres further. Had I known that, I would have shouted stop! Not that she'd have listened ...

The final 10 kilometres to Frómista were very difficult, to put it mildly. My ideal distance is around 25 kilometres, 30 at a push. After that, the soles of my feet start to give out, never mind my calf muscles. The sun was high, the temperature an incredible 35 degrees, but the landscape was rather pleasing. Much of the walk into Frómista was alongside the Canal de Castilla. It was built in the late 18th century with transport in mind, but by the time it should have been coming into its own, as it were, rail was in the ascent. The canal has proved to be a blessing in disguise, however, because for over two centuries it has been the main artery serving the region's irrigation system. The canal has meant this part of the meseta is moist and fertile and also lovely to look at. The banks of the canal are populated with bulrushes and other plants and a slight breeze takes the edge off the heat.

But 46 kilometres? We hadn't met anyone who'd walked that much in one day. I felt quite good about that ... but I wasn't going to let her know.

Frómista to Carrión de los Condes: 20.9 km in 4.5 hours

PETER: The Camino is attracting all sorts of what one might call alternative types. In Hornillos del Camino, for instance, I was writing on my little netbook portable computer when a petite, middle-aged woman approached me and said: "There is wi-fi here?"

"I don't know," I replied. "I am just using this to write on. Are you looking for wi-fi?"

"No. It makes me ill."

"Oh."

"Yes. It is why I avoid cities. I live in the Black Forest to get away from it."

"But it is everywhere, surely."

"No," she said, indicating just the tiniest irritation, "it is not everywhere. It is not in the Black Forest and that is why I live there. Wi-fi interferes with me; I feel bad when it is there."

In which case, I think, you would have known whether it was here and I was using wi-fi without asking me because you would have felt sick, no?

"But you walk through towns and cities where there is wi-fi all the time surely; you cannot escape it all the time." But there was no way I would change what was clearly a very firmly fixed view; she was 1,000% sure that wi-fi was frying her brain or interfering with her in some way.

What's unusual is often what makes life interesting. But weird is just weird, no? Today on the way from Frómista, on an awful stretch of the Camino where it runs parallel and right up against a main road with trucks and cars whizzing by all the time, we stopped for coffee at the entrance to a village named Villarmentero. The café was a wooden building looking out over a grassed area with tables. In the field behind were several tepees where, for €5 a night, pilgrims could have a different sort of experience. Inside the café there were posters and flags showing Bob Marley and various images of the weed of which he was so fond (and which may very well have been linked to what did fry his brain). Loudspeakers projecting into the grassy area played music that sounded like it was being sung by an off-duty Gregorian choir standing at the bottom of a well, accompanied by one of those stand-up, electronic organs you often find at country and western sessions in rural pubs. The resultant 'music' was vacuous, toneless and formless and amounted to musical bubblegum drone. In quick succession, musical murder was committed against *Knights in White Satin* and *Bridge Over Troubled Water*. The titles are sort of inevitable, when you think of it; the world of faux spirituality is crammed with this sort of thing. It was only a matter of time before *Imagine* wafted out from the bottom of the well.

The scene was completed when two goats ambled in.

"Do you know if you startle a goat, it faints," said Gary. This had Natasha in convulsions of laughter for several minutes. The mother goat had a bell around her neck. A Spanish man went over and, holding the goat by her two horns, rocked her head from side to side making the bell ring. "Time gentlemen, please," quipped Andrew. And we were outta there, rolling about the place laughing.

It struck me later how weird it was that a song containing strong anti-religion sentiments—*Imagine there's no countries / it isn't hard to do / nothing to kill or die for / no religion too / imagine all the people living life in peace*—should become an anthem of a new sort of religion: the religion of suburban drop-out kids in dreadlocks and rainbow-coloured baggy pants, sitting around smoking roll ups and worrying about the environment. But then, having just been to a cathedral containing live chickens said to be descended from dead, half-roasted ones that leapt from a spit, who am I to have such thoughts? …

NATASHA: I was rather pleased to begin the day with a casual start of 7.00 pm. After our disgusting 46-kilometre walk the day before, we had agreed a nice 20 kilometres would do just fine. The funny thing is that if you told me three weeks ago I would be calling 20 kilometres an easy walk, I would have laughed in disbelief.

Andrew and Gary had stayed in the town before us, six kilometres back, and had left early and were outside the *albergue.* Jesús and Tasmanian Steve joined us on our 20-kilometre journey. Unfortunately, it wasn't a very pleasant walk, as the whole 20 kilometres was beside a main road. At the half way point, there was a small beer garden café. We stopped here for a coffee. I haven't laughed as much as I did in the 20 minutes we were there, as I have the whole trip. I was already very hyper, probably from exhaustion, and a couple of goats was exactly what was going to make me laugh hysterically. When Gary made a comment about goats fainting when they get scared, it gave me an image that made me laugh for the rest of the journey.

For the second 10 kilometres, I walked with Jesús. It was the first time I talked to him properly, and how pleasant and interesting he was! We talked about everything under the sun. He is a big fan of movies, and when I go home I'm making a trip to the nearest video rental shop, as he has given me a list of movies to watch. We shared a love for the same movie, *The Notebook.* It's one of my favourites. Another of the many things we talked about was love. He was shocked when I told him I had never been in love. I explained to him that I thought a lot of people my age get love confused with infatuation. He told me about the three different people he had been in love with in his life. I also explained that sometimes I have found myself liking someone, but there's been something in the way, whether its age or country, or something else. That's when he told me, "If you love someone, those things won't stop you. You will get by anything when you're in love. One day you will understand."

I enjoyed walking with him. He's good company.

The last three kilometres, the town was in view. At this stage, it was really hot, and I badly wanted to get into the shade of buildings. Carrión de los Condes was much bigger than I expected. I like big towns. They give me space and time to wander alone, to think by myself and have a few Dumbledore moments of wisdom.

We stayed in an *albergue* run by the most delightful bunch of nuns. I don't think they could have been any nicer, or smiled any more than they did. The building was old but had been done up on the inside. A Spanish man with very good English, named Carlos, showed us to our rooms and told us where everything was. Dad had bought some bread, cheese and meat, and we took it into the garden and had it for lunch. I then took a stroll through the town. It didn't have many big shops but plenty of pubs, small pastry shops and clothing boutiques. The streets were old looking and filled with character. A large river ran through the bottom of the town, and families sat around eating lunch. A bridge went across the river, and children were jumping off it into the clear, flowing water.

After I had a nap Dad started cooking the dinner for 10 of us. He was making sea food pasta and salad. I was sitting in the dining hall writing. There was silence, then the delicate strumming of a guitar, and the soft voice of a woman singing in Spanish seeped out from the reception area under the closed doors. There was a small singing session going on for anyone who wanted to sit and enjoy. The nuns, and anyone else who wanted, played music and sang. It was such a beautiful gesture, and everyone in the room was smiling. I opened the door and popped my head around the corner to see a full room, with pilgrims pouring down the stairs, joining in the music. It was one of those lovely gatherings you could only find on the Camino.

After that we sat and had dinner. For everyone else who hadn't planned a meal, the nuns worked away busily, making sure everyone got a bowl of the traditional garlic soup that they had prepared, and some bread and fruit. We had made far too much pasta, and so Dad gave the huge red caldron containing it to the rest of the people. Everyone was sharing everything they had: food, drinks, time, and company. It was an evening that demonstrated beautifully the generosity found in the people on the Camino. While we were having ice cream dessert, a French boy, who was sleeping in a tent in the garden, passed us. We offered him some ice cream, and he joined us briefly. His name was Antoine. He was tanned and had shaggy blonde hair. He wore bohemian, hippy clothes that he probably doesn't wash very often. He is typical of the characters one finds on the Camino. He's a bit away with the fairies, and finds himself 'one with nature'. He walks extremely slowly and is always smiling dreamily. He lives in Paris and is travelling from there to Santiago, on €100. Until now, he has spent €45. He saves money by staying in donation *albergue*s, in his tent, accepting offerings of dinner from others and anything else he can find that's free.

Carrión de los Condes to Terradillos de los Templarios: 26.6 km in 5 hours

PETER: It is not true that everyone you meet on the Camino is nice and cheerful and interesting, though it sometimes seems like that. So far on this Camino, Natasha and I are agreed that we have encountered three pilgrims whom we regard as fairly nasty and unpleasant.

First there is José, a Spanish man who is known to all and sundry, without great originality it must be acknowledged, as El Loco. He is a man probably in his mid-50s, with a slightly weathered, tanned face, short cut, dark hair, and is of medium build. He is usually carrying an iPod which he is either using or clutching in his hand as some sort of prop. El Loco is travelling alone and his modus operandi in *albergue*s, or during stops at cafés, is to insert himself into the company of others, which usually means inflicting himself on them.

My first encounter was, I think, somewhere around Pamplona. I was sitting in the corner of a common area of an *albergue* typing away on my netbook when El Loco approached holding the USB plug attached to his iPod and, without saying anything to me, tried to see whereabouts on my computer he might plug it in.

"Ah, pardon, señor," I said, "non."

"My friend! Porkay non? Why no?"

"C'est mon travaille; c'est très importante; ce n'est pas possible; pardon."

"But my friend, I need ..."

"Non, c'est ne pas possible; c'est mon computer; c'est très importante, très importante to me and the answer is non; je m'excuse; sorry mais non; Okay!"

And so El Loco retired, muttering. But there was simply no way I was going to allow someone I didn't know plug something into my netbook which contained several thousand words in draft chapters, in whose quest Natasha and I had scaled the Pyrénées and walked all the way through Navarra; plus tens of thousands of words of my pre-Camino research. There could be any sort of computer virus gibberish in his iPod just waiting to invade our hard-crafted prose. So, non mate, et sorry and all that ...

A few hours later he was back again, this time employing a charm offensive.

"Eh, mon amigo," he says, palms open, turned towards me, mouth closed, lips turned down, shoulders slightly hunched up in that 'why not?' pose, "no simpatico, mais ..."

And he's eye-balling the USB ports again, iPod in hand and making to plug it in.

"Oi," I said, "c'est mon computer, et non is still non; Okay? Non! Amigo et no amigo; non est seulement non!"

And off he went muttering again. These incidents of themselves meant little, though it did strike me as odd that he wanted, with a certain degree of persistence, to get attached to *my* computer when almost every *albergue* in Navarra had pay-as-you-go computer internet access. But I didn't think too much about your man after that until we met up with the Belfast Musketeers—Gary, Andrew and Reece.

"Did ya hear about Reece?" Gary says excitedly one morning.

"No, what happened?" said Tash and me.

"There he is asleep in bed, right there last night, right? And he turns in his sleep, right? And this bloke leaps out of his bed, switches on the lights—like it's half past one and there's eight other people in the room and this guy switches on all the lights—and goes up to Reece, grabs him by the shoulders and pulls the scarf off his eyes, right?—Reece had this scarf around his eyes, right?, to get asleep—and your man pulls it off and starts roaring at Reece, roaring like a madman, and shaking him. '*El signor no respecto meo!*' he's shouting at Reece. The whole place wakes up, there's people leaping outta beds, and this other bloke grabs your man and tells him to calm down or something and gets him back into bed and turns the lights off again.

"Next morning this bloke, the one who helped and pulled your man away, this bloke goes up to Reece and says, 'Sorry about that; don't worry about the other fellow, he's just a wee bit mad.'"

"Jazus," says Tash and I, and then I say, "There was an odd bloke awhile back kept trying to get access to my computer. He kept coming over to me. Oh, there he is there," and I pointed to the man in question.

"Fuck me," says Gary, "that's him. That's your man. He's loco."

With that, we had our name. Next time El Loco was witnessed in action was at the foot pool in the back garden yard of the *albergue* in Logroño. Eight walkers, two to each side, are sitting around the pool, cooling their feet after checking in. El Loco walks up to one of them, a girl, and slaps her on the face with a leaflet, not a hard slap, more a glancing swish on both cheeks. The woman tries to swot him away like he was a fly. He ignores her, does it again and then walks away.

By this time I have become a leading member of the El Loco Observation Club, while he is the sole member of the Bloke With the Computer Observation Club. We keep a good eye on each other; I think he's wary of me, can't quite figure me out. By the time the muscle above my right ankle gives out coming into Hornillos del Camino, El Loco and I are like old sparring partners and, when he also stops at Hornillos, my enforced rest gives me the chance to watch him at close quarters for a whole afternoon.

The *albergue* in Hornillos, together with the church, a private house and the village's only café, form a square where there is a drinking fountain for pilgrims and tables and chairs belonging to the café. El Loco spends the entire afternoon going from table to table, inserting himself into the company of others and talking *at* them until they manage to effect some excuse and exit. Gradually, I begin to see a pattern to his behaviour. He will spot an individual, or maybe a cluster of people, in the near distance and throw a comment or a question their way. If they respond, he's in like a flash; if they do not or turn away, he throws another comment, this time at no one in particular, gets up and walks off in the direction of his last remark as if to indicate to the first, unresponsive target, well, if you aren't interested in me, others are! And so he walks away and lurks, maybe a little way down the street, waiting for a new target to emerge (and in the middle of the Camino outside a café, he is in a target-rich environment) and the process begins anew. In the Hornillos café that evening, he inveigles his way into the company of two Italian cyclists, dining diagonally across the room from Natasha, me and two French women. At various times I see the iPod raised in the air, hands gesticulating, pointing over to me, El Loco looking angry. The

Italians look across, a tad mystified, and I raise a glass, smile and shout "Salut!" "Buen Camino!" the Italians respond, probably even more mystified.

I have no idea what is wrong with El Loco but I know no one wants to be near him or walk with him once they have experienced his company for more than a minute or three. He is travelling alone. He seems to want to be friends with everyone but doesn't appear to have the social skills to go about it in the right way. He seems to talk *at* people, rather than participate in a two-way conversation. He seems always to be acting the expert with people, talking like an old Camino hand. Maybe he is. But there is something unnaturally urgent, manic almost, about the way he pushes himself on people. Whatever is the matter with him, I hope he gets better.

The second person of note is one Natasha has christened Disgusting Man. DM, as she has observed, has an unfortunate appearance in that he is unlikely to be the face of next season's El Corte Inglés menswear collection. DM has two specialities.

The first is, immediately after checking into his *albergue*, to strip down to his underpants, which to date and after two weeks seem to be the same pair of green boxers. He then walks about, inside and outside the *albergue*, lifting one leg of the boxers, removing what they cover and scratching the objects contentedly. Occasionally, he will roll a stick of underarm deodorant over the objects, put them away ... but not for long; out they will come again for another scratching. This may deliver a certain satisfaction to him but it revolts everyone else.

The second thing DM does with total indifference to all about him is use his mobile phone. It is not uncommon for people to speak into their mobile phones a little louder than is perhaps necessary in the view of most other people forced to listen to a one-sided conversation. When DM uses his phone, he roars, no, screams, into it. We have seen people in restaurants splutter and remove food from their mouths to stare in stark amazement as DM takes or makes a call. People on the street have literally jumped, startled, as the same process begins. And the conversation continues, with total indifference to everyone, at the roar/scream pitch until DM has finished. Then he stops, puts the phone away and carries on doing whatever he was doing before (which may well be that described in 1 above).

Disgusting Man lives in a world of one.

The final person worth mentioning is the Italian woman from Lombardy. She is a slight woman in perhaps her late 40s or early 50s. The first time I noticed her was in the *albergue* in San Juan de Ortega. There is a code of etiquette that governs how people behave in *albergues*; some elements are written down (boots off downstairs, that sort of thing) but others are not (in general, respect other people's space; like, don't invade it). One of the written rules is that you can't book a bed in an *albergue* in advance—everything is strictly on a 'first come, first served' basis, and walking pilgrims are given preference over cyclists. If people are walking in pairs and one falls behind, it is very common, and accepted by everyone, that the first one to arrive at the *albergue* books and pays for two beds, holding the other bed for the usually short period before their companion arrives. Executing this in the dormitory is generally done quietly and deferentially—"Hi! Is that bed beside you taken? No! Oh, would you mind very much if I held it for my friend? She's fallen behind; blisters! you know. Yes, oh thank you very much." And so the bed is held unoccupied for a while and everyone feels fine about it.

Well, in San Juan this etiquette was blown apart by the Lady from Lombardy. She arrived in the dorm, put down her rucksack and began walking at pace from bed to bed, disturbing the pillows and folded blanket on each and shouting "Ocupado, ocupado" as she laid claim to bed after bed as other walkers ambled into the room seeking a bed. Other pilgrims began to complain (which is almost unheard of) but your woman just shouted back at them "Ocupado, ocupado".

A couple of nights later, in Frómista in a room for six people, Lombardy Lady got out of bed at 5.30 am and, instead of doing her packing and dressing in the corridor or bathroom as everyone else does at that hour so as not to disturb, she unpacked her rucksack, repacked it, huffed and puffed, unpacked again, rummaged about in plastic bags (plastic bags at 5.30 am in an otherwise silent room have the decibel quotient of a foghorn) and generally made such a who-ha of getting up that she woke the entire room.

But the star turn came when she presented herself, first in the queue, for the opening of the *albergue* run by nuns beside the Church of Santa Maria del Camino in Carrión de los Condes, a pretty little town on the Meseta Alta rich in medieval history and pilgrimage lore. Tash and I were a few places behind her in the queue. The nuns are Augustinians and four of them run the *albergue*, helped by a young seminarian volunteer. The nuns were among the cheeriest and most helpful people we have met on the Camino. They were simply delightful and radiated goodness. It helped, of course, that three of them were unusually pretty and had a charming, coquettish way about them. The young seminarian was a serious, slightly earnest looking man of dark features. He smiled a lot and behaved in a diffident manner; he spoke excellent English, having lived for a time in the United States.

Lombardy Lady was signed in by one of the nuns who then went through a little routine—there would be an ecumenical musical gathering here in the reception area at 6.30 pm and we were all invited to come; Mass was at 8.00 pm and we were all welcome; there was a communal meal at 8.45 pm in the dining room and, again, we were all welcome.

"What we have we share with you," said the saintly nun.

The young seminarian then led about five of us, Lombardy Lady first, upstairs into a dorm of perhaps a dozen beds. He indicated to one and, smiling, suggested that she take this bed.

"Why?" barked Lombardy. "I take this one!" she said, pointing elsewhere.

The shocked seminarian tried his best to explain, in Spanish and English, that they placed pilgrims in numbered beds, according to their arrival; this way, they knew where everyone was and it was easier to manage everything.

"Why this one?" she barked again, pointing at the bed, which was like every other bed in the dorm and in a position of no disadvantage relative to any other bed. Then there was a blast in Italian, Uzi-machine gun style, as to why the seminarian only spoke Spanish and English. "Spanish English, Spanish English," she shouted.

And then the poor man really sealed his fate.

"And in the morning," he said smiling sweetly, "we open door at 6 and you leave by 8."

"No, no, no, no," shouted Lombardy. "Ees impossible; you open at 5, I leave at 5; I walk 40 kilometres tomorrow. I begin at 5."

The seminarian repeated what amounted to the rules of the house in which she was a €5 paying guest (for superb facilities, I might add); the doors would open at 6 am. At this point, I thought the poor man would start crying. He was being subjected to what amounted to verbal abuse and bullying. "This is his place, not yours," I said. "They make the rules, not you."

I don't know if she understood but I turned away because I felt that if I didn't, I'd throttle her. Later I noticed that she had taken up residence for the night in another dorm in a bed that seemed precisely the same as the one she had been offered. Next morning, the door out to the street and the Camino was opened, as per the house rules, precisely at 6 am. As various pilgrims went about their ablutions and breakfast, quietly and in deference to others, Lombardy was sitting in the kitchen doorway in a way that obliged everyone else to step around her. She was packing and unpacking her rucksack.

At the other end of the dining room a few metres away from her, one of the nuns was walking past a late-middle-aged Italian man, a lovely, gangly man with a huge smile who greets everyone warmly and chats as best he can even though he hasn't a word of another language. He always responds to the smallest gesture of recognition or friendship. He was sitting on a chair, trying to bandage his blisters and not making a terribly decent fist of it.

The passing nun paused. And then she sat cross-legged on the floor in front of him and gently lifted his limp foot onto her lap. She opened a first aid box and spent several minutes gently, lovingly, caressing his foot, dabbing it with disinfectant and applying a bandage. She did so smiling and uttering soothing words for him. It was a moment of almost biblical, saintly intensity.

But I don't think Lombardy noticed anything.

NATASHA: The walk from Carrión de los Condes is said to be the worst stretch of the meseta: the longest stretch of nothing and it was just as horrible as I expected, even though the sun wasn't strong. As soon as we left Carrión, we didn't see any civilisation for 17 kilometres. The walk was along the most horrifically boring, dusty road I have ever encountered. It was never ending, like those blasted Brussels sprouts on Christmas day. It just went on, and on, and on. There wasn't even a hump in the horizon to at least make me think that beyond it there would be a town. It was just flat and straight.

PETER: Actually, the Camino track along this part of the route did have its interesting aspects.

"Instead of concentrating on how straight and flat and long it all is," I said to Natasha, "look at the interesting bits. The sky and the different shapes of the clouds, the tone of colour in the cut wheat fields, the bulrushes in the ditches, and there are some flowers. Look over ..."

"Dad, shut up!" she snapped. "You are always writing poetry."

"I don't write poetry. I'm not that good. I write prose," I replied.

"Well then you talk it."

"Thank you for the compliment!"

There is a beauty to the apparently dullest landscape if only one looks at it with the right frame of mind. Flat land creates big skies and big skies often play host to wonderful cloud formations. At the start of our walk along the endless, flat road, there was a breathtaking sunrise that turned the sky a magical golden colour. Then in the early dawn there were brush-stroke cirrus clouds, white feather-like formations drifting across the sky. And later still, as the sun threatened to rise high and roast us, dark brooding clouds drifted over us from the Picos de Europa mountains in the north, welcome visitors saving us from the sun.

And there was lots of bird song. Shoals of linnet-like birds kept rising en masse from the stubble as I walked along, flying across my path to settle ahead of me, only to fly off again as I neared them once more.

NATASHA: Finally, after about two hours of nothing along the way, and nothing in my stomach, I smelt meat, and heard Beyoncé. I looked up, and there, perched on the side of the road was a beautiful sight. A large white van opened up into a café, with a man beside it, cooking burgers and hot dogs on a BBQ and playing Beyoncé music. If I hadn't been dehydrated, I probably would have cried with happiness. But before I could even celebrate, I see Dad in the distance walking straight by. I would have happily dined without him except he had all the money. I didn't. And he was too far ahead to shout at. Trying not to look in, or breathe, I walked by. I tried to cheer myself up by thinking of a couple of fainting goats, but it didn't work.

Eventually, I began thinking of other things. I began thinking of home. And I started to realise something for the first time. The urge to sign onto Facebook, and see what I was missing, had died. The yearning for a juicy gossip text from Andrea, or one of my other friends, had disappeared. It no longer interested me. I was feeling something different about home. I didn't know whether it was fear of change, or fear of reality. On the Camino I've been surrounded by such selfless, good-hearted, and good-intentioned people for so long, that some things about my life back home don't seem appealing. My life is filled with brilliant people whom I couldn't love more, and I wouldn't change any of them. But my life is also filled with things like *The Hills*, MTV and

Big Brother. And there are also people in my life at home I encounter that are selfish, greedy and unkind. I was feeling for the first time that I had escaped something. And the fact I didn't realise this earlier, meant to me that I was slipping into a world where this was accepted by me.

When I ask people why they are doing the Camino, many of them say to escape the bad things at home. This hadn't been a main reason for me, and now I'm thinking, maybe it should be. My thoughts along the way have changed. They are less materialistic, and I'm finding I get more lost in my surroundings, rather than my thoughts. The littlest things are making me happy and I notice small things more than ever. I'm not saying I don't enjoy hearing from home, I'm just saying I can feel the Camino is changing me. And it's changing me in a positive way. I'm really happy.

After the longest 17 kilometres of my life, I came crawling into a small café in a town, where I found Dad, happily perched at the bar, with a *bocadillo*, a *café con leche* and a very large cognac. "I've earned this," he said with a big smile as a laughing Swedish woman took his picture. I had a cup of tea and a Coke. We sat there for nearly an hour, and then moved on, with Charlie, a 31-year-old Englishman, who looks creepily like Ralph Fiennes.

In the next town, we came to a bar where we found Andrew, Gary, Reece, Steve and Jesús, the usuals. I also saw an internet connection, where I immediately Googled Ralph Fiennes so I could show Charlie. I was content for the rest of the day after my proud Doppelganger find. It was only three kilometres until we reached the place we planned to stay. Unfortunately it wasn't such a great 'town'. To put it in a nutshell, aside from the *albergue* the most that was on offer was a post box.

Terradillos de los Templarios to Bercianos: 24 km in 4.5 hours

PETER: Walking the final stretch into Terradillos, I finally have an opportunity to chat with Charlie. Charlie is Charlie Morris, a 31-year-old lay chaplain with Britain's national health service. He is attached to a major hospital in Westminster and lives in Brixton. He is a man of shortish stature, has an oval face and short curly hair going bald at the front with the effect that he appears to have a rather high forehead. Charlie speaks with one of those rounded English accents that suggests a public school (that is, private) education, which indeed he did have. He engages people in a friendly but serious way. He is very measured and thoughtful in all that he says.

We have run into each other a couple of times and exchanged hellos but have never had a substantial conversation. Now I meet him after a long, dull walk along the longest straight road I have ever walked. Sitting outside a café where I have rewarded myself with a *café con leche* and a good big glass of Spanish brandy, we fall into conversation. Charlie tells me that his family on one side (his father's) were Jews who came to Britain from Lithuania at the end of the 19th century. Somewhere along the way, the Lithuanian family name was jettisoned, as was Judaism. His mother comes from France. Charlie was raised a Roman Catholic.

"At school, it was always made clear that we Catholic boys could go to Mass if we wished. I didn't really. I never took it that seriously—first communion and then confirmation passed and I really don't remember them," he said.

Charlie went to university in Bristol and qualified as a mechanical engineer, a career in which he worked for some six years. Then he trained to be a lay chaplain. "I think it's good that people try different things, don't you?" I agree.

"During training, one of the seminars we had dealt with the difference between spirituality and religion," he said.

"This is something I have been trying to work out in my own head," I replied. "I read something before coming on the Camino to the effect that religion was for people who feared hell and spirituality was for those who had been there. I remember thinking that was quite clever but the more I think about it, the more I think it is rubbish. It doesn't actually mean anything. I think now that people who are spiritual are religious but don't want mediation, don't want an institution getting in the way."

"I think there's something in that," said Charlie, "because religion for me certainly has to be organised. I'm really getting into Catholicism now. It is so rich, so complete. I'd really like to get more into the lives of the saints."

I mentioned that I was Protestant, though a fairly detached one, but I could not see myself ever signing up for the Catholic Church. "But what is Protestantism about?" wondered Charlie. "It seems to be defined, as its name implies protest-ant-ism, by what it is against."

"Well, that's certainly true in terms of its origin," I said. "It was against buying indulgences, the selling of faith, the buying of forgiveness as it were, of entry to heaven; it was against the excesses of the Renaissance church in Rome. But I think nowadays active Protestants would define themselves in much more positive terms."

I told him of the things I had heard at home as a child, things that I later understood were part of my indoctrination as a Protestant. I would hear things about the individual conscience ("Let your conscience be your guide," my mother would say if I was unsure about a course of action), about work ("Never put off until tomorrow what you can do today"); things about personal responsibility and being charitable to others. I said it seemed to me that Protestant churches were inherently more democratic, with congregations heavily involved in choosing priests and bishops, running their parishes and their wider church. While Protestantism wasn't entirely bottom up in his approach to running itself, there was a very substantial element of bottom up.

Charlie felt that Europe badly needed to affirm its Christian roots. "I think the Church can lead that; I'd like to see that happening," he said.

I said I thought the Church could but probably not for a very long time. I said I felt that Rome was so out of kilter with mainstream public opinion in so many areas—science, medicine, family life, sexuality—that its capacity to lead was severely reduced and its moral authority was shot through because of the worldwide clerical sex abuse of children and cover-up scandal. Charlie would not share these views entirely though I think he understands them well.

In his work as a lay chaplain, Charlie is a non-medical point of contact for patients within the health system should they need one. He's not part of the medical process as such but he can be part of the healing process. He radiates decency and thoughtful engagement with difficult religious and spiritual issues. He's a little bit ascetic. He is walking the Camino in leather sandals ("They came from San Tropez," he says slightly detracting from the effect), wears a smock-style loose top and shorts. He has a fairly large crucifix on a leather thong around his neck. He's walking with a crooked staff given to him by a little Korean boy doing the Camino with his Mum and Dad. Charlie has been improving the staff by carving off the rough bits. He carves a notch on the shaft for each place he spends a night on the way. And he's made a tiny hollowed-out place near the top of the staff for a little statue of St Jude.

"Ah, the Patron Saint of Hopeless Cases," I say.

"Hopeless causes," Charlie corrects me, laughing.

If I was ill and in hospital, perhaps trying to come to terms with bad news, I'd like to have someone like Charlie to spar with.

On the way to Bercianos, I also have a long chat with a small woman I had christened Peru—simply because that is from where she comes and I was calling her Peru to her face, affectionately, to break down what I saw as her shyness. I noticed her in church once, apparently praying, and so I took her to be religious. Natasha saw her in a church crying. Peru is a tiny woman who beetles about the place and approaches one at first with a seeming awkwardness. She will do something in a slightly jerky manner—"Here, I think this is yours," handing you something and walking quickly away before you can engage her in chat.

"Hi Peru, how are you?" I say as I come alongside her walking.

"I'm fine. How are you," she says with a smile.

Peru looks slightly shambolic. She wears baggy, half-length fleece-type trousers and her money belt sags on her hip as though not fastened properly. Her rucksack is a little ill-fitting and she has a floppy white canvas hat with a black band on it. I ask her real name: "I can't keep calling you Peru."

"My name is Johanna; it's German but I am from Peru."

"Whereabouts?"

"Lima but I live in Lausanne in Switzerland."

Johanna is about to begin a Masters in chemistry at Lausanne University. Her father is a farmer; he makes a tequila-type drink and other produce which he sells. His wife works on the farm with him. I get the impression that Johanna's family are of modest means. An aunt is paying for her education in Switzerland and Johanna supplements this by teaching mathematics to chemistry students. I asked her why she was doing the Camino.

"When I was a little girl," she said, "I read a book …"

"Paulo Coelho's *The Pilgrimage*?" I guessed.

"Yes, Paulo Coelho. Have you read it?"

"No. I bought it but did not get around to reading it before I came but I will when I get home."

"Well, I read it and I said to myself, 'One day, I'm going to do that'. And so here I am! I also like walking and nature and meeting people and talking."

"And you are religious?"

"No, not really."

"But I have seen you in church," I say.

"Yes. Before the Camino, I go to church once, maybe twice, a year. But now, I have been on the Camino and I have been to church and I have cried. I don't know why but I cried. It's weird."

I tell her about the people—friends and work colleagues—who are bemused at me going on the Camino for the third time (once on motorbike didn't really count but it was a Camino of sorts; the second time, in 2008, was real, León to Santiago 300+ kilometres with Natasha). Some of them think I'm getting very religious; some think I'm about to convert to Catholicism! I tell her that I find much of the Camino very emotional, especially sharing the observances and devotions of others.

"Yes, I am the same," she said.

"Do you believe in God?" I ask her.

"I don't know. One part of me, the part that cries, wants to believe in God. But I am a scientist. I look at evidence and science, not at this ..."

"I think I'm the same; I listen to some of what comes with religion, what's said in church and think to myself, 'This is bonkers!' But at the time, I find it very moving, very attractive. The rational in me wins out each time, however."

And so we walked on, kicking about such matters, solving nothing of course, but sharing time, sharing thoughts ... Johanna is a lovely woman and I like her very much. This is so much of what the Camino is about: talking with a complete stranger who quickly becomes a close friend, thinking, walking together and sharing. Pilgrimage is a journey of discovery—the find may be inside oneself, it may be a fresh appreciation of nature, or the pleasure of opting out of the real world for a while; it might be the delight in making new friends in a very random but quite intense way. And it can be—nearly always it, I think—about having time to process things. That's certainly part of what I'm doing, processing. Working through thoughts about my Mum and Dad. Is that religious? I don't know. It seems spiritual ...

Brooding on chatting to Charlie and Johanna, it strikes me that however convincingly people like Richard Dawkins argue their case, they will never win over a majority of people because, fundamentally, humans are emotional and have a deep-seated need to believe in something beyond themselves. People have an evident need to believe there is a power outside themselves which is greater than them. You don't have to be a creationist to think this way or believe the literal word of Genesis. But the problem for Dawkins et al is that we are not all cousins of Mr Spock; we are not a species that lives by logic alone; we also live by emotion.

NATASHA: I have noticed the weather has been more or less the same each morning, and gradually forms into the same warm evenings, with a cool breeze. Rather perfect for the Camino, actually. This morning, leaving Terradillos, I had my arms wrapped tightly around my body, trying to keep warm from the coldness of the night. Then slowly, as we clocked up a few kilometres, the sun began to rise and leisurely heat the day. The familiar breeze came with the sun, and I thank it every time.

I was glad to be leaving Terradillos. No offence to the people who live there. I'm sure you are lovely, but your town is horrible. It was so uneventful and deathly boring that I could imagine the passing by of an outsider, such as a pilgrim, was incredibly exciting. I could imagine the families behind the shutters: "*Quick!* Children, come! Here comes another pilgrim," shouts the mother, munching on some popcorn, looking out onto the street.

Dad and I were the last to leave, as Dad had to apply a dressing to a nasty blister that was causing him some problems. Of course we caught up with the others in no time. After our first stop in a café, I walked ahead of Dad, and walked alone for a good while. My thoughts were racing away with my feet as I walked towards to next town. My mind was on something in particular this morning: my Leaving Cert exam results coming out on the 18th, and it being the 12th. I wasn't quite sure what I was worrying about the most: the fact that if I come up short of a few points, and will miss the course I really want, or, the fact that if I come short of a few points, I could ruin the next week of my Camino. Dad has told me, over and over again, not to worry about disappointing him or Mum, but I can't help it. I badly want to make them both proud, and I know they will be, regardless of the digits on my results page. But I can't help it.

Everyone I have met has asked me if I'm a student and I say yes. Then they ask me what I'm doing, and I explain to them that I don't actually know yet, but I'll find out on the 18th. So a good few people are aware of it. Before I came on the Camino, and realised I would find out my results here, I was devastated. Now, being here, I can't think of anywhere

I would want to be more. I'm surrounded by amazing, caring people, and not one of them is a Leaving Cert student. I won't have other people asking me what I got, and comparing their results to mine, or judging me. Another thing is, not many people will understand my results; it will only be a number to them. And since I'm the only Leaving Cert student here, I've been promised a good night of celebration. We have also worked out that we are likely to be in Astorga on the 18th, which is one of my favourite cities, so I'm delighted.

But for now I need to push it out of my mind and concentrate on other things. For the last six kilometres of the walk I walked with Andrew. We had a brilliant but simple conversation. We talked about what was the first thing we were going to do when we got home. My answer was that after talking to Mum, Patch and the dogs, I will go upstairs. I will put my bag down, and observe the changes in my room. Usually, Mum will have changed the sheets, and got one of my teddies, usually the ferret Dad bought me, and will have sat him perched on my bed. There will also, probably, be some fresh flowers from the garden, scattered around the place, which I love. After that I will quickly check the post to remind myself I actually have no friends and never get post, but insist on checking it regularly. Then I will scan the fridge, take a snack if anything interests me, hop into my car and drive down to Andrea.

PETER: Eh, you mean your and Patrick's car, young lady!

NATASHA: Andrew said that when he gets off the bus in his town, Saintfield, in Co. Down, he's going to walk home. He usually wouldn't. It's only a mile, but it would be the best mile to walk, through the town, with his rucksack on his back and with the biggest smile on his face. A smile that's come 800 kilometres.

After that, we talked about what we would do, on a normal day, at home. I went through mine. He went through his. We laughed at similarities. We talked about our Mum's best home-cooked meals. I mentioned Mum's brilliant chicken tikka sandwiches and her unbelievable raspberry cheesecake. I missed things like that. We talked about the things we do for fun at home. I told him about Andrea and my various daily activities, and then nights out with the girls. He mentioned his versions with Craig and his other friends.

I was curious about his life, after hearing so much about it. When we reached Bercianos, I was relieved. Even though, yet again, it was small, it had one shop and one bar, which compared to the last, was fantastic.

We had it set in our minds that we were going to stop here and it is very difficult to move on after that psychological end. The *albergue* was closed, but we only had an hour to wait. The *albergue* was standing on its own, nothing but orange land on either side, in the distance. There was a fenced-off sitting area and washing facilities. When it opened, the inside was surprisingly nice. It was run by volunteers and built upon past pilgrim memories. The men behind the desk explained the rules and the timetable of the day. They had a number of activities scheduled out for us, which was all lovely and thoughtful. I know that not attending things is awfully embarrassing but as a pilgrim who had just walked 26 kilometres, sometimes you just want to rest and so Andrew and I remained upstairs during Mass.

One of the nice things about the *albergue* was a little table on the landing, on the way down the stairs from the bedrooms. There were six small baskets, each one labelled a different language. I went to the English basket. Inside were a number of notes from pilgrims who had stayed here. I read a number of them. "I pray that my grandmother survives cancer, recovers and gets to see many more grandchildren, for years to come;" another read: "I pray for many years of happiness to my friends and family and to all those who complete the Camino." My favourite read: "May the person who carries this message have a happy complete life. Buen Camino."

I thought this was lovely. Later that evening I left my own, for Dad and me, a poem I had written earlier in the trip.

The fiery sun creeps up over the horizon,
Like a fox hunting through the day break.
Our aching bodies carry us along the winding roads,
Our boots tell our journey with the collecting dust.
Strangers' footsteps print the roads together,
Stories are shared, friendships are made.
When coolness lingers like a fog,
Darkness puts our shadows to sleep.
The Pilgrims' dreams are cast into the night,
To be forgotten along the morning path,
And we will see them again in Santiago.

BERCIANOS DEL CAMINO

PETER: Pity poor Bercianos. It's a one-horse town and even he has checked out. Bercianos' one obvious asset, the church of San Salvador, a substantial structure on a ridge at the edge of the village on the Camino, collapsed in a heap some 20 years ago. All that is visible today is a huge pile of rubble—mud, bricks, mortar dust and splintered beams—and the arched entrance. The good beams have been dragged from the rubble but are still, 20 years on, in a pile beside the collapsed house of God. And with it, the life has gone out of the village, or so it seems to the passing pilgrim.

Some 250 people live in Bercianos. So says a sign at the entrance to the village. It is 858 metres up on the Meseta Alta, surrounded by wheat fields and not a lot else. Most of the buildings in the village are made of mud: mud mixed with straw, rounded pebbles, broken tiles—anything essentially that will bulk out the mix and give it a bit of strength. In most instances the deep-brown mud walls are not plastered and so the matrix is clearly visible—as are the wooden lintels above windows and doors. Bockedy tiled roofs overhang the walls, affording a degree of protection from eroding rainwater. The streets are largely empty, devoid of people save for the occasional, almost always elderly person shuffling along to the tiny grocery shop or the bar where a TV blares out football news to an almost empty room. The clientele when I peer in include two late-middle-aged Japanese pilgrims standing at the bar. God knows what they make of this place but to me, much of the village, and the atmosphere within it, are like parts of a film set from one of those classic Sergio Leone spaghetti westerns starring Clint Eastwood and featuring, somewhere along the way, the treacherous looking Lee Van Cleef. All that's missing is tumbleweed blowing aimlessly down the empty streets.

But the *albergue* turns out to be a delight. It too is a mud brick structure, the façade of which has been lined with brick. Inside the wide, square, ancient, wooden front door there is a large entrance hall, paved in patterns of small cobble stones. Upstairs the rooms have timber floors and the walls are all plastered with a mix of mud and straw, exposed wooden beams within the mud giving added strength. The building was given to the Augustinians in Madrid some years back by the parish of Bercianos and it is now a nightly refuge for pilgrims on the way to

Santiago. The reception is manned when we arrive by two young men and Father Antolin Javier, an Augustinian. They are all volunteers and accept only a donation of an unspecified amount for a bunk bed and a warm reception. Father Javier normally works in the Augustinian provincial bureaucracy in Madrid where he is also an assistant parish priest and a teacher of philosophy. He is very much in charge of events in the *albergue*. At 7.00 pm, he and two of the young people lead about 25 pilgrims across the village through the streets to Mass in the still relatively new parish church, the Church of St Roque. They sing as we walk, and as we pass some of the village menfolk playing bowls and skittles they smile and acknowledge us. Even though this is a daily ritual, it must be the single most visible thing to happen in the village every day. Apart, that is, from the morning ritual of the Pan Van, the small bread vans that announce their presence in each village by careering about the streets blowing their inevitably high-pitched horns to alert would-be customers.

The red-brick, rectangular village hall-style church of St Roque is, sadly, utterly unremarkable, but Mass begins with Fr Javier symbolically washing the feet of four pilgrims. There is some singing and praying, Mass is said and there is also, of course, the Eucharist. And in a homily in Spanish, Fr Javier kindly breaks into English to say two things: firstly, he urges us on our pilgrimage to contemplate that we should love all mankind; secondly, that Christian marriage is made with God, lasts forever and cannot be broken. After Mass, we stroll back to the *albergue*, this time individually rather than as a group led by guitar-strumming young people. There is a communal meal. Everyone was told to bring something—a baguette, a head of lettuce, spaghetti, ham, whatever—and it was all made up by volunteer pilgrims working in the kitchen. Oddly enough, grace was not said, but after the meal there was a final blessing of day on a hillock beside the *albergue* to coincide with the setting sun.

As the great flaming orange orb dipped beneath the horizon and we all watched and took photographs, Fr Javier moved among us and, with his wet thumb, marked each pilgrim on the forehead with the sign of the cross and lay a hand on our heads as he uttered a blessing.

We sat, largely in silence, as the sun set and the day was done. I think Boheh Stone man would have felt entirely at home.

NATASHA: I attended the final blessing of the evening and was glad I did, having skipped Mass. It was amazing. All of us gathered to the side of the *albergue*, looking out to the horizon, watching the sun go down.

Music was played gently and Fr Javier came around to each of us, and blessed us, and gave us a little scallop shell with a message on the back. Mine read: *The limits of love, are love without limits.*

As the music stopped, and the sun was at its last wink, I looked around at the others sitting. I was touched at what I saw. A Spanish couple I have talked to a few times before sat on the bank. Their faces glowed with the colours of the sunset. He had his arms wrapped around her; she looked out onto the horizon, tears streaming down her face. He kissed her every now and then, and whispered in her ear.

Later that evening I asked her why she was crying. She replied, "Because I have never been so happy in my life as I am now."

Bercianos to Mansilla de las Mulas: 26.5 km in 5 hours

> *There is no experience like having children. That's all. There is no substitute for it. You cannot do it with a friend. You cannot do it with a lover. If you want the experience of having complete responsibility for another human being, and to learn how to love and bond in the deepest way, then you should have children.—Morrie Schwartz, in* Tuesdays with Morrie *by Mitch Albom (Doubleday 1997).*

PETER: The Camino today passes through two small villages and skirts around several others. All are unremarkable, as is the landscape immediately surrounding the Camino as it wends its way to León, the second great city on the way to Santiago. Here the wheat is long harvested and few of the fields have been ploughed again for next season's sowing. Even this surface change exposing the rich, brown-red Spanish clay would relieve the visual tedium. There are no other crops, just a few stray vines, one tiny field of vines, and just one good-sized field of sunflowers. But, in the far distance northwards, the Cantabrian Mountains and the Picos de Europa rise majestically to 2,600 metres. This morning in the early dawn, they are painted a Paul Henry slatey-grey and look inviting.

When I am walking, I am writing in my head so that by the time I reach the next *albergue* and I have showered and rested a few minutes, I am ready to put my thoughts down without much further ado. Walking this morning this is what I was thinking …

Dear Natasha,

I was there the moment you came into the world. I saw you lifted from your Mummy's womb, all blood-covered and squealing, placed gently on a weighing scales under the warm glow of a lamp, checked that everything was where it should be and then wrapped up. I was overcome with joy—a little girl! A beautiful little girl! And as Mummy was wheeled out of theatre after her stitching and brought out of her sleep, she opened her eyes and I said, "We have a girl, a little girl and she has red hair!" And Mum smiled and fell back to sleep, happy our family was complete—a little girl, a sister for Patrick!

And since that day you have kept us smiling and with Patrick have brought joy untold into our lives with your presence, your personality, your love, your writing, your painting and everything you do. When you were leaving school for the last time recently, one of your teachers, who has been with you since first year, recalled her first class with you. She said, "I looked down at all my new pupils chattering away to each other, or looking about the room anxious and curious, or rummaging in their bags, and there in the middle was this one big happy smiling face beaming up at me ready to learn—that was Natasha! And she has been like that almost every day since, a joy to have about."

You respond to love and affection and return both a hundredfold. I have watched you grow and your character develop into the wonderful young woman you now are. You and I have a special bond that holds us close to each other's heart; our personalities chime, we have overlapping interests; and you know how to make me laugh, how to keep me in check.

Now as we walk to Santiago together, you are also walking away from me. This is as it should be; you must be your own person, make your own way in the world. You are growing stronger, more independent by the day, more sure of yourself, more your own person, more willing (and able) to question what I say, more willing to take an independent stance. This too is as it should be. Now you are about to make your own way in the world unaided, unrestrained. Soon you will go to college and a whole new world will open before you; you will learn things beyond what I can teach you, and you will start teaching me.

Here are some thoughts of mine I hope will help you and which you will carry with you …

Happiness comes from inside you; it comes from being able to sit on the grassy bank of a river watching the water flow, listening to lark song rising higher and higher in the sky, as we do in Mayo; it comes from watching the sun set behind Clare Island and knowing that you are loved and love in return; it comes from lying on your back staring up at the night sky and seeing shooting stars, as we have been on the Camino.

Money is great but it is only a means to an end and not an end in itself. Enjoy simple pleasures in your life such as observing the delicate beauty of a flower, the rustle of small creatures in the undergrowth, or the unexpected joy of seeing a Pine-Marten gambolling along a path, stopping and turning to watch you in return, as we saw in the forest in Navarra. In these things is richness that no money can buy and they are worth more than all the money you will ever have.

Enjoy solitude; take time out to be on your own. Know yourself and learn that people count; the things people buy and squabble over do not. If you seek happiness from objects only, you will find that your life is hollow.

Never be afraid to stand out from the crowd. Never be afraid to stand alone when standing alone is the right thing to do. You will know what the right thing is, and when to live by it. If you have doubts, listen to that small voice inside your head and be guided by it. This is your conscience and it will not let you down.

… strong in will
To strive, to seek, to find, and not to yield …

Be an optimist because the optimist knows things will get better and that knowledge alone helps make things better. Optimists are intrinsically happier and happiness breeds further happiness. Light a candle rather than curse the darkness and do not wait for someone else to light it; do it yourself.

Wear your successes lightly and accept your failures gracefully. You will judge yourself by the former; others will judge you by the latter. Be kind to those who are less successful than you and generous to those who will never experience success as you do.

Learn to love great music because it will bring you happiness for all your whole life. When you walk the countryside, or sit alone, or ride on a train and hear Grieg or Sibelius, or Vivaldi or Elgar or Beethoven or Tchaikovsky, you will understand what I mean. When you know wonderful music and are lonely, you can play it in your head and it will comfort you.

Be ambitious but not ruthless; strike out into the unknown and leave your comfort zone. Take risks but do not be reckless; test yourself, not others. You have a wild streak. It is a wonderful part of your character; use it to good advantage. Do not rest on your laurels.

How dull it is to pause, to make an end,
To rust unburnish'd, not to shine in use!

Never let anyone tell you that you are less than them but never act as though you are better than anyone else; you are the equal of all and let no one tell you otherwise.

Choose your life partner wisely; find one who makes you laugh and smile, who shares your interests and loves you for who you are, not what they want you to be; choose a partner who is strong but gentle with it; choose a partner you want to wake up beside every morning for the rest of your life. Choose a partner who would walk the Camino with you.

Live life to the full and see the world. Enjoy your life for it is yours to enjoy and it is the only one you will ever have. Go, but come back.

There lies the port: the vessel puffs her sail:
There gloom the dark broad seas.

And when you have done all that, never forget from where you come; honour the things in which you believe and live by them. Know that when you are away, there are those back home who love you and will be thinking about you every day you are gone.

Mum and I and Patrick love you more that words can measure,
Dad.

NATASHA: When we arrived in Mansilla de las Mulas, in the late morning, we went straight to the *albergue.* We had half an hour to wait for it to open at 12.00 noon. We sat on the ground outside. Dad and I hadn't a bead of sweat on us and we both agreed we could happily carry on to León, a further 20 kilometres away. However, when one plans a destination for the day, it's very hard to walk further as you have stopped, physically as well as in your head. I'm extremely glad we didn't walk on, as Mansilla was a beautiful town, and the first large one we had seen for a couple of nights. I was getting really sick of small villages with nothing but the *albergue.*

The *albergue* was situated in the heart of the old town, on a little narrow street, scattered with cute pastry shops and small bars on either side. The *albergue* itself was quite small. There was a large kitchen, and a computer room, and a lovely courtyard with tables and chairs. The rooms were upstairs looking out onto the courtyard. Dad and I shared a room with the usuals: Gary, Andrew and Tasmanian Steve. Reece's bed was robbed by some guy that Steve had been walking with.

Reece had been a bit quiet walking into Mansilla. Later, Andrew told me that he had received bad news from home. His Granny was very sick, and Reece's family told him that the news in the coming days might not be good. Reece spent all day looking at bus times from León to Santiago, trying to find a way to get home. In the end, he decided to stay. I haven't spoken to Reece about it, but I think he's going to complete the Camino for his Granny. She would be proud of him for what he's doing.

I went out and bought some bread, meat and cheese, and Dad and I ate in the courtyard with Steve and Gary in the heat. After that, Andrew and I went wandering. We walked through a little cobbled square, bordered with boutique shops, down the main street, and towards the river. There was a massive stone bridge going over the river leading out of the town. We scaled down a grassy bank and walked through tall, skinny trees to the river bank. We walked down along the river, further away from the noisy city. The river was very wide, very clear, and flowing fast. It was beautiful. We found a tree that had fallen and was hovering out over the edge of the river. We sat on the trunk and dangled our tender feet in the cold, flowing water. The sun was shining down onto the river, casting sparkles along the surface. 'Jesus bugs' skimmed the water, hopping upstream. Green, hair-like weed danced on the river floor with the current. We looked at small things floating towards us in the distance, and watched as they became larger and showed their forms—a Coke can, a stick or a cluster of leaves. As soon as you got to see what it was, it would be gone down the river, out of sight. The river reminded me of life. One minute something is here, and before you know it, it's gone, and moved on. Things pass you by in life, as time goes by. And it all happens very quickly. As quick as the current of the river. I wanted it all to slow down. I don't want my life to race ahead and for things to pass me by without seeing them properly.

I didn't want to reach Santiago for the pure fact that it would mean the end. The Camino is moving so fast, and it's not going to slow down unless I'm willing to slow down, which means losing our friends, and watching them go by. We have less than two weeks left, yet it feels like I only left St-Jean a week ago.

Some of the best things in life are brief, so you have to take them in while you can. I want to take all of the Camino in and remember every step along the way. I don't want to lose the people I've met just because the walking is over. I want that part of the Camino to stay with me forever.

Later on, Dad, Andrew and Gary went out to buy things for dinner. I stayed in the kitchen and wrote. We had a tortilla made by the boys. We drank wine. Steve and Reece joined us. And yet again, we had a lovely evening full of conversation and laughter. Dad went to bed at around 10.00 pm. Andrew and I went up next. As I was lying in bed, I could hear music coming in the window from a nearby club. It was a good song, Edward Maya, *Stereo Love*. The bed above me started moving with Dad's tossing and turning; this was followed with a: "Tasha. What the hell is that noise? That's bloody ridiculous. They're all going to hell!"

Of course Dad didn't know what I was talking about when I reminded him of his cursing the next morning.

Mansilla de las Mulas to León: 20.5 km in 4 hours

PETER: It is strange and wonderful how walking 20 kilometres has become something of a doddle; a mere trifle of a stroll! We arrived in León at 10.30 am without even breaking sweat and now there is a whole day to enjoy the third great city of the Camino, and the last one before our destination is reached.

León began as a Roman city, founded by them in 70 AD to exert control over gold mines against the Asturians and Cantabrians. It was home to the Seventh Legion, hence its name Le[gi]on, and it was from here that Rome set out to conquer Spain's north west. Five hundred years later the Visigoths took control of the city but then lost it in 712 to the Moors, who managed to hold it for a mere 134 years until 846 when Ordoño I of Asturias took it back and booted them out. There was never any hesitation in affirming León's importance as evidenced by the fact that the first cathedral was started by Ordoño II in 916. León's wealth was based mainly on produce of the meseta surrounding the city—grain, meat (from sheep) and wool also. And while the city prospered and grew, the 10th century was not peaceful. Kings, princes and would-be rulers squabbled among one other and at times sought alliances with the Moors to the south to gain strategic advantage against a rival within their own kingdom. In some instances we can surmise that the epithets attached to rulers—Sancho I the Fat and Ordoño III the Evil (who was also a hunchback)—were indicative of how they were regarded by their luckless subjects. Both the Fat one and the Evil one were among León kings to pay protection money to the caliphs of Córdoba but the peace thus bought was not always sustained. In 988 Vermudo the Gouty made an alliance with Almanzor the Moor but Almanzor, far from propping up Vermudo, invaded León, raised much of the city, including the cathedral, and occupied it until his death.

After the destruction of the first, Romanesque cathedral, it was twice rebuilt in Romanesque style. But at the end of the 13th century building began on the current Gothic cathedral. And what a building it is—a real treat. Built like Burgos in the French and Germanic style, it has none of Burgos' arrogance; nor does it seek to project power in the manner of that vast structure. León's cathedral is a statement, of course, but of an altogether more gentle nature. What truly marks León Cathedral out from others is its glass—an astonishing 1,800 square metres of medieval stained glass; hundreds of thousands of pieces, each one (bar those inserted during restorations) individually cast and crafted up to 600 years ago to create an uplifting celebration of the glory of God.

To this end, the people of León, and a goodly measure of pilgrims also, crowded into the cathedral at 12 noon on the Sunday of our arrival in the city for sung Mass presided over by Bishop Julian Lopez Martin. I went with Johanna, my Peruvian friend. We had no idea that a bishop would be presiding and so this turned out to be *the* Mass of the day, the bishop being assisted by six priests and three other men wearing what appeared to be vestments but whose status seemed to be somewhat less than that of the priests. They may indeed have been priests but sadly my capacity to distinguish is limited by my background. The pews between the altar and the choir were filled to capacity and many more people were standing in the side aisles. The organ went full tilt, always guaranteed to make for a good service in my book. Of course I would have loved to hear the congregation give a lusty rendition of the Irish hymn *Be Thou My Vision* or *Guide Me Oh Thou Great Redeemer*, the great Welsh anthem also known as *Bread of Heaven*, but I was in the wrong church, let alone the wrong country, for that … No matter, a cathedral filled with people, all of one purpose, has its own enriching and uplifting dynamic, and it was so. The bishop's homily was one delivered by an old man going through his paces—without great feeling, it seemed to me, and with words a tad slurred and mumbled. When it came to the moment to share a sign of peace Johanna and I embraced spontaneously and hugged each other. And we shook hands, rather stiffly and formally, with the good burgers of León in whose midst we were sitting. I went up to receive the Eucharist. Johanna did not.

Even though it was Sunday, the city was alive with people—families strolling about the old town, Sunday lunch in snazzy cafés. In the early evening, walking alone, I was attracted by the hubbub in one particular crowded bar and went inside. Everyone was drinking wine and eating slices of meat from small plates. I asked for some *vino tinto* (the most basic Spanish red wine in terms of quality but almost always excellent in my experience) and pointed to one of the saucers of meat. Soon I was holding a glass of fine rioja and eating a selection of five different salamis and bread. The price? €1.20. I had seconds. And thirds …

Natasha said she would treat me to dinner and when we settled on a modest-looking place near the cathedral, we ended up having the best pilgrim menu meal of our Camino to date—starters of spaghetti bolognaise and salad with tuna and asparagus; main course of delicious garlic fried chicken and potato wedges; a little tub of crème caramel for dessert; half a bottle of white wine, bread and water—all for €9 a head. Tasha also had some calamari. Most guidebooks don't say it, but a bed for €5 a night and dinner such as this is part, a good part, of the reason why hundreds of thousands of people do the Camino each year, sprinkling a little wealth in their wake as they make their way across northern Spain.

NATASHA: I was looking forward to our arrival in León. It would mean that, technically, Dad and I will have completed the whole Camino as this was where we started our first Camino in 2008. Also, I loved León, and the fact that it was only 20 kilometres from Mansilla. It would be a mere stroll to the shops.

The last six kilometres were like any six kilometres outside a large, industrialised city. We passed car showrooms, petrol stations and kitchen wear shops. Over every little hump in the path, Dad and I would expect to see the explosion of León spreading out before us. The Camino was lined with dry nettles and weeds, and with every step a rustling noise would follow from the scurrying of small mice and other rodents.

Finally, unexpectedly, it appeared, sitting there in all its glory, peeking out from behind a mound of land. The cathedral wasn't in sight yet and for us that was the centre of the city. As we followed the path around the mound, the towers of the cathedral appeared into view. It looked magnificent.

It was strange arriving in a familiar place for the first time in three weeks. Of course everything was as I remember. We arrived at 10.30 am, and thought we would have a while to wait for the *albergue* to open.

We went to the same *albergue* as last time, one attached to a convent, and to our surprise it opened at 11.00 am. Dad and I sat in a café, 20 metres away from the *albergue* doors, in a little cobbled square, warming in the morning sun. Gradually, one by one, pilgrims staggered around the corner, left their bags at the *albergue* doors, and came to the café. Everyone who was expected came, apart from Tim and Louise. We hadn't seen them since Burgos, and we didn't think we would see them again. But of course, in usual wonderful Camino fashion, as Dad and I were checking in, we heard the little squeak of an Australian girl. Standing there, with two huge smiles on their faces, were Tim and Louise. I was very happy. "Tash! How are ye!?" asked Louise, arms open and looking even more beautiful than I had remembered. We hugged and chatted. It had been Louise's 32nd birthday the day before and so, as with Tim's birthday, they treated themselves to a hotel. They looked very fresh and bushy tailed; one could have confused them for new pilgrims beginning in León. I was happy; our whole Camino family was back together.

Another thing that made me very happy was the news Gary gave me on his arrival. There was a Burger King 100 metres from our *albergue*. I think I was as happy as I was when I thought Dad had lost his hat back in Estella.

At 12.00, Dad and Johanna, and Gary and Steve went to Mass in the cathedral. Andrew, Reece and I stayed in the café waiting for their return, so that we could make our trip to Burger King. Gary had been wishing for one since the day I met him. There we were, at 1.30 pm, Gary, Andrew, Reece, Steve, Louise, Tim and I, sitting around a table in Burger King, in León, eating Whopper Burgers and chicken fries. It was brilliant.

At 3.00 pm, I went wandering León with Andrew. We went to the main street. The sun was shining down the crowded street right onto the cathedral. Cafés and restaurants mobbed the area. Talk and laughter filled the air. The sun was extremely hot, and I was glad not to be walking in it. We sat in a café looking at the cathedral, drinking mojito slush puppies.

León Cathedral is unbelievable. The outside is magnificent, but the inside is what makes it. The building is covered in stained-glass masterpieces, and the colours shine brilliantly as the sun hits them. I took Dad out for dinner that night. I was absolutely over the moon to see calamari on the menu. I had to have it. And I did. It was amazing. Then we got the pilgrim menu—the best yet. It helped that it was served by a delightful little lady too. Of course, there was one place we had to go to. Two years ago, when we were in León, Dad took me for my first tapas experience, and boy was it one to remember! He brought me to a bar just around the corner from the little square outside the *albergue*. It was small and ugly. It was a washed-orange colour with brown window sills, protected by black bars. Inside, a loyal local man sits at the bar, proud builder's bum on display, hunched over the tapas, smoking. The floor is covered in sunflower seed shells and receipts. There was a dog asleep on the floor and another old man sitting at a table, staring at the TV with lost eyes. The barmaid looked unfriendly as she leaned against the bar, smoking. Dad ordered what he thought was marinated chicken, and brought it over to the table. An orange and red oily mixture was plonked in front of me. I'm always up for trying new things and so I took a large bite of whatever it was. It was slimy in my mouth, not particularly nice, but swallowable.

"Dad, what is this?" I asked as I stared at the little portion.

"Eh, oh, it's tripe, sheep's stomach, I believe," he replied after tasting the 'chicken' himself.

Well, that experience went down so memorably that Dad decided it had to be revisited. We found the place and went there. The only thing that had changed was the barmaid. It was a man. Everything else remained, just as we had left it. Our tapas was even just as interesting—squid and mussels in vinegar and vegetables. As least we knew what we were eating this time.

León to Hospital de Órbigo: 32 km in 6 hours

NATASHA: Leaving León brought back very vivid memories. The town was asleep and dark, just as it had been two years ago when we left for Hospital de Órbigo. We both remembered the journey, so knew exactly what to expect. Road. Lots of boring road. Turns out, there was even more boring road than we had thought. We all left the *albergue* around the same time, and the journey was spent mostly with our little Camino family members. It was a hot day, very like our last time walking, but thankfully I didn't get horrifically burnt, as I did two years ago. Walking out of León, the path was scattered with a few unfamiliar faces. This had been expected. León was a starting place for many pilgrims.

The walk there is unfortunately not enjoyable. It is basically only road. A couple of times, one will pass through a tiny stretch of corn field for a few minutes, but is quickly brought back to the side of the road.

However, apparently there are two routes from León to Hospital, and one, the route we didn't take, is supposedly beautiful. Our Italian friend Enrique said it was her most pleasant journey yet.

Towards the last 13 kilometres we walked through a little village that both Dad and I remembered. We remembered it because there was the cutest little pastry shop where we had bought our lunch last time, to eat by a bench looking out to the fields. This time I was with Andrew, Gary and Reece and just bought an icecream to take me along the rest of the way. Surprisingly, my walk from León to Hospital was one of my favourites, purely because it was the most I laughed on the trip so far. Andrew and I spent a majority of our walk hunched over in fits of laughter, so I was distracted from the ugly scenery.

The last five kilometres of the walk was the hardest, as often it is. The sun decided to gives us a hard time as we continued along the roadside, heading towards a constantly empty horizon. Nothing could be seen in the distance, and it was rather frustrating not knowing when you were going to be there. But when we did arrive, at around 12.00 pm, the town of Hospital de Órbigo was much more beautiful than I remembered. It was larger, and cuter. Unfortunately, the wonderful, long, medieval bridge that brings you into the centre was being restored, and it didn't look its best with builder's rubble and tape everywhere.

PETER: The bridge over the Río Órbigo is a wonderful, long. medieval arched structure. The river here is quite wide and made to seem even more so by the very wide flood plain on one side of it. The bridge spans everything, the river sand flood plain. As we walk over, workmen are dismantling the wooden posts and seating arrangements for what was clearly a mock medieval jousting arena. I am very sorry that we missed it as it is held in honour annually of a tournament here in the Camino Holy Year of 1434 that is worth recalling.

Suero de Quiñones was a knight from León whose advances were rejected by his chosen lady. To show that he loved her nonetheless and would remain loyal to her, he wore an iron collar around his neck permanently. In July 1434 he decided to stage a huge tournament in the hope of impressing her by challenging the best knights in Europe to joust against him at Órbigo. An arena was built on the flood plain. It was 146 paces long and lined with a palisade and spectator galleries. The area was covered by brightly coloured tents and penants fluttering in the breeze. At dawn on 11 July the knights paraded to Mass through Órbigo, led by musicians and dancing ladies as the church bells rang out. In the ensuing tournament, Suero and his companions are said to have broken no less than 300 lances in jousts. In one, a Catalan challenger wary of Suero's fearsome reputation is said to have donned double-thick armour; Suero allegedly mocked him by putting on a woman's blouse and prancing about the place jeering him.

At the end of July, Suero proclaimed that his bravery at the tournament proved for all that he really did love his lady, even if she did not return his affections, and so he took off his collar, returned to León and from there, went to Santiago de Compostela as a pilgrim. There he gave the cathedral a bejewelled bracelet which today may be seen only in a painting of Santiago Alfeo in the cathedral museum.

Suero went on to take part in many other battles but, 24 years after the famous tournament, he ran into one of his former opponents, Gutierre de Quijada, who was still smarting from the humiliation visited upon him. De Quijada challenged; both men lowered their lances and ran at each other; in a moment, Suero was dead. Next time I am in Hospital de Órbigo, I must be sure my visit coincides with the re-enactment of the tournament. I bet it's great fun …

NATASHA: Over the bridge and into Órbigo proper, the main street welcomed us with busy people trotting about the place on their way to lunch, or just relaxing in an open café, enjoying the sun. The river was flowing gently, looking very inviting as we struggled over it. Children below played in the clear water by the bank. A swimming pool was visible to the left of the bridge, so relaxation time was sorted. Dad and I wanted to stay in the same *albergue* as we had last time, so we walked through the town, almost to the other side, but still central enough. The *albergue* is a simple terraced house on the main street with an entrance door that is small and a little misleading. You are welcomed by an old, withered atrium, with a mini-blossoming garden situated in the middle.

PETER: And we were also welcomed by a familiar accent, a Northern Ireland lilt from Celine, a warm, smiling woman from Newtownards no less. She had done the Camino with her daughter and, clearly moved by it like myself, she volunteered to do a stint as a *hospitalero*, one of the army of volunteers who operate the length of the Camino helping *albergue* owners or the church authorities where they run *albergue*s. Celine books us in and I watch her later padding about the place, cheerily helping people to their rooms.

NATASHA: The atrium is paved with smoothed pebbles, and the walls are painted in blues and greens to show a mountain scene, part of the Camino to come, it appears. The upstairs bedrooms look out onto the atrium through a blue-painted wooden balcony. There is a relaxed atmosphere to the place. Through the atrium, past the doors for the rooms, you come out into the garden. It appears uncared for, yet holds character and charm. The grass is naked in areas where the dry, orange dust comes through. A couple of inviting picnic benches in the sun tell us it's a homemade dinner tonight.

After a quick nap, Tim, Louise, Andrew, Gary and I trot down to the village swimming pool, and I finally get to use my bikini. The swimming pool is there for anyone to use at the small price of €1.60. It is completely empty as it's siesta time. The pool looks untouched and almost sinful. The sun is high in the sky, and hot on our skin, so jumping in was bliss. It was a sensation I had forgotten. A couple of beers made it even better.

We stayed there for a couple of hours; then I left to go see Dad and prepare some dinner.

That evening was my favourite moment on the Camino so far. I felt such happiness it felt unreal. Our little Camino family was sitting outside on one of the benches. Bob Dylan was playing softly, glasses were never empty of wine, and conversation was never dry. Everyone was happy to be there and in each other's company. I didn't want any of it to end.

It came to 10.00 pm and Dad decided it was time for him to go to bed. It was getting dark. Empty bottles of wine filled the table, and Dad took it upon himself to dispose of them. Looking like a little hunched-over creature with large claws as he waddled away, six bottles in hand, he seemed to sway slightly. There was silence back at the table as we watched. Unfortunately for Dad, the large row of bicycles parked against the *albergue* got in his way, and he walked straight into them with a little bang. We watched and gasped, expecting the smashing of bottles to wake the sleeping pilgrims but, steadily on his feet, Dad carried on and disappeared into the *albergue*, like a trooper. Of course, in Dad's usual fashion, he dismissed such antics, and protested his innocence next morning.

Hospital de Órbigo to Astorga: 16 km in 3 hours

NATASHA: I was sad to be leaving Hospital as I had really enjoyed our time there, but I was also very excited to reach Astorga, as I labelled it my favourite town of our last trip. Also, our journey promised to be easy. It was a small 16 kilometres.

Leaving the village, we are presented with a choice. Two Camino roads, two distances to Astorga. One said 15 kilometres, the other said 16. One would assume the decision was easy. The longer route disappeared into a field of vines and maize and, said Dad, hops; the other veered towards the main road. Dad announced he was going the longer way. I immediately went against him and said I was taking the shorter route. After one of Dad's best puppy-eye faces, I gave in, and took the longer route. And I'm glad we did. It was most enjoyable. We had avoided the mistake we had made walking to Hospital de Órbigo by taking the nicer route.

The first kilometre or two is through rich, cared-for crops of vines, barley, apple trees and many other foods. Then we are met by a tiny village, which is completely silent. We have our morning coffee there, and realise this is going to be a very relaxed walk, and that's just fine with me. As our path continued further into the rural landscape soaking up the sunrise, the noise of the motorway became fainter and fainter and I was very glad not to be walking beside it. Things soon become very familiar as we reach old farming towns where the road is trailed with tractor marks, and the air is filled with the cries of hungry animals.

Disappearing over the hump in the land, the rest of our journey is on a dusty road, weaving through mini-forests and large yellow fields. My city peeks up over the horizon every now and then to say hello to me. I like it when we get a glimpse of our destination, like a little tease and then it's gone again.

Dad had said we should stay in the same place as last time—the *albergue* San Javier. It is privately owned and we had enjoyed our stay there last time very much. When I arrived there two years ago, I was seriously burned. My skin was tight and it looked raw. A horrified lady, who checked us in, immediately took me out to the courtyard and began covering me in tomatoes. Instantly the sting was gone. Entering Astorga this time, the city was packed with people who had come for the open-air market that was being held in the centre. Squeezing through with my fat rucksack was a challenge but soon enough we were outside our *albergue.* The same woman was sitting at the desk. I looked at her, with a beaming smile. Dad tried to aid her memory.

"Eh, deux année, ago, we stay here," he said, constantly making ridiculous hand gestures. She is lost. He tries again.

"Le soleil, burned her. You, tomato."

"Ah!" she exclaimed, realising who I was. "You! Non?" She examined me thoroughly, noting how much I had grown in two years. I was happy she remembered our last encounter. She had been so caring to me last time, and nothing had changed. We christened her Señorita Tomato. She liked this. We laughed about it, and then we went to our rooms.

The *albergue* was just as I remembered it. Nothing had changed, and this was good. It was perfect the way it was, even the ridiculously squeaky floors. Nearly everything was made from old wood: the stairs, the ceiling, the floors and the bunk beds. The downstairs is completely open; it's one huge room that includes the reception, a good kitchen, and a relaxing area with mattresses which are used in the evenings for massages. The dining area is off the kitchen, and includes computers. There is a washing area outside in the terrace, and tables and chairs for sitting.

PETER: Astorga is the sort of place that I would love to come back to for a weekend break. It's a manageable size, in terms of walking about, and is full of history and interesting buildings. When we were here two years ago we went to Mass in a convent church facing the *albergue.* You entered the church in the middle, as it were, and naturally your eyes went immediately to the altar. After sitting for a time I turned to see in the rear wall a window opening with jail-like bars across it. Behind the bars were several nuns, members of a closed order never allowed more contact with the outside world than what they might observe through the bars. It was a strange and unsettling sight.

Astorga has two interesting monumental buildings—the cathedral and the Gaudi Palace. The second wins hands down, for me. The cathedral is ordinary enough, although it is a cathedral. There are 13 chapels, some of which are little more than *retablos* in alcoves. The altar *retablo* is devoted to Mary, and the panels, which are in Georgian style, tell various biblical stories. The choir and organ are in the centre of the main aisle (there are two side aisles) with the organ boasting both vertical and trumpet-like horizontal pipes projecting out over the stalls. But it is Gaudi's legacy that attracts me.

His palace, commissioned by the Bishop of Astorga in 1889 and finished in 1913, is a bright granite building that combines elements of gothic, art nouveau and the style of the arts and crafts movement. Overall, it looks like something that central casting at Disney might dream up—a magnificent fantasy palace in pale granite, gleaming in the sunshine, smaller than the adjacent cathedral but complementing it. Inside on the ground floor, granite pillars support a vaulted, gothic-style ceiling. The nerves, the spine-like ribs that flow up and across the ceiling from the tops of the columns, are lined with glazed bricks. The walls are oak-panelled to half height; plastered walls and ceiling are painted plain white. The overall visual effect is strangely like that of a mosque. Upstairs, however, there is a magnificent small chapel, ablaze with coloured light from stained-glass windows. There is parquet flooring and more glazed bricks.

The palace is now a museum of the Camino and contains many artefacts of interest to the pilgrim. These include a facsimile of the *Codex Calixtinus* or *Liber Sancti Jacobi* by Aymeric Picaud, the original of which is in the cathedral in Santiago, and numerous statues of pilgrims and St James. There is also a 'book of privileges' noting the granting of permission to open an *albergue* in Foncebadón and a reference to an 'Ermitaño Gaucelmo'.

NATASHA: I didn't get to explore Astorga as much as I would have liked, as it was extremely hot outside—well over 30 degrees—and I was tired. I only made it as far as the nearest *panadería* to get myself a tasty little pastry. The city was bustling when I left for the *panadería* at 2.00 pm, but walking back to the *albergue* at 2.30 pm, the streets were empty and the bedroom shutters were down to bring darkness to siesta sleepers.

I went back to the *albergue* and was met by an excited Steve, informing me that he was going to show the boys some of his photos from his home, Tasmania. He said he would wait until I was ready to begin the slide show on one of the computers downstairs. Within five minutes of meeting Steve, you will learn he is from Tasmania, an island off the south of Australia that's home to around half a million people. He is extremely proud of where he comes from, and talks enthusiastically of his home, and takes pleasure at how other Australians look down a bit on Tasmanians. For Steve, this is a badge of honour.

Stephen's second name is Gill. He's a tall, well-built 27-year-old and one can tell he is into his sports by just looking at him. His body is covered in freckles and bronzes gradually, as Tasmania is the coldest part of Australia, not like Tim and Louise who are extremely tanned.

Tasmanian Steve is very into his hiking, and regularly plans weekend mountain hikes with his friends all around Tasmania. He had hundreds of photos from his various trips and they advertised Tasmania very beautifully. He had pictures of the western plains, showing every mountain standing, and was able to name each one, and say he had climbed it. He seemed to have a solid group of climbing friends. One of them went by the name 'Green Giant'. We had thought Steve was big, but it was nothing on his friend Green Giant. I asked him if he often went to the mainland and he said he had been a few times. He explained that he didn't really like the atmosphere in Canberra, and that, as a Tasmanian, he felt out of place. He prefers the character and closeness you find within places like Tasmania.

The more I get to know Steve, the more I see he is a well-brought-up boy, who has his morals in place very well. He can also cook a brilliant basil and black olive pasta dish, as he did for our dinner in Astorga. He cooked a whole feast for 12 of us. It was brilliant. After our dinner, a few of us sat outside in the garden area. We were accompanied by our Spanish friend Roman, and Dirk from Germany, who had his guitar with him. They played music for hours. It was lovely. It calmed me right down for a well-needed sleep, to prepare me for the next day—

Leaving Certificate results day. The night ended with a call from Mum and Patch, wishing me luck.

Astorga to Foncebadón: 26 km in 5 hours

NATASHA: Waking up this morning, there was only one thing on my mind: finding out my Leaving Certificate exam results at 1.00 pm. It didn't bother me that I was going to get mine later than everyone at home, because I wasn't at home, so it didn't matter. I was glad I was where I was, because already everyone was being nice to me about them when I started to talk nervously. Nobody else here is a Leaving Cert student, so there is no worry about competition. But I had six hours to kill before I got them, so getting in 26 kilometres beforehand would be a good way of distracting myself.

The walk, again, was familiar. It was also promised to be a nice walk.

Coming out of Astorga, onto the first flat stretch of the Camino, we were welcomed by a shocking sight. The path was flooding with pilgrims, all with unfamiliar faces. The crowdedness was beginning. One of the things that made me angry was the regular sight of pilgrims passing energetically, without rucksacks on, as they were being carried by a helping van. They would be the people to leave me bedless one night.

Dad and I raced through the first 15 kilometres of the walk, to avoid the crowds and find our Cowboy Bar to have our morning coffee. When we had passed through cute little villages such as Murias de Rechivaldo, we reached El Ganso, location of our bar, the one that gave us a good photo two years ago. Of course, all the places we come across where we have a good photo from two years ago, we get another taken, for this trip.

As we sat outside our bar, having our tea, and for Dad a coffee and a cognac, the crowds of pilgrims came pouring around the corner, telling us it's time to keep moving. Our journey intertwined on and off with Tim and Louise. I walked with Louise who spoke to me about life back in Melbourne, which she hadn't experienced in nearly three years. She told me she and Tim were getting two dogs when they got home, to begin their family. Walking through Rabanal del Camino, and not stopping for the night, was difficult for Dad. I know he wanted to stay there, like we had last time, but I wanted to walk on to Foncebadón, to be with everyone else for my results.

PETER: This was Natasha's day and so there was no way I was going to force the issue and stay in Rabanal. But she's correct: I would very much like to have stayed there. I have a soft spot for the place since 2007 when my friend Tony and I passed through on our motorbikes and attended vespers in the tiny Benedictine church. It is opposite an *albergue*, the Refugio Gaucelmo, named after the 12th-century hermit who promoted monasticism in the region and where Aymeric Picaud, he of *Liber Sancti Jacobi* fame, also stayed. The *albergue* is now run by the English Confraternity of St James, two of whose middle-aged women volunteers were exceptionally kind to Natasha and me in 2007 when we came in from the snow, freezing and wet like two drowned rats. They lit a fire for us and plied us with hot chocolate. Vespers is a delight—two monks sing beautifully and the ceremony is intimate due to the smallness of the church. But not today, not this day. I sit outside the *albergue* for a few minutes munching a nectarine before we set off again for Foncebadón, high in the mountain range that separates León from the Bierzo region beyond.

NATASHA: As the day crept on I was receiving texts from friends and family asking how I did. I read a lovely text from my friend Andrea in the morning, wishing me luck. One of the less expected good wishes was from my history grinds teacher, Gráinne Leddy, who rang me to wish me luck. All the other texts from fellow students, asking me what I got, I blocked out of my head and tried to forget about.

The last seven kilometres from Rabanal was beautiful. We were cast out from the road into the protection of the mountains. We were surrounded by tall growing gorse and purple, pussy willow bushes, that grew out of control, spitting onto the Camino path. The sun was shining strongly, but there was a constant breeze about that kept us from sweating. We arrived into the collapsed and ghostly, almost unoccupied town of Foncebadón, at 11.30 am. We were the first to arrive because of our fast morning pace. We settled ourselves into an *albergue*, after checking it had internet access. I had time for a sleepless hour-and-a-half nap. My phone was constantly beeping, and I wanted it to be the others, informing me that they were here, but it was a nervous Mummy back home, reminding me that I had to call her as soon as I read my results online.

Finally, with only half an hour to go until logging online, my phone started to ring. It was Andrew, telling me that he, Gary, Reece,

Tasmanian Steve, Tim and Louise were outside one of the *albergues* and he wanted to know which one Dad and I were in, to be sure they were all with me for my results. They were all being so nice to me. At 1.05 pm, Dad and I went upstairs to log on. I hadn't really thought about the online process, and presumed it would be fairly straightforward. Unfortunately, I was wrong, and there was a dramatic bit of panic to the whole process as we had to telephone my school, St Andrew's College in Dublin, to get my exam number and pin code. After a really helpful lady on the switch got them for us, I typed them into the website and my grades popped up on screen. I started to cry and cover the screen. Dad got out his notebook and assured me it was going to be okay. All eight of my subjects were onscreen, blunt and unchangeable. Both of us began translating the grades into points and adding them up furiously. On the last subject, the number stood there on my phone calculator, and the same number on Dad's notebook that he had been calculating—405. I burst out crying horrifically. Dad started crying too, followed by a "That's very good, Tasha," and he hugged me.

"No," I cried, "it's not good. I've missed my English and philosophy course by five points."

After seeing I was upset, Dad recalculated my results. Still 405. The number wasn't changing, and neither was my reaction.

"Get me out of here! I want to leave!" I was devastated, and all I was aware of was the crowded room of pilgrims checking into the *albergue*, who would see me crying my eyes out. I didn't want anyone to see me, I was that embarrassed. Dad brought me straight outside and we sat on a bench looking out over the mountains we had spent five hours earlier that day, climbing. I had to ring Mum as promised. "Hello," a worried little voice answered as I called her. All I could do was cry.

"Tasha?" she asked.

"I got 405, Mum," I blubbered,

"Oh darling, that's brilliant!" she shrieked.

"No, I've missed my top courses of English," I continued to cry.

I wasn't upset about getting 405. I knew this was a good result. It was the fact I had missed the four courses I wanted the most, and by five points. Mum immediately began reassuring me I was going to be fine. She began telling me how wonderful it was to read what Dad had been sending her about the book, and that she was so proud of my writing. She made me forget what I was crying about within 10 minutes. She was brilliant. I was very happy to talk to her. Dad was brilliant too of course. He comforted me by telling me all my other options, and that we could get a few papers rechecked, and hope that my points would go up 5 points. Auntie Jane also suggested I do a writing workshop in Dublin for a year, and reapply to college next year, with a different selection of choices on my form for the CAO, the Central Applications Office.

As I sat on the bench with Dad chatting about it all, Louise popped out from behind the *albergue* with Tim and a little bouquet of flowers she had picked.

"Hello, my beautiful girl," she said as she handed me the flowers and gave me a big hug. Dad had informed the others I was a little upset. The two of them had come out to me to see if I was okay. They were sweet, and kind and lovely. I was ready to go back into the *albergue* and face everyone else. I also needed to shower very badly. The others reacted just as kindly as Tim and Louise had, and they all cheered me up. It was wonderful, and I was happy to have been on the Camino when I received my results.

For the rest of the evening I sat outside with Andrew, at the same picnic table, looking out onto the mountains we had achieved, munching on a large bar of chocolate and a packet of crisps and drinking a cold Coke; just what I needed. Later, the celebration included several bottles of wine upstairs in the restaurant after dinner.

PETER: I was desperately sorry for Tash—just five points off the mark. But Miss Leddy, her wonderful history grinds teacher, was adamant: the English and history results didn't accord with Natasha's track record and what she, and I, knew of her performance in the exam. There was nothing to be lost by seeking a re-check, and maybe a lot to be gained. We had six days to go online and make the request.

Foncebadón to Ponferrada: 28 km in 5.5 hours

PETER: Foncebadón is a tiny hamlet on the Camino, high in the mountains of León. Looking back along the Camino to the east, one can see the great plain spreading out to Astorga and, beyond, to León itself. The meseta is at last behind us and we have climbed through woods, the path lined by heather in full flower. Most of the houses in Foncebadón are wrecks—stonework buildings whose roofs have long since fallen in, taking walls down with them. The Camino through the village is unpaved, an uneven path of rubble and dust. The glory days when privileges were granted for an *albergue* and the place had the attention of the hermit Gaucelmo, are long gone, though in recent years something of a renewal has been happening. Foncebadón now has no less than three *albergues*, each of them apparently prospering, and two separate restaurants, but there is no shop and the facilities in general are a bit grim. As we leave in the half light of dawn, pilgrims are pouring from the *albergues*.

We trek up the mountain to the highest point on the whole Camino, at 1,500 metres, higher than the Pyrenean crossing. And up here is the Cruz de Ferro, a cross atop a tall wooden pole around which has emerged an enormous pile of stones. Pilgrims leave them, one by one, as they pass this spot.

Like so much about the Camino, this tradition long predates the trek to Santiago to honour St James. Before the Romans left their mark on Spain, the Celts were in the habit here, as elsewhere, of marking the tops of mountains with piles of stones, or cairns. The Romans themselves adopted and adapted this custom, doing the same but in honour of Mercury, their god of travellers. Our friend the hermit Gaucelmo erected the first cross on top of the pile, thereby 'Christianising' an existing custom.

I doubt if many contemporary pilgrims know this as they pick up a small stone, or maybe bring one with them from their home, and lay it at the base of the wooden pole. Apart from stones, the pole itself is festooned with objects—they include shoes, a straw hat, numerous handwritten notes of both the silly and highly personal, emotional kind, bicycle tubes, scallop shells, scarves, socks and other items of clothing including, weirdly, underpants and knickers, flags, T-shirts, a water can (presumably punctured), a fox tail, beads, business and personal cards, and photographs of children and other, usually older, people, all presumably ill or passed away. It's an eclectic, not to say odd, collection of personal flotsam, and the nearest I can think to anything that matches it are the flag poles high in the Himalayas where contemporary travellers are also wont to leave some token behind them. The pile at Cruz de Ferro now includes three small rocks from Croagh Patrick, including a piece of clean white quartz that Natasha and I deposited at the base of the pole, left in the hope that Mercury will grant us safe passage to Santiago and beyond ...

NATASHA: We set off this morning at 6.00 am, in the complete darkness. The boys, Dad and I, were the first pilgrims on the road. The sky was completely clear, and every star was out to wish us well. After a short two kilometres, we met the Cruz de Ferro. I was worried my experience was going to be ruined by the darkness, but if anything it was enhanced.

Walking towards it, it looked like a pile of darkness, and the silhouette of the pole made it like a spear into the night sky. As we got closer the things people had left over years became real and I was able to make out things. Dad brought me to where he had left his two stones from Croagh Patrick, so that I could leave mine beside his. I took mine out of my bag for the first time, examined him, and placed him gently beside Dad's two stones. My stone represented Mum and Patch. I wanted them to be with us, and it was my little body of their presence that I was leaving at the Cruz de Ferro. We left with a brilliant photo of the place in the darkness.

Without a doubt, the walk into the first town, eight kilometres along the way, was the most beautiful walk we have done out of the whole 600 kilometres so far. I had forgotten about it, so it came as a pleasant surprise. We are already high from our walk yesterday, so the gradient wasn't difficult. We climbed gently up a rocky road and suddenly were thrust into a bowl of mountains reflecting every colour of the sun. It was breathtaking. Every hump and hill of the mountains across the valley was picked out by the rising sun behind us, and cast a purple shadow horizontally across the mountains. Our path was on the top of a mountain ridge, hugged by wild flowers projecting pinks and purples onto our boots. Looking forward, a sleeve of cloud slipped through the valley, covering the land below. The beauty of everything in sight was indescribable.

As I walked downwards, looking out onto everything, I realised I was learning something. I was learning something that couldn't be taught in school, or aided with a book, but only by firsthand experience. I was learning to appreciate the beauty of things around, in the landscape, and in the people around me. I was learning something I had seen in Dad for a while. He appreciated beauty in nature from an early age, he got it from Granny, and it was something I was noticing in me as I walked through the mountains, down into Molinaseca.

PETER: Before Molinaseca, we pass Manjarín, the first settlement after the Cruz de Ferro. It is an abandoned village of wrecked, rough-stone houses and farm buildings. For years only one has been occupied—by a man obsessed with the Knight Templar, a crusader outfit dissolved by the Vatican in 1312 after their career of excessive zeal against the Moors grew into obsessive secrecy, and because they introduced a form of banking, great wealth and political power thereby generating fear and envy of them in equal measure. But the man of Manjarín, and his sidekick Paco, keep the flame alive. In a tumbledown wreck to which they have added awnings and extensions so that it now looks like a shanty, they entertain pilgrims with a strange, almost tai-chi style dance in faux Knights Templar garb. Inside their lair the walls are covered with information about the Knights and the Virgin Mary. Dogs and cats roam freely. The walls are also covered with newspaper clippings about them. One suspects this attention is the reward they crave. You can stay here as Dirk, a well-spoken, slightly hippy-ish German boy with a guitar did the night before we passed by.

"Yeah," he said to me, "it was fun but a little strange. They had all sorts of rituals and rules you had to obey."

Paco stamps our pilgrim passports and I recall for him how Natasha and I spent time with him two years ago, sharing tea with him inside the lair. His face lit up and he scuttled inside, emerging with two 'coins', which had unspecified significance but were presented to us with a certain solemnity.

Further on are two delightful small villages, both at least Roman in origin, if not earlier. El Acebo and Riego de Ambros. In the first, we all gorge on the best *tortilla y jambon bocadillos* and coffee of our Camino so far. The third town is a major one, Molinaseca, a little jewel in a valley after the dramatic and extraordinarily beautiful early morning scenery of the mountains following the Cruz de Ferro. There is a wonderful, strong-looking, medieval arched bridge into the town from the mountain. Like El Acebo, Molinaseca is a classic Roman town astride the Camino: a single, straight, narrow and paved street, with lesser streets branching off it at right angles. The houses, mostly of cut stone, bespeak a prosperous little place, and this morning as we pass through it is bathed in sunlight.

NATASHA: We stayed here on our last Camino and it was a pity we weren't staying there again, as it was incredibly beautiful. The town is on a bend of a gently flowing river of clear water. The houses on the main street are cute little things with flowers tumbling from balconies, and there are tiny food stores and pubs full of character. I remembered, from last year, I had the best paella ever here, and as I passed the restaurant I ate it in, the picture menu made me hungry. Ponferrada was only eight kilometres more, and I remembered the way, so it wasn't too bad, until the sun decided to blaze heavily down on us, on the last stretch into Ponferrada.

As we all strolled into the town together, Gary gasped at the litter: "A McDonald's bag! There must be one near."

"Oh god, we have to find it for lunch time," I replied. Reece, Tasmanian Steve, Gary and I had the idea in our heads, and there was nothing that was going to satisfy us otherwise. We had to find it. Andrew stayed in the *albergue* with sore feet, but once we checked in we prepared for our McDonald's hunt. We thought it would be a stroll, but unfortunately it was a gruelling two-kilometre walk, completely exposed to the sun, which was incredible at this hour. "We must earn everything on this trip, lads," Tasmanian Steve would remind us as we groaned in the heat. Thankfully, we had a Spanish lady escort us to the doors of the shopping centre, where it was, right outside the city in the industrial area. We were hot and sweaty on arrival but never slowed down as we climbed to the food hall.

"Can I have one Big Mac, nine chicken nuggets, one large chips, one large Coke and an Oreo McFlurry please," I said, finished with one of my best smiles. A rather shocked Spanish man gave me my order and watched as I trotted happily away to devour my reward. It was much better than I ever imagined. I was content.

I spent the rest of the evening typing. My beastly lunch held me through dinner and I only joined the others at 8.00 pm, when they had enjoyed a homemade chicken curry, courtesy of Gary. Wine and nuts scattered the table and darkness fell quickly. German Dirk and his Austrian friend, Michael, filled the night air with beautiful music, and soon pilgrims gathered round the two tables and began to sing to all the songs.

Tasmanian Steve brought home the gold with his rendering of *Down Under* by the Australian group *Men at Work*. His deep, hard Australian voice blasted through the night, and he was rewarded with cheers from all around. It was brilliant. Then it was off to bed, to prepare for a 27-kilometre walk in the morning.

Ponferrada to Villafranca del Bierzo: 23 km in 5 hours

PETER: This is one of the loveliest parts of the Camino. The Bierzo is a rich, wine-producing area west of Ponferrada, sandwiched between, on the north, the Sierra de Ancares of the Cantabrian Mountains, and to the south, the Sierra del Caurel. To the east, there is Ponferrada and the mountains peaking in the Cruz de Ferro. To the west, beyond Villafranca, these two in effect come together where the Camino traverses the Cantabrians at O Cebreiro and enters Galicia. But before that, the delight of the Bierzo!

The valley floor is incredibly fertile; the soil is a rich alluvial created by regular river flooding. This also allows for a substantial network of irrigation channels. We began walking late—7.30 am—and it was half light already. Early coffee in a very trendy café opposite the big strong walls of the castle at Ponferrada set us on our way and soon the suburbs are behind us. We enter a wide, flat area of intensive market gardening. Individual plots contain a huge variety of produce: onions, tomatoes, peppers, beans of every imaginable variety, melons, cabbages, maize, and flowers. There are fruit trees aplenty—plums, apples and pears are common. The village of Fuentes Nuevas is where most of the people who work this land live. It is another of the single, straight-line street communities that dominate the rural Camino. The tiny Church of the Ascension is open. It is filled with flowers and their perfume; but the religious artwork is fairly poor. An alcove *retablo* sits beneath a domed ceiling which has a fresco showing the last supper. It is dated 1742, the year the church was built, the lady on the door manages to tell me.

The Camino rises again and proceeds through a large area of vineyards. The hedgerows are now looking plentiful as well—filled with rosehips not yet ripe enough for picking; sloes that are plump and luscious but, sadly, picking them to take home for Christmas sloe gin is impractical; but the blackberries are, at last, ready for picking and a pilgrim may feast for free. The vineyards roll up and down the landscape; there are both red and white grapes. The red look almost ready for harvesting but a sneaky nibble at a few reveals they are still tart and have a way to go. Three tiny villages emerge from amid the vineyards. They are neat and well kept; the unpaved Camino track becomes a paved road while it passes through each. Cacabelos is the first major town since leaving Ponferrada. The entrance is not promising: a street lined with traditional brick and plaster homes, all with first-floor bays supported by timber pillars that provide some shade but most in a very poor state of repair. A small church standing alone in the middle of a street appears to have been given over to housing an eclectic collection of religious artefacts of no particular significance: there are statues of Christ on a donkey, a Roman soldier, a Virgin Mary, various paintings of highly questionable quality and a small *retablo* showing St Roque in characteristic pose—lifting his cloak to display his wounded thigh, knee pointed forward. He looks like something from a *Little Britain* or *Black Adder* comedy sketch.

But then Cacabelos comes into its own. A little further along the Camino, a delightful old town emerges—a warren of little streets, small squares and all that comes with them, shops, bars and restaurants. The town has existed since the 10th century. An earthquake destroyed it but it was rebuilt in 1108 by a bishop who had it as his personal fiefdom, and in terms of church governance the town was part of the Compostela diocese until the 19th century. The heritage is strong. Over the river as one exits the town is the Church and Santuario de las Angustias. Since Navarra, I have got into the habit of wandering into many of the open churches the Camino passes and just sitting there in the quiet. It is invariably rewarding. First there is the solitude, the time spent gazing at what is on display and simply thinking ... about whatever one wants to think. It might be what is on show—in this case, a huge *retablo* covered in gold leaf and devoted to Christ and the Virgin Mary and showing, weirdly, the child Jesus playing cards with St Antonio of Padua (What were the stakes? And who won? I want to know!); it might be something on one's mind, one of the many and varied reasons why people do the Camino, taking the time necessary to process some difficult matters. Either way, time spent like this in a church always seems to me to be time well spent.

I wander the church, examining the sights, and the volunteer manning the door comes over to me. Am I a *peregrino*, a pilgrim, he asks? "Sí," I reply in my flawless Spanish, and he's off! A full guided tour of the church ensues but I really have very little idea what it was all about. But it was a typical Camino moment—someone taking time out, for no pay or obvious reward, to share enthusiasm and knowledge with a stranger. In due course he stamped my pilgrim passport and bade me "Buen Camino", telling me Villafranca was but another 5.5 kilometres along the way ... 5.5 kilometres of delightful Bierzo wine-producing countryside.

The day's walking ends with the news that the municipal *albergue* is closed. No matter, another just beside the Church of Santiago is operating; we queue and are admitted. It is a slightly hippy-ish sort of place—lots of timber (good) but mixed with faux spirituality stuff, such as wind chimes and so-called dream catchers; all very dodgy. Not long after we check in, word reached us of a bedbug infestation back along the Camino. As events transpire, this place is infested as well (or at least one dorm of it) and several pilgrims fall victim.

NATASHA: Every time we have a late start, I feel guilty. I hate it. This morning, leaving Ponferrada, we were late. But a stop in a café that gave us our midday break on our last Camino had to be revisited for breakfast. Finally, a place that served me a large cup of tea, just how I like it at home. And to top things off, they were playing the one and only Michael Bublé. After a quick breakfast of coffee and tea, we were off.

The Camino out of Ponferrada was very fresh in my mind. We don't veer down the industrial end, towards McDonald's; instead the Camino takes the old town way, skirting along the side of the city's huge castle, and we escape the city within 15 minutes. We approach a few odd things along the first 10 kilometres. A creepy 'C' shaped building of bungalow apartments surrounds a tiny church. The area looks like it was originally a military barracks. There isn't a soul in sight. Then we pass through more ghostly towns that whisper into vision very quickly and disappear just as fast. However, once you have broken through the suburbs and away from the city, you hit beautiful countryside. Flat stretches of the Camino travel along quiet roads with well-kept crop fields on either side. All the vegetation is growing successfully, apart from the odd patch of abandoned vineyard.

As we pass through one of the many housing streets, we notice a small dog up front, trotting along with a beat, as though he has some urgent business to take care of. Whistling and clapping does nothing to catch his attention. Eventually I catch up with him, and he is delighted to see such company. He is a fluffy, fox-type mongrel with characteristics of Buster, my little Jack Russell at home. We have a little moment together. After a couple of minutes tickling him and playing, Dad and I carry on along the Camino but the little dog wants to come too! Thankfully, a man walking towards us recognises the dog as we ask him if he is his.

"Ah, Toby!" he exclaims, and picks up my little friend, carrying him off down the road tucked under his arm.

We hadn't stopped for breakfast yet and my stomach was rumbling. Dad hadn't said he was hungry and there was no sign of an upcoming pit stop. As Dad stopped to look at a church, I carried on. As I walked along the narrow street out of the town, I was surrounded by a glorious fruity smell. I looked around me and there were dozens of wild apple, pear and plum trees, all seemingly ripe. I was delighted—free breakfast. I picked one of each, and enjoyed them all thoroughly. The only thing better than fresh fruit for breakfast, is fresh fruit for breakfast that you find yourself.

I lost Dad at that church but was content with my own company. The walk was pleasant until the Camino went off the rough road and alongside the main road. I found Tasmanian Steve, Andrew, Reece and Gary along here, and walked with them. The sun was getting incredibly hot, and we were dying to get under the shadow of the trees. Eventually a big fat yellow arrow was painted onto the road, pointing diagonally across, towards a cute farm road. Slowly but surely, Andrew and I began to slip behind the others, who were marching up the hill. Panting and moaning and turning to every bit of shade we could find, we thought we were going to pass out with thirst. And then we were saved. "Thank god for you, little man in the blue hat," I whispered. "What?" said Andrew looking up.

And there, perched on the top of the hill, was a little man, who had a table set up with boxes of fruit, and a cooler full of cold drinks. I bought a bag of small, green, plum-like fruits, grown locally, and we got a couple of Cokes too. The last leg of the journey flew by with our little treats. Before we knew it, we were walking down along a grassy path, into the town of Villafranca del Bierzo. The sun was getting unbearable, and I couldn't have been happier to arrive there. Tim and Louise, being crazy Australians, decided to walk on a further seven kilometres and got caught in the heat with no cover.

Strangely, the municipal *albergue*, which was the first building on the right, was closed. We later learned that it had to be closed down due to bedbugs. This seemed to be a growing concern along the Camino, and we were hearing more and more of it. One Irish woman we met, Madeline from Donegal, had caught them just after Burgos and was only getting rid of them here in Ponferrada. It's a difficult process of fumigating everything you own by washing them. Also, people don't want to be near you or your belongings in other *albergue*s if they think you have bedbugs.

I remembered briefly walking through Villafranca del Bierzo last time and I was glad I now had the opportunity to explore the city further.

We placed our bags outside the next *albergue*, a private one, and were first in the queue. It seemed lovely from the outside. It was right beside the stone church that is immediately on your left as you arrive into the town. It looked like a trendy bar from the outside. There were large wooden gates on the side, which were open, and showed the cute hippy-styled garden. It was made up of loads of random little things, tables and chairs to relax in, and an open washing area. Everything was very relaxed here, and lots of little paintings and quotes coloured the walls. The bedrooms were off the garden area, in little chalet-type wooden huts, attached to the dining and reception areas, and they were delightful. The bedroom was one big open space, with a tiny stairs that led up to another small, raised space, where mattresses lay on the floor. The roof was old and had little star-shaped windows cut out.

After showering and settling in, Dad wrote, and I went for a cold Coke with Andrew. Unfortunately, the temperature had reached 38 degrees, and walking was unbearable. On top of that, just as we were walking down the cobbled street, Andrew's knee went and he groaned in pain. But he insisted on carrying on. We walked down to the centre of the town, where there was a large plaza, bordered with cafés and restaurants. It was very inviting. We sat and had a cold Coke and watched the world go by. After a trip to the shop for some snacks, we went exploring for a spot to sit and nibble on some nut mix and sweets. Down in a dried-out river valley, just outside the plaza and near the *albergue*, we found a playground in the shade. Perfect. I don't know whether it was because we were tired, or just giddy, but the bench we were sitting on gave me laughter I thought would never end. When we laughed the bench squeaked, ever so slightly, like a small monkey. But the more we laughed, the more the bench squeaked, and the louder it squeaked. At the bench's peak squeakiness, it sounded like a large squad of monkeys, and was impossible to stop as our laughter was causing it. We spent the rest of the time we had before dinner here, mostly laughing.

Sometime in between laughing with Andrew at the squeaky bench, and having dinner, I got a text from home that reminded me of the wonderful friends I have waiting for me when I get back. It was from

Aoife Leggett, one of my best friends. She wanted to say hello, and had heard from Mum that I was upset that I hadn't got my English and philosophy in Trinity College, Dublin, or University College Dublin, and was reassuring me that I was going to be fine. It made me happy.

On our return to the *albergue*, Gary, Reece and Tasmanian Steve were hungry. We decided a pilgrim's menu meal down town would be nice. Dad and I joined them and we ate where Andrew and I had had our Cokes. Proving that the closer you get to Santiago, the better the meals get, we had brilliant food at the price of €9 each. I had pasta salad to begin, followed by pork knuckle, finished with a cinnamon rice pudding. The following morning was sure to bring a difficult day, the most difficult of the Camino promised, so it was off to bed after dinner.

Villafranca del Bierzo to O Cebreiro: 29 km in 6 hours

PETER: Lombardy Lady re-emerged last night and, as we readied to leave the *albergue* in the half light of dawn, she's at it again. The *albergue* does not have kitchen facilities for pilgrims. There is a small kitchen but it is only for the people who run the *albergue*. Lombardy Lady is having none of it: she wants in there and, in characteristic and charmless fashion, she is demanding access, apparently to fill her water bottle. The helper on duty explains that there is a tap for pilgrims just over there, a place to which he points that is perhaps five metres away. But no, that's not good enough. She wants into the kitchen area and starts screaming at the man, ranting her demands until she flounces out in a temper, slamming the door behind her.

"There's really something wrong with Angela. It's no wonder she's alone," says Steve as we walk through the town. "I think she has a problem with authority and she was probably also hurt by someone, a man I'd guess by her behaviour, sometime in the past." That, perhaps, and maybe she's also just a spoilt brat who can't control her temper.

There is a distinct change to the landscape once you leave Villafranca. Even though you are still within the province of León, the architecture changes, as does the land use and the way people seem to lead their lives. After a while, it strikes you that it feels like Galicia, which does not officially come into existence until just before the Camino scales the heights of O Cebreiro. The Camino here follows the valley of the Valcarce River. We are just above the river, maybe three metres or so, following what is clearly the old road, a perfectly good road but one now made redundant by the highway above us. It is several hundred metres up the side of the valley, through which it sheers, rather gracefully, on giant stilts. It looks at times rather like a giant anaconda, snaking its way through the valley. As we plod along, one step at a time, rucksacks on our backs, looking at the stars and waiting for the dawn, listening to the river and the first birdsong, I am struck once again by the parallel but utterly separate worlds of the Camino and the world we have left behind temporarily. Trucks and vans and cars and motorbikes whizz along the new highway on stilts, occasionally hooting at us encouragingly, part of another world, another time zone. We move at our own pace, a pace that somehow seems more in tune with everything around us and one that allows us to notice things like plant life, how people are leading their lives, what the buildings are made of.

As we progress up the valley and the mountain peak becomes more distinct in the half light, owls hoot in the distance. The forest becomes more dense: the trees are oak, beech and poplar, Chinese chestnut and walnut and hazel. The forest is worked; everywhere there is evidence of logging—piles of rough-cut timber are by the side of the road, and there are occasional sawmills. The village houses are made of rough stone and seem quite dark, a little like Welsh villages. There are some sheep but cows become more plentiful as the amount of dairying increases.

One of my favourite villages along this way is named Vega de Valcarce. It is one of the last before the valley runs out and walkers hit the incredibly steep climb to O Cebreiro. What I like here is a small bar on the main street named the Bar Refugio del Cazador. It is the drinking haunt of the local hunting club. The walls are lined with mounted boars' heads; one of the beasts on show weighed a hefty 104 kilos. There are several photographs of hunting parties returned triumphant to the bar, the kills of the outing displayed proudly on the pavement outside. In one photo, 17 men with shotguns are lined up behind a display of seven dead boars. The woman behind the bar explains that the hunting takes place from September onwards in the woods on either side of the valley and that all the huntsmen are local. I'd really love to join them one day …

Suddenly the valley ends and the mountain presents itself. Cyclists stay on the road which veers off to the right and up; walkers go down a dusty mud path into the forest. Soon, it enters a very steep climb which lasts for about six kilometres. It is grinding, draining, endurance-testing stuff—sweat blisters out of the top of my head and trickles down the back of my ears and temples and down my neck onto my chest and back. I stop every 20 metres or so to catch my breath but there is no alternative to going forward. Respite comes at the tiny hamlet of La Faba and its tiny church of San Andrés, the last parish church of Astorga. After La Faba, more steep climbing, though the forest gradually dies out as the mountain breaches the tree line and timber gives way to windswept grass and gorse.

NATASHA: It was an early enough start this morning, for a challenging day to O Cebreiro. We left in the dark, all six of us. The Camino went down the town and exited over a river and almost straight onto a path that ran along a wide road, separated from it by a concrete barrier. I remembered this walk very well from last time and nothing had changed. Walking under alien-like motorways on stilts, with enormous green tree forests around us. We even had our first coffee break in a bar we stopped in on our last trip, that had pennies stuck to the wall from other visitors. Early on Dad mentioned he had a bad ankle. We kept going, but we were both aware of it, and I didn't mind stopping at any time to take a break. I was feeling very tired myself, as the bedroom last night in the *albergue* in Villafranca had been roasting.

Also on our previous Camino, we stopped in this bar that was smothered in stuffed boar and pigs that were shot by the local hunting gang. Dad wanted to revisit it, and so we did. After a fright of thinking we had lost our camera memory card, the boys passed us. Andrew's knee was really getting to him; he told the boys he would slow down and walk with Dad and me. I was up for taking it easy, as Dad had my pilgrim passport, so I could let him carry on and book me in, while I walked slowly with Andrew. He too had given his credentials to Gary, Reece and Tasmanian Steve, so he would get a bed. Andrew was in a lot of pain, and we walked the slowest I've ever walked, but I didn't mind. After the last of the small villages, the gradient of the road became really steep, but uphill was easier on Andrew's knee. Things only got steeper, and soon the Camino disappeared under the forest and turned into a monster of a climb. Until we reached the very top, we hardly spoke because we were out of breath.

At the top, we saw Dad and had a Coke with him. He carried on while we recovered for a bit more. We only had three kilometres to go, and I wasn't worried. But I had it in my head that it was all straight and pleasant. Unfortunately I was very wrong as it was uphill on an exposed road. This is where we found the most difficult. Sweat was dripping down my head onto my face and stinging my eyes. I could feel my feet swelling and new blisters filling with liquid. I tried to ignore the pain and kept pushing on. I wanted to at least be able to see O Cebreiro in the distance, so I could have some sort of motivation. But there was nothing, and it was impossible to even guess where it was, as we could see far around us, but only green fields. If I hadn't been exhausted, I would have chatted about the beautiful scenery. Thinking back on it now, it was gorgeous, and very like Ireland. Rich green fields layered on the valley. Winding roads disappearing behind humps and hills in the distance and slug-shaped rows of gorse and heather.

The only other people in front of us were two Italian men. Off the road to the right, there was a very Camino-looking dirt path climbing steeply over the hill and beyond our right. It seemed like it could be the Camino, as it would make sense if O Cebreiro was just over the hill. The two Italian men asked a car driving past if that was the Camino, and they said yes. Trusting them, all four of us turned up this incredibly steep, rocky path. My face felt like it was going to explode I was so hot and red. After about one kilometre, but feeling like it was five, my head was lifted by something blocking my path—a wire fence. We had taken a wrong turning. I turned around to see Andrew trooping up behind me, and with great reluctance I had to tell him to turn around.

"Stop walking! Turn around!" I shouted beyond Andrew to the two Italian men.

All four of us were completely drained and this was the last thing we needed. Without saying a lot, we all turned around, back down the steep, rocky road. This was what did the real damage to Andrew's knee. He was in serious pain at this stage and I didn't know what to do, or how to help. I thought my best option was to walk ahead as fast as I could, dump my bag in the *albergue* and come back to him. It was 2.00 pm and the sun was cooking the earth in 32 degrees of heat. Once we got back down onto the road, I was determined to get there as fast as I could. The Camino followed the road and twisted along the valley to the opposite side. I could see tiny pilgrims' heads bouncing along behind the heather bushes on the other side. It was horrible to think I had to get there. I started to run. I really needed to see this town and tell Andrew it wasn't far. Finally, a small stone wall hidden behind trees was visible; I knew that had to be the beginning of the village. I ran straight through the main street, following the yellow arrows. I reached the entrance to the *albergue*, and to my surprise it was only just opening, and Dad was in the queue. He saw me and waved me over. I just dropped my bag and turned back. I half expected to see Andrew lying dead in a ditch, but instead I met him 50 metres away from the *albergue*. We had made it. I have never been as relieved to reach our destination as this.

The evening was spent quietly. We had dinner in a restaurant near the *albergue*; Tim, Louise, Tasmanian Steve, Gary, Reece, Andrew, Dad and I, and two Germans, Thomas and Sascha, we met in Astorga.

PETER: O Cebreiro is a cluster of stone buildings 1,300 metres above sea level, about 200 metres lower than the highest point on the Camino, the Cruz de Ferro. O Cebreiro has become a Mecca for tourists, with its huddle of trinket shops and bars and fine views into Galicia. The Romans settled here and used it as a vantage point to defend access to Galicia; around a thousand years later, the pass was defended to prevent Norman pirates from entering Castile from Galicia. But it was not until the 9th century and the growth of the pilgrimage to Santiago that O Cebreiro developed the status it has had ever since. The Benedictines built a hospice which ran in good order from 1072 until 1486. Christian legend has it that the Holy Grail, the cup from which Christ drank wine at the Last Supper, was hidden in O Cebreiro and used at communion. In the 14th century a sceptical priest attacked a priest saying Mass for claiming the cup to be the Grail, at which point the bread and wine turned literally into flesh and blood, a miracle 'confirmed' by Pope Innocent III in 1487. These days, bread and wine and much else is polished off by the procession of pilgrims and tourists passing through.

The church at the highest point in the village is dedicated to Santa Maria la Real, a modern structure dating from the 1960s, but built on pre-Romanesque foundations. It is very plain inside, which probably appeals to the Protestant in me, but along one wall, under a small statue of a crowned Mary, there are rows of candles. I light one for friends, acquaintances and family members who have died recently and take a few moments to enjoy the quiet before exiting into the tourist hubbub once again.

As we enter the *albergue*, our first in Galicia, we note approvingly a sign on the door. Place preference will be given, in this order, to walking pilgrims with injuries; then able-bodied walking pilgrims; next pilgrims on horseback, followed by those on bicycle; finally pilgrims with back-up vehicles carrying their luggage.

Proper order, we all agree!

O Cebreiro to Samos: 28 km in 7 hours

PETER: Tip-toeing quietly out of the dorm, then the *albergue* itself, we are soon strolling under the stars at 5.10 am. This is the sort of thing the Camino is about—solitude, quietude and a bit of adventure. It's amazing just how much light you can get from the glow of the screen of a mobile phone. Activate the phone every few metres and enough light is cast on the trail to avoid any potholes or rocks as it winds its way through the woods that cover the mountainside falling away from O Cebreiro. And then, as the Camino leaves the woods, and the silhouette of the mountains further into Galicia appears on the far horizon, there's a finger post with two directions indicated, neither of which illuminate for us which is the correct way to go. But the Milky Way is to our right and points in one direction, according to the flow of its stars. Another star, a very bright one, is to the left of the Milky Way as we have walked it before, heading west. So I'm guessing, but following the direction of the Milky Way in relation to that bright star has to be due west—the way to Santiago. The pagans used the stars in this way to guide themselves to Finisterre, and what was good enough for them will have to do us too.

And so it proves; after about another two kilometres we come across Camino signs. We chose the correct way. When you are doing up to 30 kilometres a day, there's little worse than making a two-kilometre wrong turn that becomes four by the time you have retraced your steps. But I also get a considerable kick from knowing that something people were doing two, maybe three, thousand years ago—using the stars as their guide—still works for a fellow from the 21st century groping his way through a forest with the help of the glow from a mobile phone!

The difference between the Galicia in which we now are, and the Spain through which we have just passed, is apparent almost immediately there is sufficient dawn light to survey our surroundings. And Natasha notices it too, once daylight starts to reveal the countryside. "It's so much like Ireland," she says. And it is: fields are divided by slightly unkempt hedgerows of shrubs, small trees and brambles. There are rough stone walls too (soon we will see field walls made of vertical stone slabs, very much Galician style) and the Camino at times meanders into hamlets—clusters of farm homes, farm buildings and farmyards in which it is impossible to tell public space from private property. But no one seems to mind; the farmers and their families go about their business as pilgrims wander through their farmyards and everybody exchanges greetings. "Buenos días!" say the pilgrims; "Buenos días—Buen camino!" come the replies.

Dairying is a very significant part of farming in these parts, unlike most of the Bierzo on the other side of the mountain, and cow pats spatter the side roads. Alsatian dogs are used to herd cattle and many of them hang around the farms, lazing in the early morning sun, or approach passing pilgrims, tails wagging, hoping for an affectionate pat or twirl of an ear. Occasionally, a farmer's wife has turned one of the otherwise disused outbuildings into a small café that, for a few pence, sells beer and coffee and tea and soft drinks and *bocadillos*, the delicious Spanish bread roll sandwiches of ham and cheese and tomato, and also provides the invariably welcome early morning loo stop. In one, there's Galician folk music playing. A CD cover reveals it is a group named *Brañas Folk*; other CDs are of Carlos Núñez, the Andy Irvine-Paddy Moloney-Christy Moore of Galicia. Yes, this is different. Castile Spain is behind us.

As we walk down the mountainside to the hamlet of Fonfría, the foliage also reminds of Ireland: there's bracken and broom and gorse and hellebores; ash and rowan, beech and birch, Chinese chestnut and walnut trees and hazelnut shrubs. A column of electricity pylons provides launching and landing spots for two birds of prey, probably kestrels or harriers, who seem to be at play as much as hunting. We find a hesitating hedgehog on the road and help him away out of danger; later I hear and then see my first Blue Jay of the Camino, squawking and arguing with nobody in particular but making a lot of early morning noise. The sun is now well over the horizon to our rear but, because we are in the lea of the mountain, the slightest elevation over our right shoulder, a hedgerow or a tree on a bank, provides shade. How different it all is from the last time Natasha and I walked here two years ago in 2008. Then, we battled through an early April snow and sleet storm to find refuge at last in an *albergue* with our new friend, Dan McCarthy. We had met Dan sometime after León but lost touch until O Cebreiro after which we walked together to Fonfría. A communal meal with the other half dozen pilgrims in the *albergue* led to a night drinking wine into the small hours, with Dan, Natasha and I solving all the problems of the world and a few others besides.

Dan comes from Rhode Island in the United States and was then 74 years old. In his younger days he had been a Roman Catholic priest, working in the Amazon and finding inspiration in liberation theology. But he later decided he had other needs as a person and left the priesthood. He married and had a daughter, a huge joy in his life. He also joined the Anglican communion and became a counsellor. Dan is a man of strong liberal values, both socially and politically, and it was a delight for me to see a then 16-year-old Natasha connect with him—she listened intently as he spoke and engaged her, and she made her own contributions to our conversation. Next day, as we trudged in silence through the rain and mist towards Triacastela, Natasha stopped dead in her tracks all of a sudden and said this, "Dad?"

"Yes," I replied.

"When I'm 74 I want to be just like Dan."

It was when telling that story some months later to friends after dinner and being overcome with emotion that I realised there was something really special about the Camino. It had got under my skin, inside my head, however you want to put it, in a way that I did not understand but was sure that I liked. Since then, Dan has visited our home in Ireland after a subsequent Camino. He left his hat behind and for months I kept it on my office desk, always meaning to post it to him, always forgetting. And then this year, when Dan set off on his annual Camino, this time the Via de la Plata from Seville to Santiago, I cursed myself for not having sent it back to him in time. "Don't worry about it," Dan emailed me. "Keep it."

Shortly before we left on our Camino, he sent me an email from the Via de la Plata in which he gave just one of the reasons why the Camino was important to him. "This walking life really does make prayer come more easily. I just spend the day thinking about all of you I love, and miss and lift you up in prayer. As one of the poems I sent at the beginning said, the Camino is about learning about all the things you can do without. It's also about learning about how one treasures the people one does without while walking."

And so today, and every day on the Camino, I wear Dan McCarthy's hat. Dan is a wonderful Camino man and I admire his simple, uncomplicated, quiet faith.

Suddenly around a corner and far below us is Triacastela, a finger of mountain mist atop her like a wig. So named because of the three early-10th-century castles destroyed by Normans around 968, Triacastela today does not really have a lot going for her. Prince Felipe II of Spain spent one of his last nights there as a single man in May 1554 while on his way to England to marry Mary Tudor. Just off the Camino, as one enters the town, there is the Church of Santiago, part of which is probably Romanesque but most of which is late 18th century. The bell-tower has a large statue of St James as a pilgrim, and inside, the altar *retablo* is also dominated by James, pilgrim staff in one hand, bible in the other, scallop shell on his pilgrim hat.

The Camino out of Triacastela initially is the hard shoulder of a modern road—a dull road although it passes through a fine gorge with raw dramatic escarpments of schist and shale. But it is still a modern highway. It is not until the Camino falls down further into the valley, leaving the modern road to its own devices and tracks the course of a river, that we are once again in delightful countryside. Lush pasture dominates fields carved out of the river flood plain; then villages hug a hillside that is so wooded with oak and beech and Chinese chestnut and other species that it looks almost Amazonian. The river is beautiful and crystal clear. Moments spent on bridges gazing at the flow of water refresh in a way that staring at no other thing can. My left foot now aches. Twenty kilometres plus seems to be its limit. Since the blister on the right foot healed and the bandage padding on the inside of the boot prevented the lace eye hook doing further damage, the left foot has taken up the cause. Just where the shin part of the front of my left joins the ankle, tendons have been in revolt for two days. A small dull ache turns into searing pain at around 25 kilometres.

"That's it," says left foot. "I've had a-bloody-nuff."

"Not long to go, not long to go," I reassure it and me through gritted teeth and implement various stratagems.

First, find a slight ridge on the road; it might be where a bit of grass verge meets the gravel or tarmac and is raised above it slightly, or it might be where a wheel impression has created a little unevenness. Then walk on the edge of the ridge to the effect of either bending my foot a little this way or that. But either way, it redirects the pain slightly and allows for another few hundred metres of pain-reduced walking. Then, simply repeated as necessary. Fools left foot every time. The second stratagem is to find a hill and walk up it. Remarkably, this helps a lot because of the angle of the calf part of my leg to the foot, but seeing as since O Cebreiro the entire Camino is on a gradual downward trajectory, I'm in trouble.

The third stratagem, my favourite, is to stop and have a beer or a cognac. And as Samos with its vast, stolid looking monastery looms around a corner and out of the trees, it is this one I think I will implement pronto.

SAMOS

PETER: Samos is dominated by the monastery of saints Julian and Basilissa, a huge complex of buildings that almost overwhelms the small village that sits on a bend in the Ouribio River valley. The monastery, which dates from the 6th century, is a series of rough-stone square blocks and inner courtyards and cloisters, and rises in height to between three and six storeys. It is big and lumpy and parts of it could pass for an 18th- or 19th-century prison block. In the 12th century, when Samos became part of the religious empire spawned by the French abbey at Cluny, it controlled no less than 200 towns, 105 churches and some 300 other monasteries, and was much favoured by royalty. Two great fires, one in 1536, the other in 1951, destroyed much of the building, the latter engulfing the library. On one side of the main building there is an *albergue* beside, oddly, a lone petrol pump. I have long wanted to spend a night here and learn more about the monastery and now finally have the opportunity. Getting booked in takes an eternity as the *hospitaleros* take their task very seriously, explaining in great detail to each pilgrim queuing at the desk just when the Masses and vespers and tours of the monastery take place.

The tour takes me on a journey around a corridor above the cloister of Friar Benito Feijoo, an encyclopaedist and polymath who was a hugely influential 18th-century figure within the monastery and was largely responsible for building the cloister, said to be the largest in all Spain. The square around which it proceeds contains an imposing statue of the man together with lawns and flowerbeds laid out in a simple, geometric pattern. The corridor walls are covered in murals, painted between the mid-1950s and 1960s, narrating aspects of Benedictine life and that of the saint himself. The abbey church is a wonderful Baroque edifice with main aisle and two side aisles. The barrel-vaulted nave and transepts meet in a crossing, capped by a huge dome. Each of the four spandrels (the triangles created between the outer curve of an arch and the rectangular pillars that support it) houses images of four great Benedictine doctor saints—Rupert, Bernard, Ildephonsus and a decidedly sinister-looking Anselm wearing what appear like goggles or, as one guidebook notes, a bit like Elton John with big, outsized 1970s glasses. The main altar piece depicts the monastery's patron saint, Julian, standing on a cloud and dressed as a nobleman. He is flanked by his wife, St Basilissa (holding a lily to signify her virginity, lest one has any notions to the contrary, it is hastily pointed out), and St Christine holding a martyr's palm.

Vespers in the church is at 7.30 pm and I go with Thomas Reiss, a new companion on the Camino who hails from Germany. Thomas is a strikingly handsome man of 58, which pleases me as I am now no longer the eldest member of our walking group. He has Harrison Ford good looks and the sort of appearance that if someone said he ran a safari park in east Africa, or was chief engineer on a drilling rig in the Gulf of Mexico, you would think to yourself, 'Yes, he looks the part'. Thomas also speaks excellent English, which helps friendship develop in a relatively short time. He laughs a full, hearty laugh when he likes a joke and quickly endears himself to us all. He is a music teacher in a secondary school and is also the master of several choirs. Unfortunately, he is not greatly impressed by the music of the vespers, and so afterwards we repair to a couple of seats across the road from the *albergue* for wine and chat.

Thomas has been walking the Camino in stages for an extraordinary eight years, during which time he has carried the same walking staff, one that he made for himself in Germany. He began in 2003 by walking from his home in Mauer, near Heidelberg, to Mont St Odile in France. In 2004 he resumed his walk and continued on to Grand Ballon; 2005 saw him reach Vittel and in 2006 he arrived in Dijon. The following year he reached Le Puy, one of the great starting points of the Camino. In 2008 he got as far as Aire sur l'Adour, just north of the Pyrénées, and in 2009 he reached Hornillos, 20 kilometres west of Burgos. This year, 2010, his target is Santiago itself and then on to Finisterre.

I asked him why he was doing it.

"I got seriously ill in 2000; some sort of virus that attacked my nervous system. I was in hospital for weeks and then in rehabilitation. I had to relearn so much—how to play the piano, how to walk. First I walked one kilometre. The next day I walked one kilometre out and then back again; the next day two kilometres and so on. I discovered that walking was good for me and that I liked it. Then a friend said, 'Have you heard of the Camino?' and so for me it started."

Walking the Camino is also a way of getting one over on his doctor. Thomas has had three major operations on his left knee, the result of a childhood mishap that went un-noticed. Something went wrong with his kneecap, causing bone splintering under it. The first operation diagnosed the problem and removed the debris. Two subsequent operations were designed to repair the damage and create as functioning a knee as possible. Thomas wears two bandage strips on either side of the kneecap that are applied in such a way as to promote muscular support of the knee. "My doctor said to me, 'Thomas, with this knee, you will never walk the Camino,' but here I am!"

Thomas is not overly religious but he is spiritual. He was in Guatemala some years ago and became interested in ancient religious observances there. As a result, he carries on the Camino a sort-of belt with Guatemalan god dolls stitched onto it; he plans to bring it to the end of the world with him. He expects to find Finisterre very moving and was earlier moved by Cluny. But for him, Conques in France was his most extraordinary Camino experience.

"[The Abbey at] Conques for me was like coming home. Immediately I went inside the church, the tears came. It was like coming home," said Thomas.

"How do you mean, coming home?" I asked.

"I had been there before," he said, meaning in another life.

"As what?"

"A priest."

On another occasion, while walking early in his journey, Thomas got lost and anxious in a forest. His late mother came to him. "She said to me, 'Don't worry, it will be okay,' and it was okay."

Thomas has been walking for a while with Sascha Thieme, a 42-year-old father of two who comes from Berlin whom he met on this leg of the Camino. Sascha works in the advertising and marketing division of Mercedes Benz and is responsible for promoting trucks in Germany. I ask him why he's doing the Camino.

"I have work since I am 18. I was very fast with my exam. I was ambitious; I got to the top and go to the next top and I work for 25 years. I have a family and an apartment. So who am I now? Somewhere on the way, I lost myself. And so I told everyone before I go on the Camino, that I go on holidays with someone I don't know. And so the question is, 'Is he someone stupid or boring?' I am good at assimilating in a new group. So the question is what do I compromise at work or in the family or the sports and what is really me and I don't compromise?"

The catalyst for what seems to me to be some sort of crisis in Sascha's life turns out to be events at work.

"Eighteen months ago I failed an assessment test for promotion to department leader. Before this I was acting head while a colleague was promoted into my old job," he said.

At Mercedes Benz, it seems, internal promotions at certain levels are decided by external review panels of applicants. And so Sascha went before a group of external assessors who, over 36 hours and based on half a dozen different tasks, probed and tested his aptitude and suitability for the position he was seeking, indeed was already doing, albeit on a temporary basis. But the assumption—Sascha's and his colleagues'—was that he was already a shoo-in. When he failed, it was like a bolt from the blue—for him and the colleague filling his old position.

"When I failed, she was fired and had to leave the company. This angered me very much."

Sascha is looking for a way out of all this and thinks he will have it by the time he reaches Finisterre.

"On the way down from El Acebo, I find one of my ways. Trust things as they happen and be an optimist; I must not be a pessimist and have fear; when I can be an optimist I can have internal calmness. In Germany we say the Camino has two ways—the first is to search for God and find yourself; the second is to search for yourself and find God."

Is he finding God?

"Yes," he says. "The beginning of trust is the beginning of finding God."

Sascha's wife Julia gave him a scallop shell before he set out. On it she wrote: "Every step you do, I am with you."

Thomas thinks Sascha will do fine when he relaxes a bit more. I'm with Thomas …

Samos to Ferreiros: 25 km in c.5 hours

PETER: Today is a day from hell that ends in heaven. It is a Camino day that defies expectations and also defines what special Camino days are. Before this day, I have read so many stories, so many memoirs replete with improbable Camino coincidences and happenings, that they have blurred into an overall Camino impression—an impression of a linear, constantly moving place where weird and wonderful things happen all the time. Here's one more …

We rise as usual between 5.30 and 6.00 am. All is dark and silent and slow moving as the early risers shuffle about the place—washing and packing quietly so as not to wake others in the Samos monastery *albergue*. I take all my belongings into the bathroom area, which is sealed from the dormitory and therefore can have lights on without disturbing anyone still asleep. I wash and pack as usual, check I have everything, and then Natasha and I step out into the pre-dawn darkness and start walking. No stars this morning, unfortunately. The road out of Samos to Sarria is completely unremarkable but soon the Camino veers right, across the road and up into woodlands. Once again we are in a lovely Galician forest of oak and beech and pine and Chinese chestnut and a trail of packed brown mud and forest debris that is gentle on the feet. Gradually, a walking party of the usual suspects forms. There's Gary and Andrew and Reece, together with their pal Steve from Tasmania, who has now booked a flight to Dublin with the lads and will be going to Croke Park for the All-Ireland semi-final between Down and Kildare. He's mad keen on Aussie rules football is Steve and so a great day in Croker is almost guaranteed. With us too are Sascha and Thomas. As the dawn brightens gradually into day, Thomas stops at a bend to admire a view across the valley and take a picture.

My camera! My left hand dives in a flash to the spot on my belt where it should be. Empty space. Oh God. Of holy fuck. No. Please don't tell me … I drop my rucksack and empty it on the spot. No camera. Jesus. Six hundred pictures—gone. Within seconds I am in a panic; a cold white terror grips me and I feel sick in my stomach. I repack and start walking faster and faster to get to the next village or a main road; the fastest way back to Samos is the only thing on my mind. I left it somewhere, right? Yes, by the bench opposite the *albergue* where we were all drinking wine last night. I took it off my belt because sitting down with it on it is awkward and uncomfortable. Sure it was there; sure you took it off there? Yes, sure. No, I'm not sure. Oh fuck, fuck, fuck, fuck—600 pictures! How do we illustrate the book now? We can overcome that one; Gary has loads of pix, Steve as well, not to mention Tim and Louise. I'm sure they'll all copy me a few …

The next village is a tiny place named Aguiada but there's a café bar. A middle-aged woman behind the counter agrees to call me a taxi to take me back to Samos and it comes in about five minutes. Louise gives me a big 'good luck' hug. "Many people on the Camino know you and Natasha," she says. "If a pilgrim has found it, you might get it back."

"This will be a big test of the Camino," I say.

"Certainly will," she says as I get into the taxi.

The 10 kilometres back to Samos is the longest 10 kilometres I've ever travelled. All the time in the car I'm trying to rewind last night, replay where I was and when; what I did next; where was I sitting? What was the last photo I took? If I could remember that, I'd be close to maybe where I left it. What if it was stolen? Then I'm sunk. But that wouldn't have happened in the *albergue*, would it? If I lost it and someone found it, they'll look at the pix and see that the camera is owned by a pilgrim, but how in God's name would they get it to me, even if they wanted?

The taxi arrives outside the monastery *albergue* at 9.00 am. I run across the road to the bench. Nothing there and the place hasn't been cleaned from the night before—the café's red plastic table is still covered with cups, glasses and empty bottles. Thinks: if it was here, someone has found it and maybe handed it in to the café or across the road to the *albergue*. The *albergue* doors are closed and the place is empty. Open 12.30 says a notice. Inside the café, a young woman behind the counter looks around under the shelf—nothing there. Over at the *albergue* there's a window open and I can just about see my bed from last night. The place looks swept and cleaned. I go back across the road and check the bench area again. Still nothing; all the time I have this eerie feeling that I will see it suddenly—look! there it is, waiting for me and nobody else noticed. But of course that doesn't happen. One of the monastery monks, a tiny man in his early 70s, I guess, ambles along the footpath by the petrol pump and I grab him. I communicate by sign language that I was in the *albergue* last night and left my camera inside. He reaches under his cassock and produces a great bunch of keys and goes towards the *albergue* door. Brilliant! I'm getting inside ... The tiny reception office by the door is open; I look about it frantically, certain that any second now my eyes will light upon the camera case. But it's not there. I rush to my bed; nothing there either. The monk indicates he understands my loss and that he's sorry. Then he goes off, leaving the *albergue* door open and goes into the monastery proper. A few minutes later the very nice *hospitalero* from last night appears. I apologise for disturbing his breakfast rest and he takes me back inside the *albergue* again, to a cardboard box—everything that was found when the place emptied a couple of hours ago is there. A mobile phone charger, some odd socks and a few T-shirts. But no camera. He sympathises with me and takes my details just in case it turns up. I go over to the Guardia Civil and ask them. No, says the very helpful officer on duty, who happens to have excellent English, no one has handed in a camera. He too takes my details.

So that's it, it's gone; 600 pictures; the complete visual record of my and Natasha's Camino. Then it really hits me: it's not the book, it's my personal record, our record; it's what I wanted to show Moira; there was the shot of Natasha standing shoulder high among the sunflowers, her face beaming out. It is the second worst thing I could lose—Dad's little silver box would be worse. The computer would not: I could get the words again, they're in my head. But the images; they are irrecoverable. The devastation is total; I am beside myself with the loss and angry with myself also. You said you should post home the memory card and get a new one; why didn't you? You thought about copying the card onto the computer in case anything happened; so why didn't you? This is your fault, 100%. Yes it is …

I try hitching a lift back to Aguiada, without success. Eventually I see another taxi and he stops. Back at the café, Natasha has secured a safe place for my bag and gone on, carrying the computer herself. I thank the woman behind the bar and write a note: "Canon camera lost," write down my mobile phone number and the word "reward" and tape it to the café door. Well, you never know, stranger things have happened. Information moves up and down the Camino, and if the word is spread I just might get lucky. Walking on to Sarria, I can't help but dwell on the enormity of my loss: all my photos, every single one, from Croagh Patrick to the Pyrénées, down into Navarra, Pamplona and Estella, the bull running, the Meseta Alta, all the churches with their *retablos* and stained-glass windows, all those shots of the Camino itself and the flowers around it, and of Natasha walking, all the people we have met—Gloria and her Italian fan club, the Belfast Musketeers …

The phone rings; it's Moira. Natasha has received an offer of a college place, according to something from the Central Applications Office. But she thinks it's a mistake. "DN012, it says," says Moira. I tell her I'll check it my end, either on the CAO form, which Natasha has, or online.

"Is anything wrong?"

"Well, I've just lost the camera and all our pix."

And I start crying as I'm walking and telling her how devastated I am. But if it is true that Natasha has a place at college, this is wonderful news and I cheer myself up a bit.

"Don't text her or say anything just yet," I say to Moira. "Let me check first so we don't get it wrong."

We finish talking and a few minutes later, after further checking her end, she says she thinks it definitely is an offer of a place in UCD. "Id luv to see her face when you tell her," she texts me. "Id take a pic 4u if I had a camera," I reply.

Natasha falls asleep on the pavement outside a grocery shop in Sarria while waiting for me. I arrive with no good news and the import of our loss is now apparent to Natasha as well. We walk on a bit; I suggest stopping for a Coke. In the meantime Tash tells me she got a text from the CAO to say she had been offered something. She doesn't know what it is but assumes it is one of her choices far down the list; something she is really not interested in. When we sit down for our break, I ask to see her CAO application form. "What's that one?" I say pointing to her third option. "UCD arts; English and philosophy," she says. I can't speak because I'm so happy for her; I just give her a thumbs up and nod. She bursts into floods of tears and so do I. And we're there, two emotional wrecks hugging each other for joy.

"See?" I say eventually, "there's always good news around the corner. Feck the camera!"

And so we walk on, Natasha still a little wary of believing truly, fully, that she has got the course she probably wanted more than any other. She wants to go online to check and see it in writing for herself. And we chat about how we should try to get word out about the camera along the Camino ahead of us. "Has anyone got Jesús' number?" I ask. "If we could text him, 'cus he's about a day ahead of us he could get the word out."

I'm thinking back on Samos. Where was I during the evening? I went to the grocery shop at about 6.45 pm for bread and salami and a carton of wine. We ate on the bench. Then I went to vespers in the monastery at 7.30. I sat with Thomas and Sascha, left side of the main aisle, about halfway up the church. Then I went back to the bench and we all sat chatting and drinking wine until about 10.00 pm and then went to bed. I hadn't checked the shop or the church! There's a chance, I guess, it could be in either of them. I remember that a pal from Dublin, Elaine Byrne, an adjunct lecturer in politics from Trinity College, has come on the Camino and is about a day behind us. She should be coming into Samos in a few hours; maybe she could have a look. I text her Natasha's good news, my bad news and then ask if she's in Samos yet. "There n 30. Let me no what to do," she texts back.

I reply: "Gr8 if u cld ask in small shop on right as camino enters town, it is 1st shop; also monastery shop and in church where I at vespers at 7.30 last night, in left pew half way up aisle. Camera is canon compact in hard lozenge-shape black case. Big reward! Xx"

"Will do my best," she texts.

"May Santiago himself guide you!"

"Feck off oh st peter wit ur religion!"

A while later: "Not in church r first shop. Where is monastery shop? Can't find it. Will check wit police. Sure not anywhere else?"

By this time, Tash and I have arrived in Ferreiros, having set a blistering pace after Sarria. I just wanted to walk, and walk through a lot of pain; my left little toe was being crushed again and had been joined by my right little toe as well. At Ferreiros, no more than a crossroads with a bar/restaurant and a tiny *albergue*, we catch up with Gary, Andrew and Reece, as well as Tim and Louise. Sascha and Thomas are there too. They, and we, have missed a bed in the *albergue* but there's a covered picnic area opposite the bar/restaurant and I resolve to sleep rough there. I haven't the energy, emotional or physical, to walk a single step further. They are all supportive and kind. Reece buys me a beer immediately; Louise gives me another hug; Gary and Steve offer me all the photos I can take from their collections. I'm just a wreck at this stage; I just want to drink some wine, probably rather a lot of wine. It's only €3 a bottle and I'm in no mood to hold back …

Andrew reveals that, as he was last to leave the bench area in Samos, he dropped his cigarettes and, bending down to pick them up, he saw absolutely nothing else on the ground. Sascha shows a photo of the bench area and there's no sign of my camera anywhere in his picture. Then Thomas shouts: "Ah! You had it in the church. I remember! You took it off to kneel down to pray and you put it under the seat."

Well, maybe … We'll see. I tell them about Elaine—my last chance saloon option! And the red wine is very good …

Elaine texts again: "Not in church r first shop. Where is monastery shop? Can't find it. Will chek wit police. Sure not anywhere else?"

I explain and a little while later she calls because she still can't find the shop.

"You know the monastery church, the big one with the big main door with steps up to it, the one where they have vespers every evening?" I say; yes, she replies. "Well, to the right of that main door as you are looking at it, and on the lower level, there's another door. (See it! she says.) Well, through that is the monastery shop."

A little later, comes a text: "Found m shop but not open till 4.30. Fingers crossed. Let me know if anything else can do. Will check vespers again and give ur details at monastery."

But by this stage the wine is taking over and I've all but given up hope. Then a while later (at least one bottle of wine later), the phone rings. It's Elaine.

"Hi, it's me. How are you?"

"Been better; how are you?"

"Grand. I'm holding your camera in my hand!"

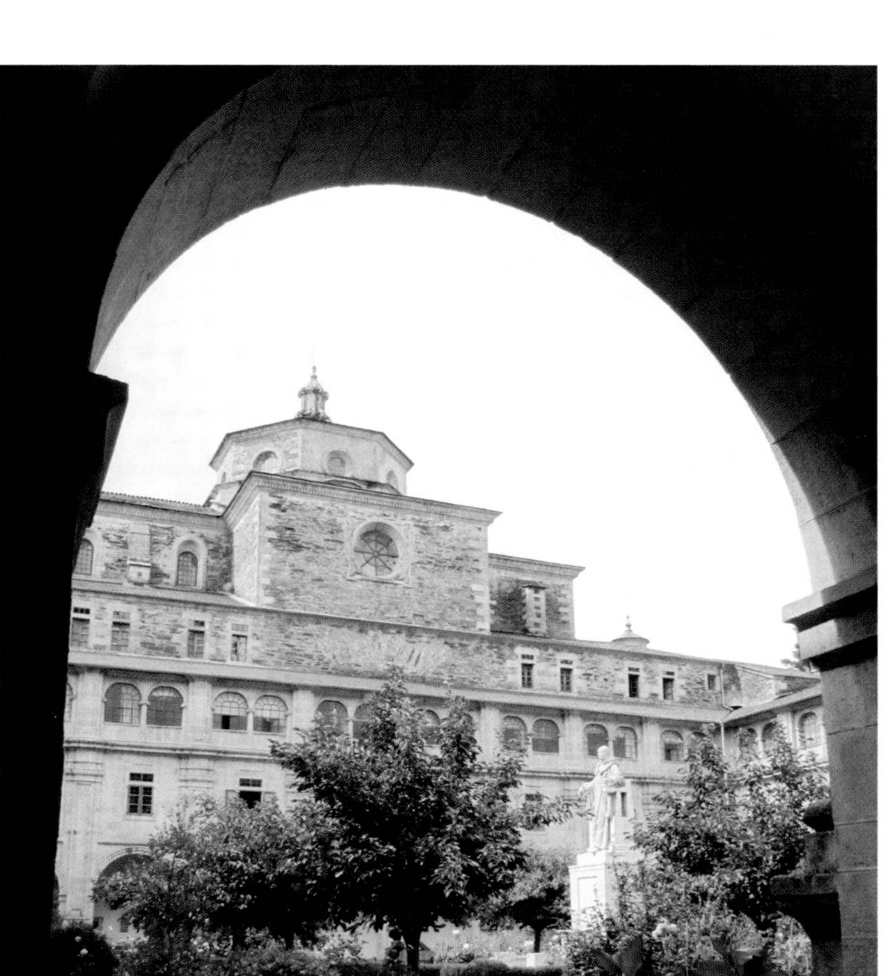

The monastery at Samos. The great cloister and rear of the Baroque abbey church.

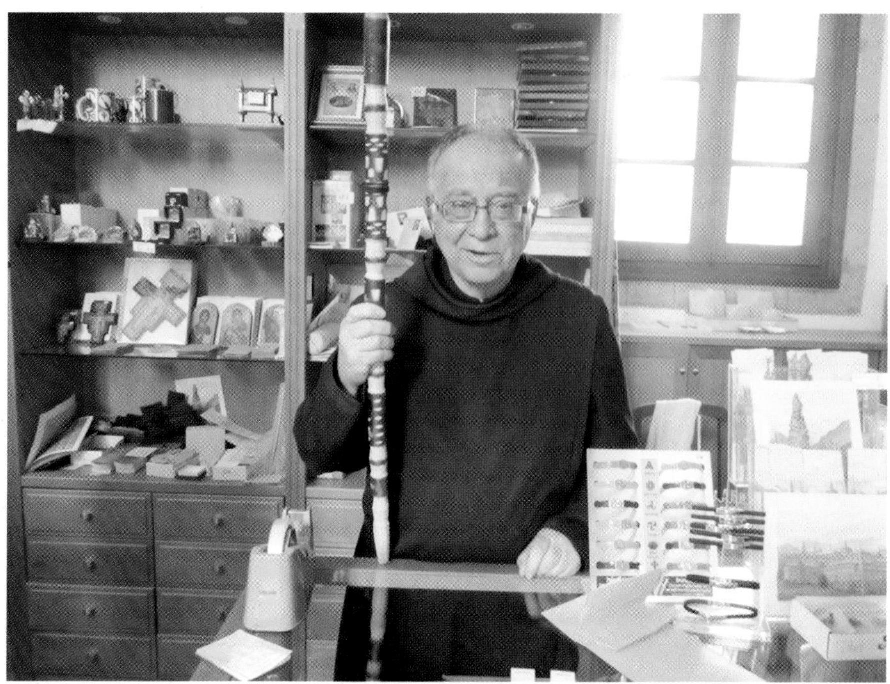

Padre Augustine in the monastery shop. (*Elaine Byrne*)

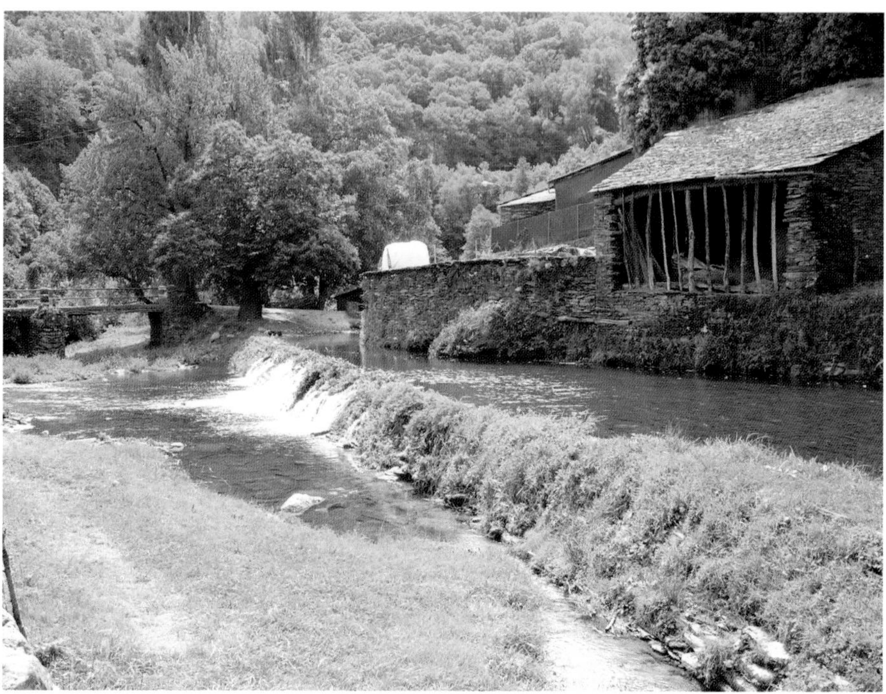

The beauty of rural Galicia. (*Sascha Thieme*)

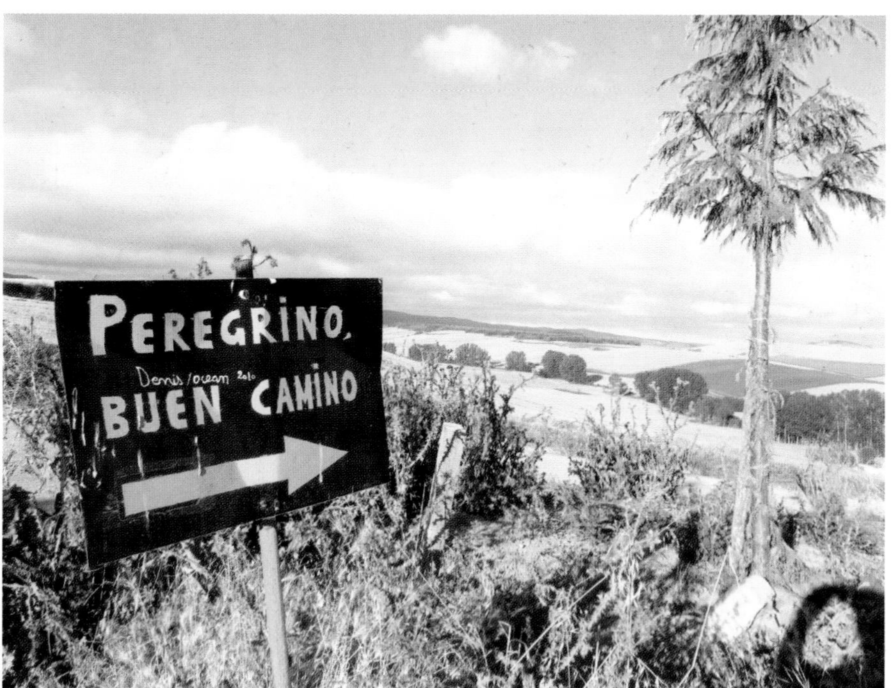

Locally made sign showing the way. *Peregrino* means pilgrim.

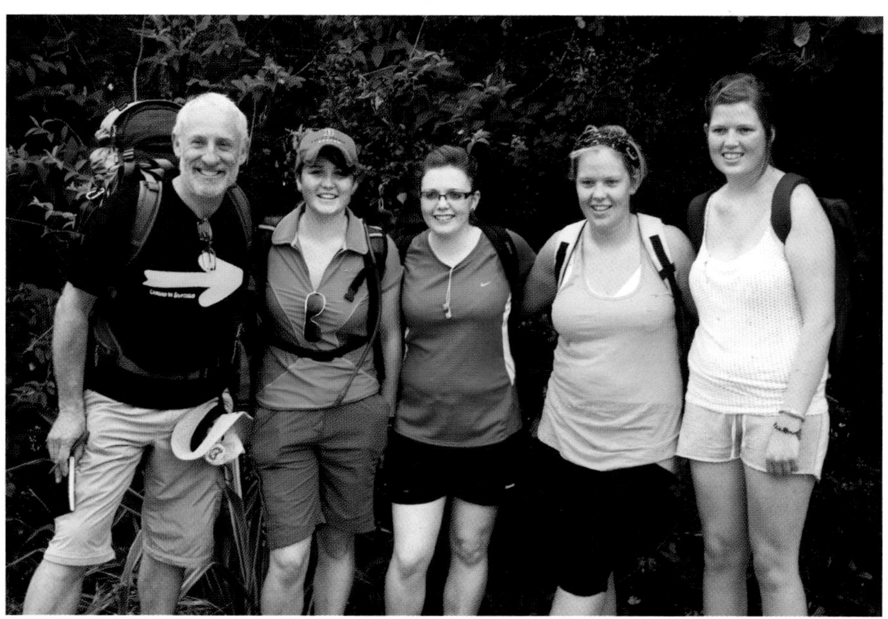

Peter with (*left to right*) Aoife Smeaton, Aideen Kinsella, Claire Collins and Mary Collins. (*Tim Hesse/Louise Tilley*)

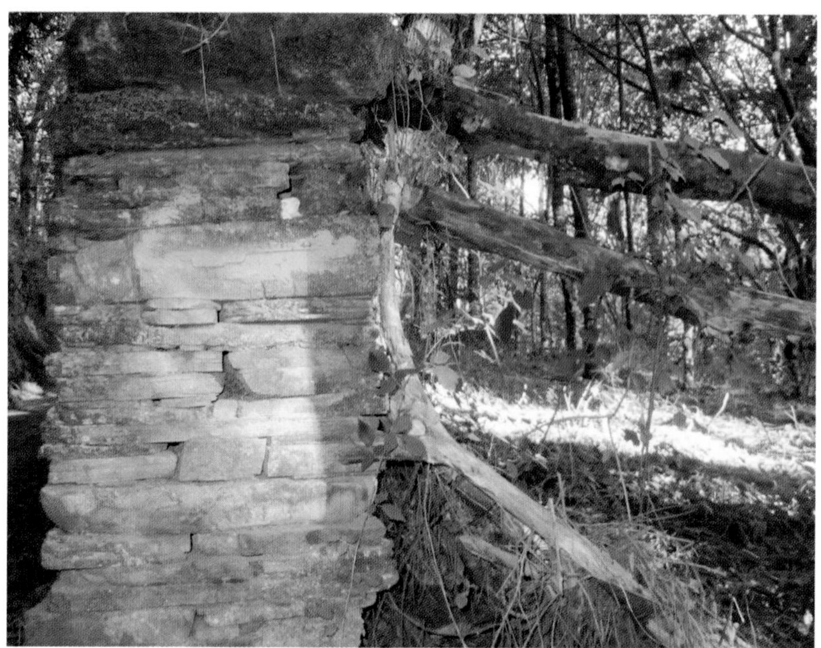

Always on the Camino, the yellow arrow—here in Galicia—points the way to Santiago. (*Elaine Byrne*)

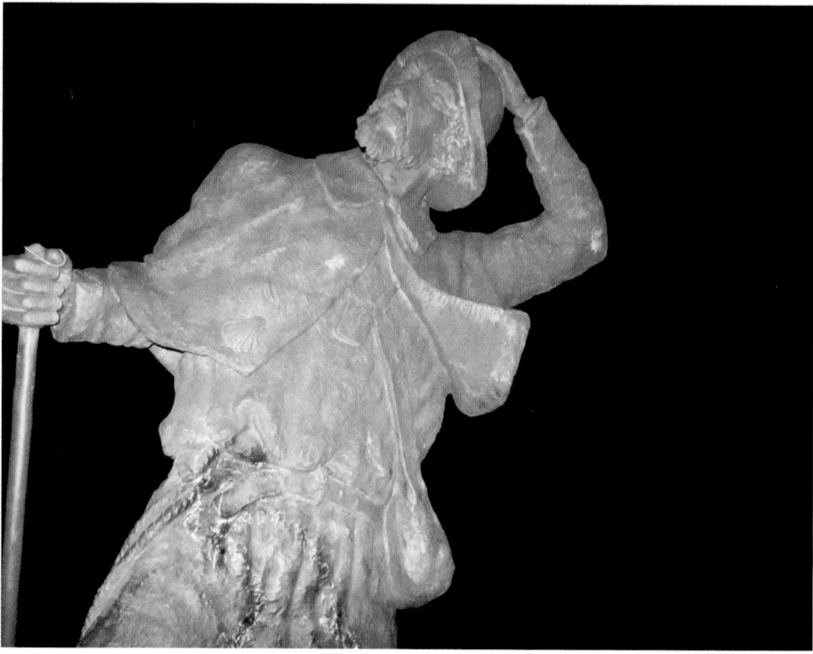

Bronze statue of Santiago at Alto de San Roque, a 1,270-metre high mountain pass after which the Camino drops down to the beautiful town of Triacastela.

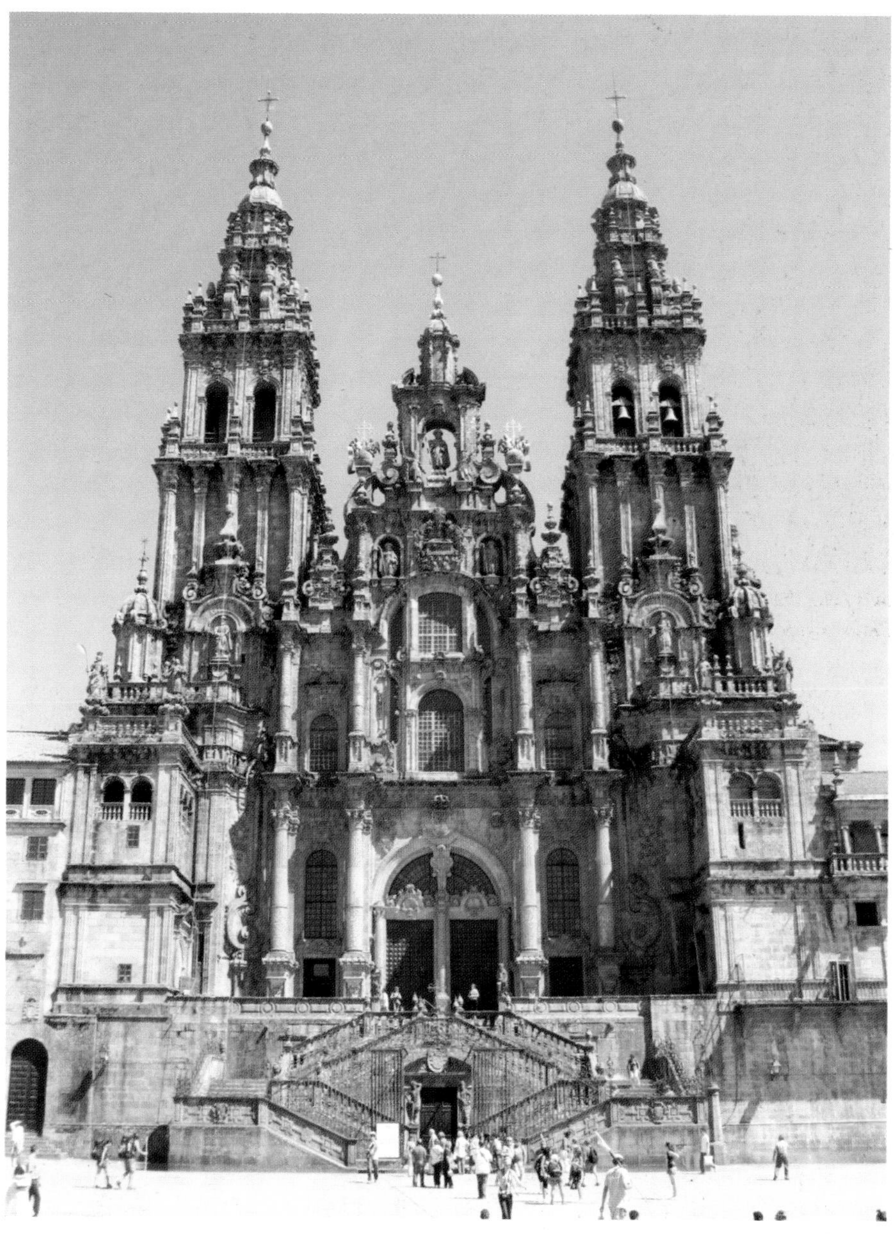

Santiago Cathedral from the great Praza do Obradoiro, showing the twin staircase leading to the main entrance, the Portico de la Gloria.

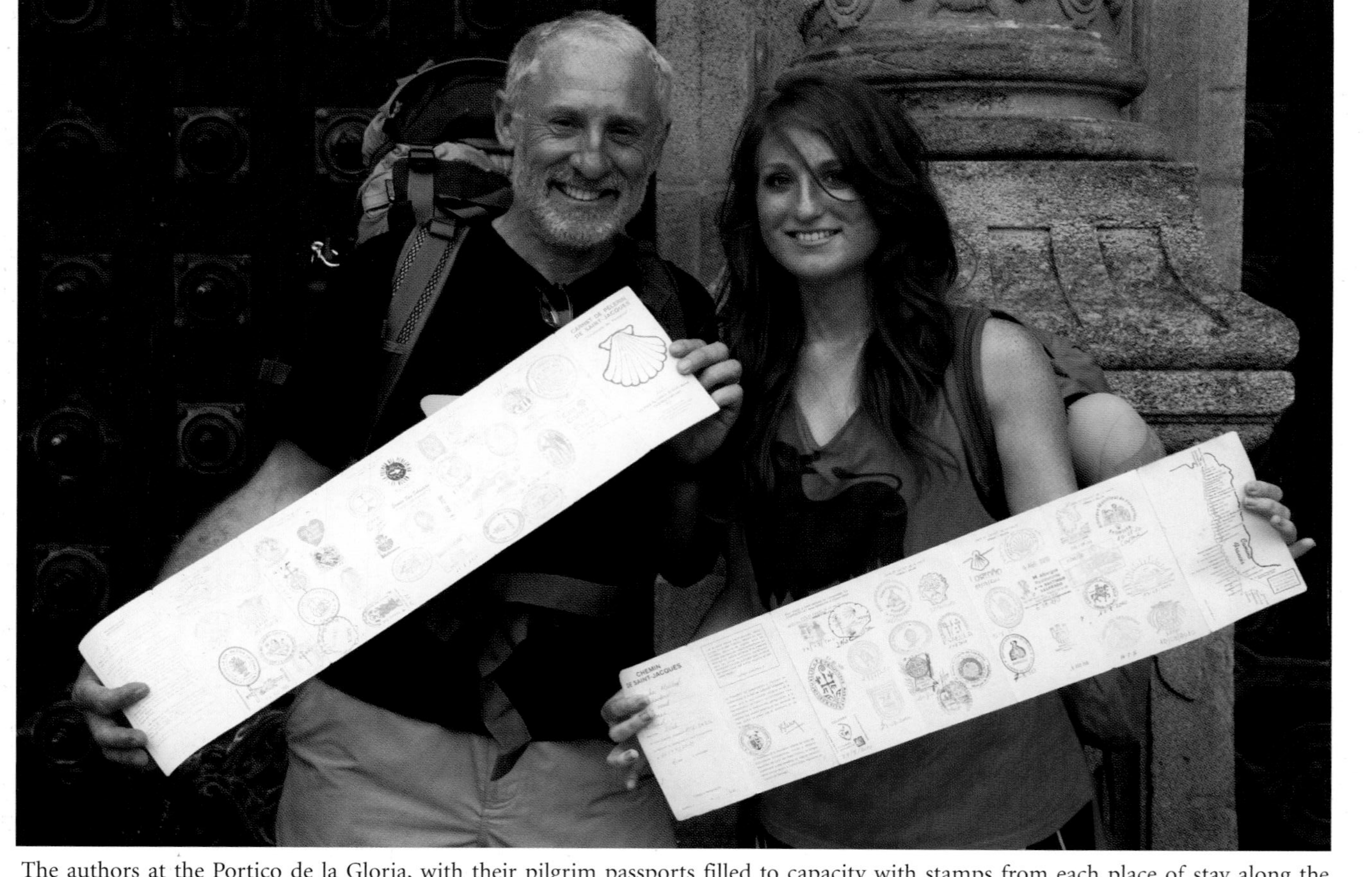

The authors at the Portico de la Gloria, with their pilgrim passports filled to capacity with stamps from each place of stay along the Camino. (*Tim Hesse/Louise Tilley*)

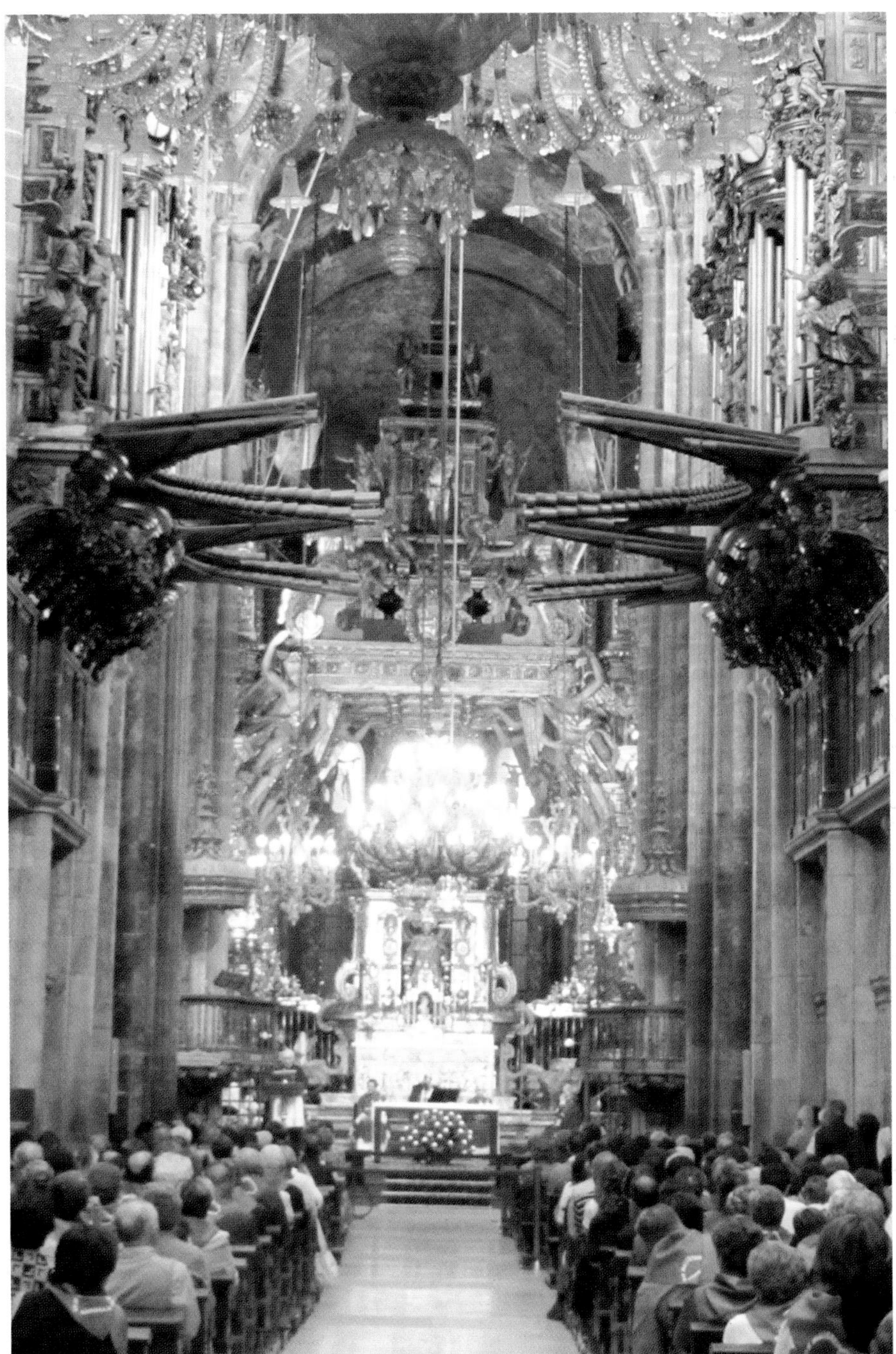

The main aisle in Santiago Cathedral leading to the altar and the wonderful, extravagant, over-the-top Baroque, gold and silver baldachin, or ornamental canopy, held aloft by rows of flesh-coloured angels, limbs flailing like synchronised swimmers.

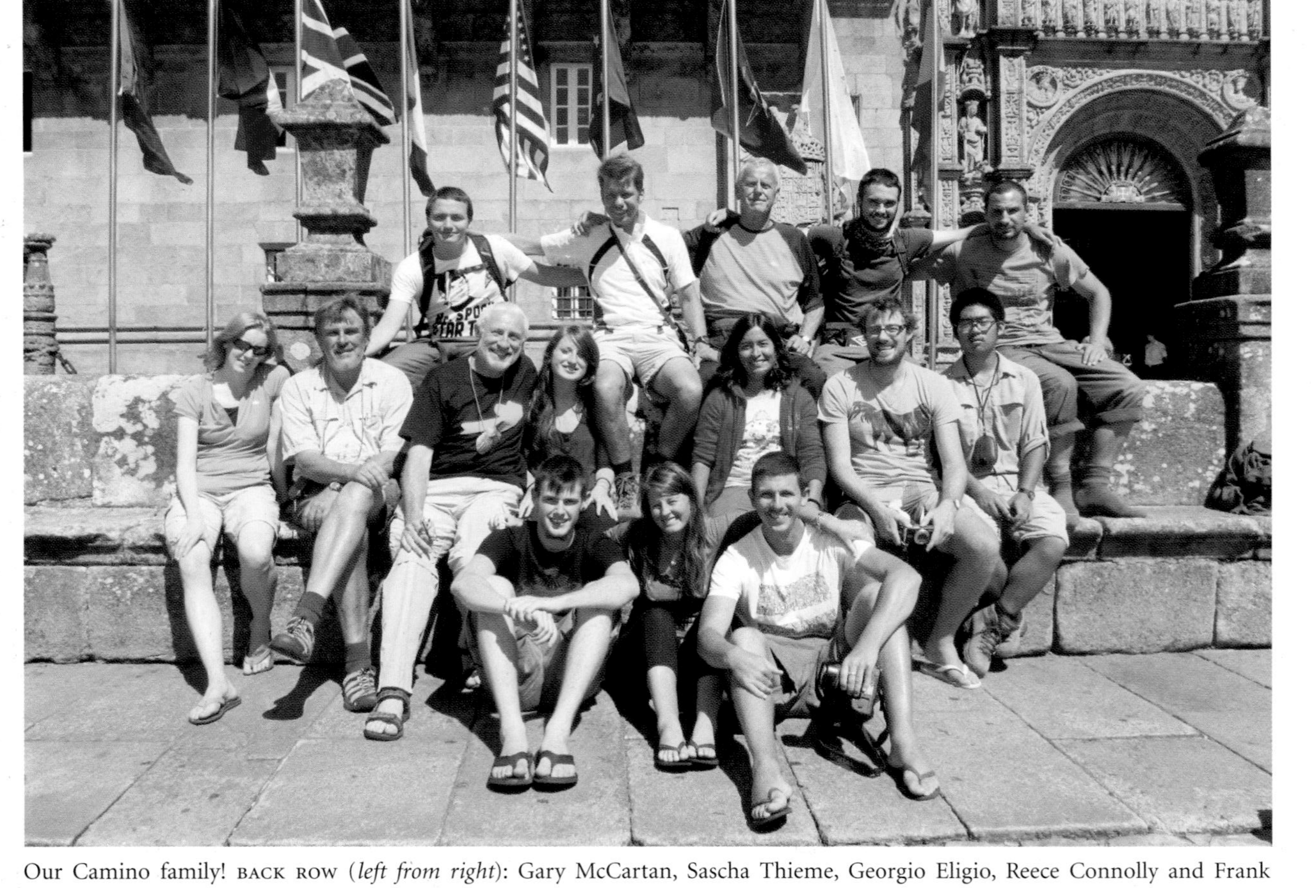

Our Camino family! BACK ROW (*left from right*): Gary McCartan, Sascha Thieme, Georgio Eligio, Reece Connolly and Frank Fernandez, a pilgrim from France. CENTRE ROW: Elaine Byrne, Thomas Reiss, Peter and Natasha, Johanna from Peru, Steve Gill and Mike, a pilgrim from Canada. SEATED: Andrew Lee, Louise Tilley and Tim Hesse. (*Photographer unknown*)

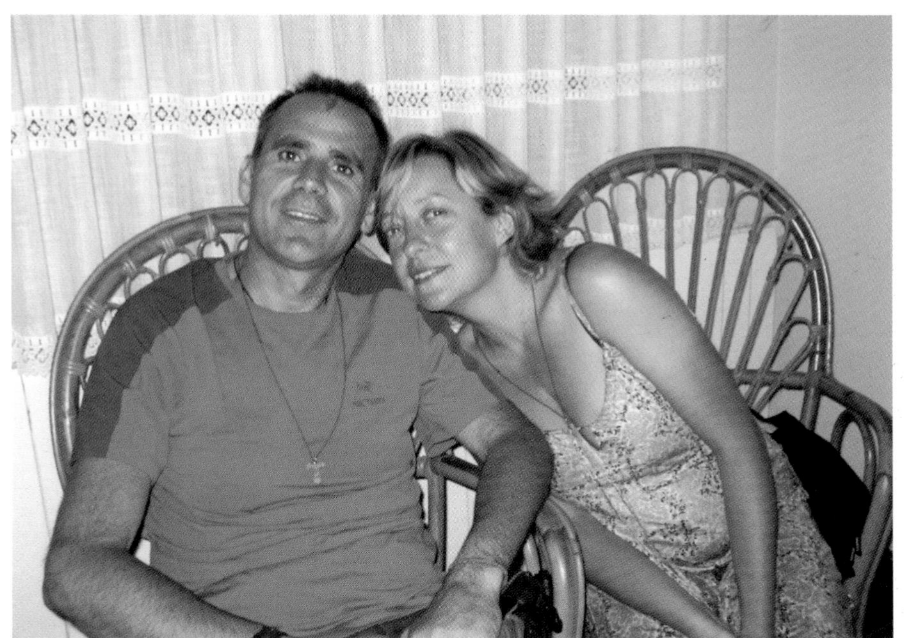

Giancarlo Enna and Gloria Baizan. (*Antonio Cebrián*)

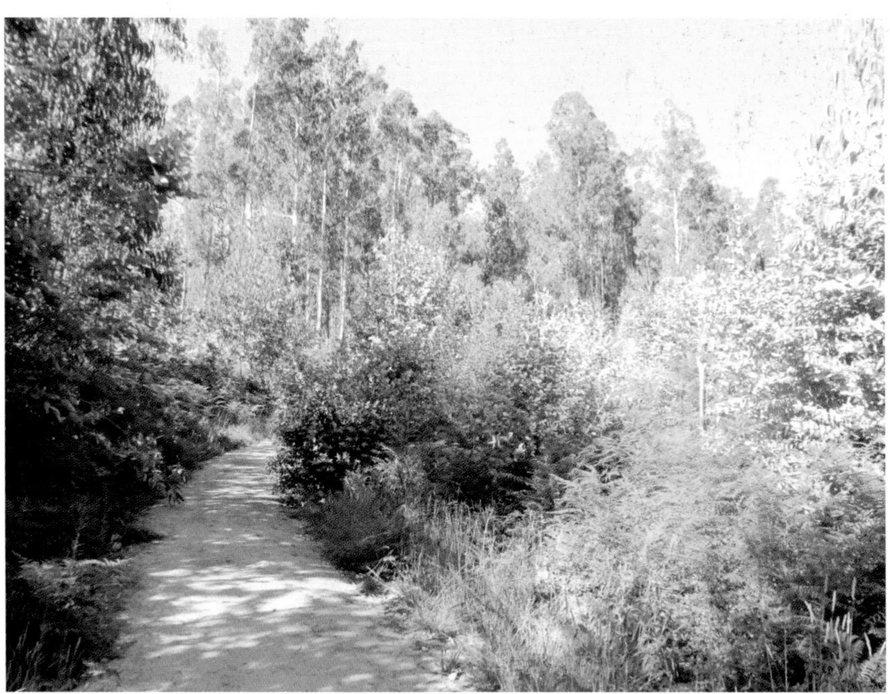

Leaving Santiago for Finisterre, the Camino wends its way through eucalyptus woods.

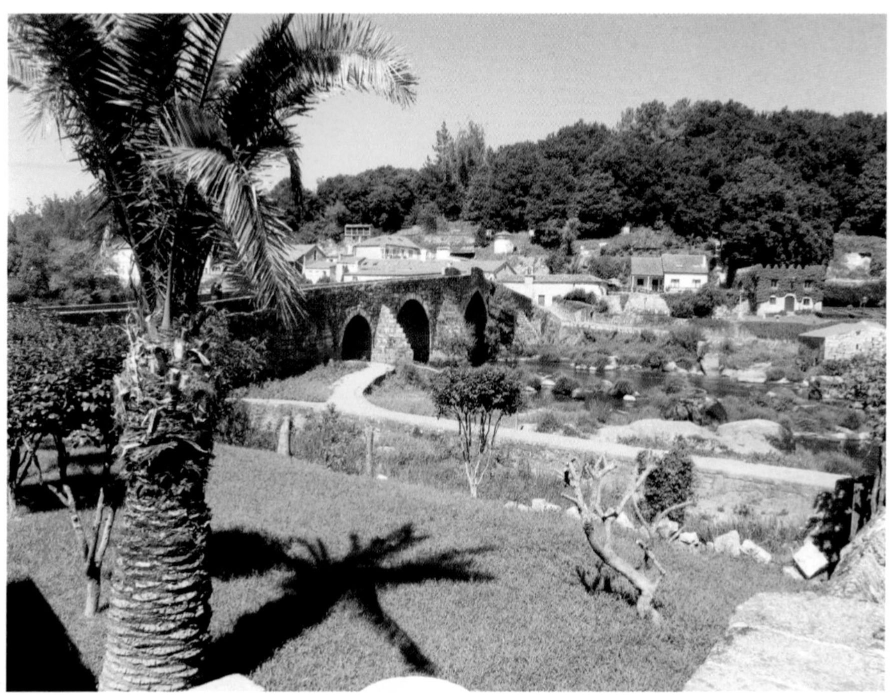

The pretty medieval village of Ponte Maceira, the most beautiful by far on the way to Finisterre.

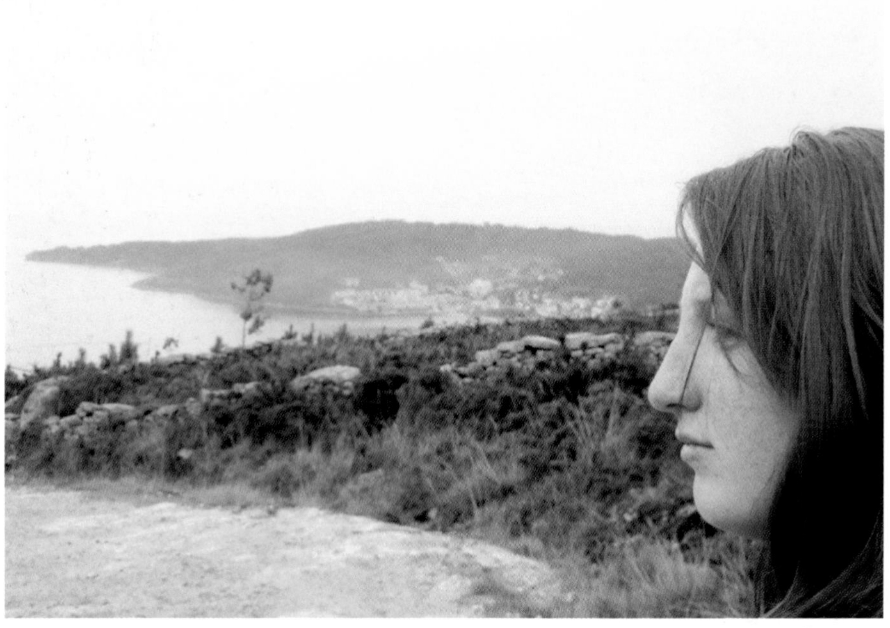

After nearly 900 kilometres, the Atlantic Ocean and the Finisterre peninsula come into view.

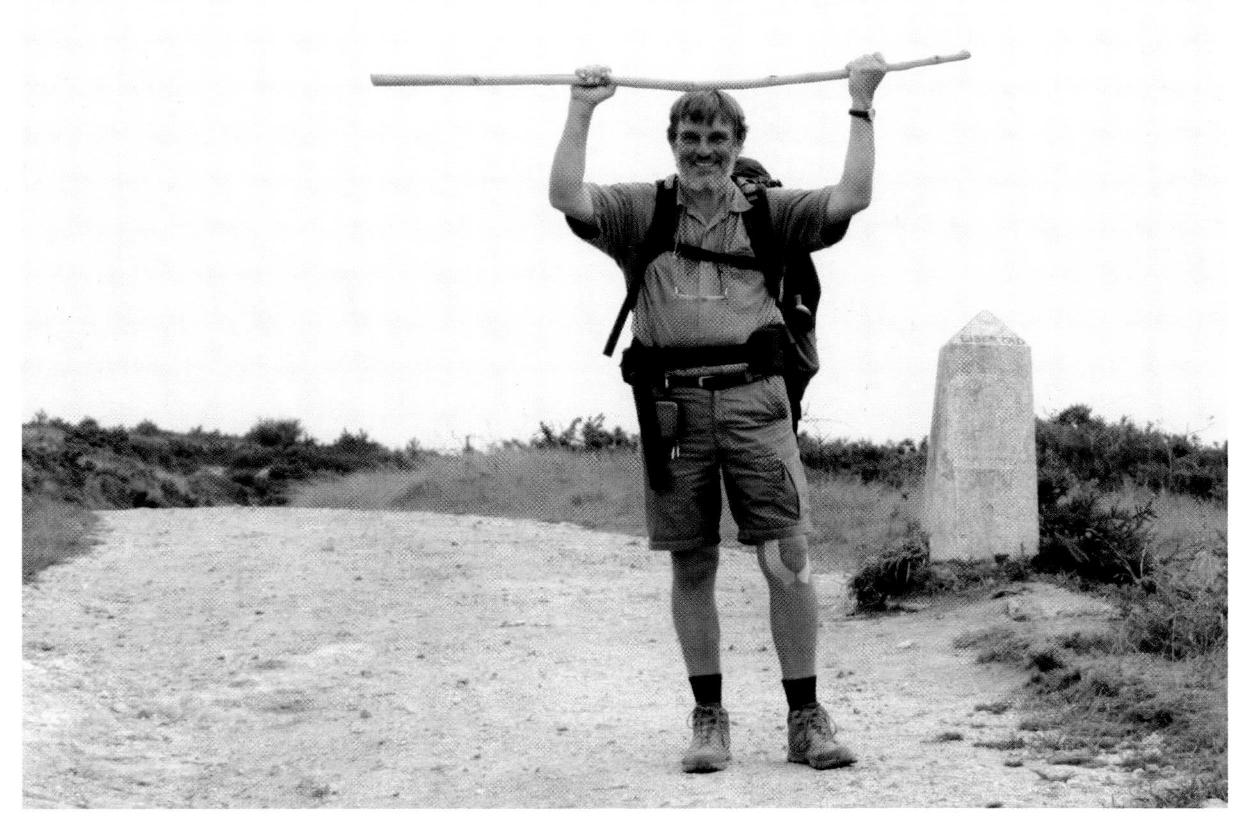

Thomas Reiss, elated at the sight of the sea … after walking 2,800 kilometres over eight years from his home in Germany.

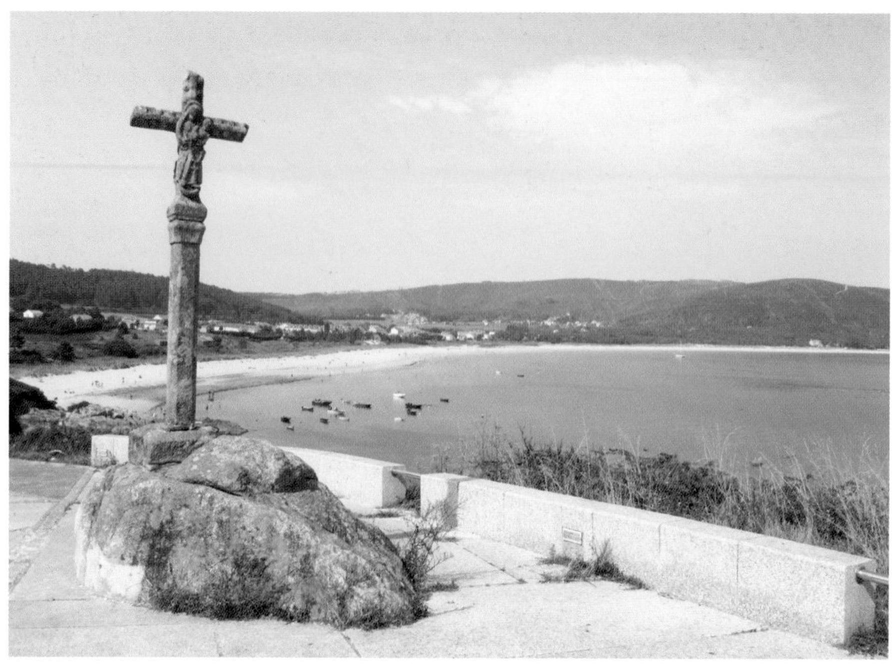

Pilgrim cross overlooking the Praia Langosteira at Finisterre.

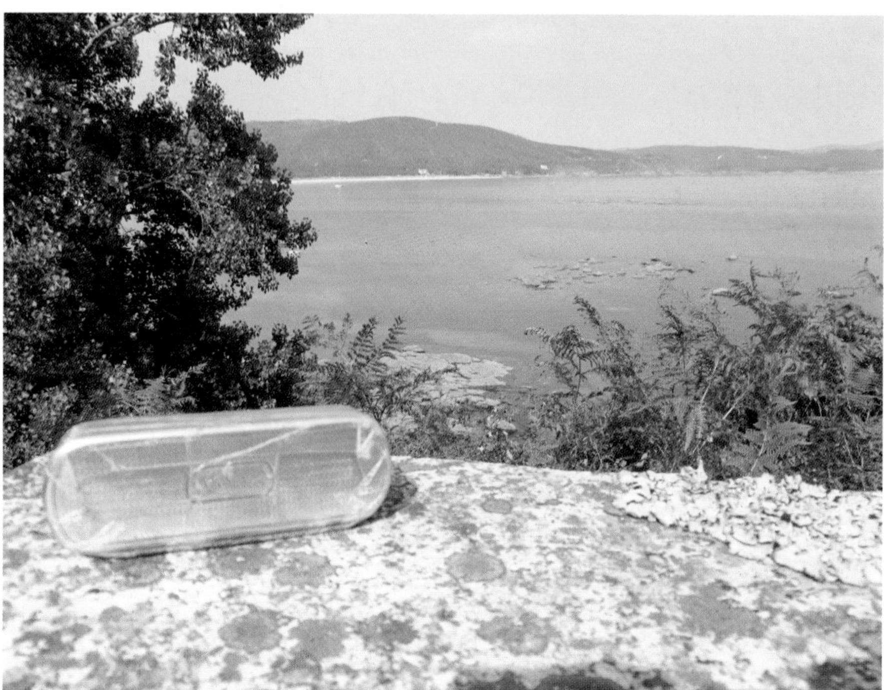

The little silver box.

The scallop shell points the way.

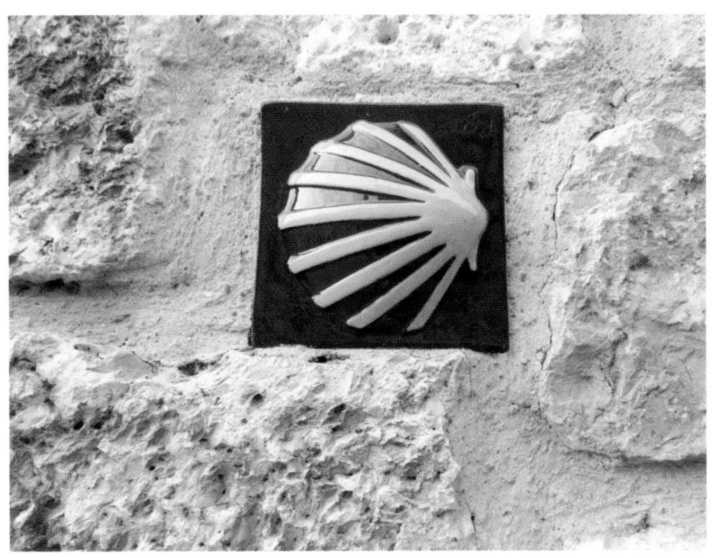

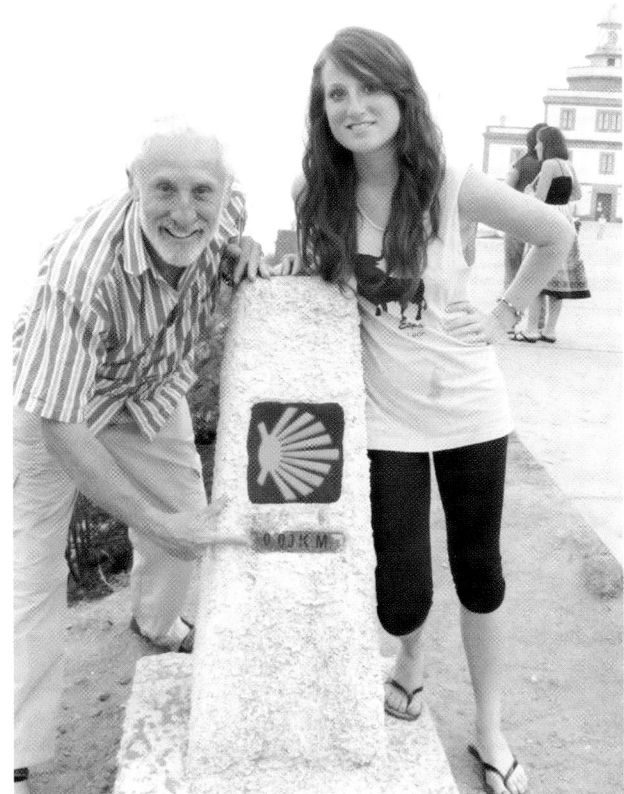

The final Camino milestone at the lighthouse in Finisterre showing zero kilometres left. (*Thomas Reiss*)

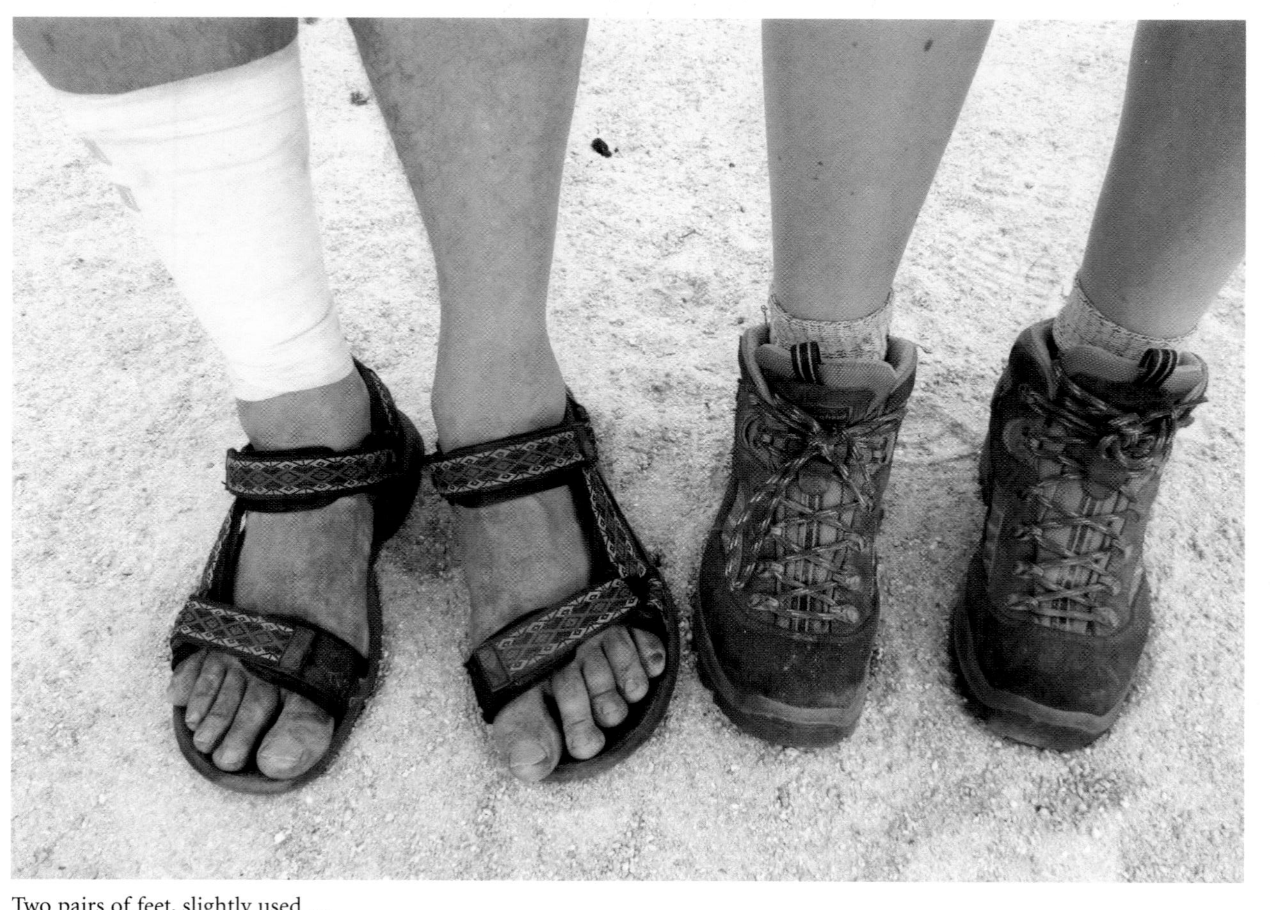

Two pairs of feet, slightly used …

Natasha watches the sun set at the end of the earth, the final moment of our Camino.

And then …

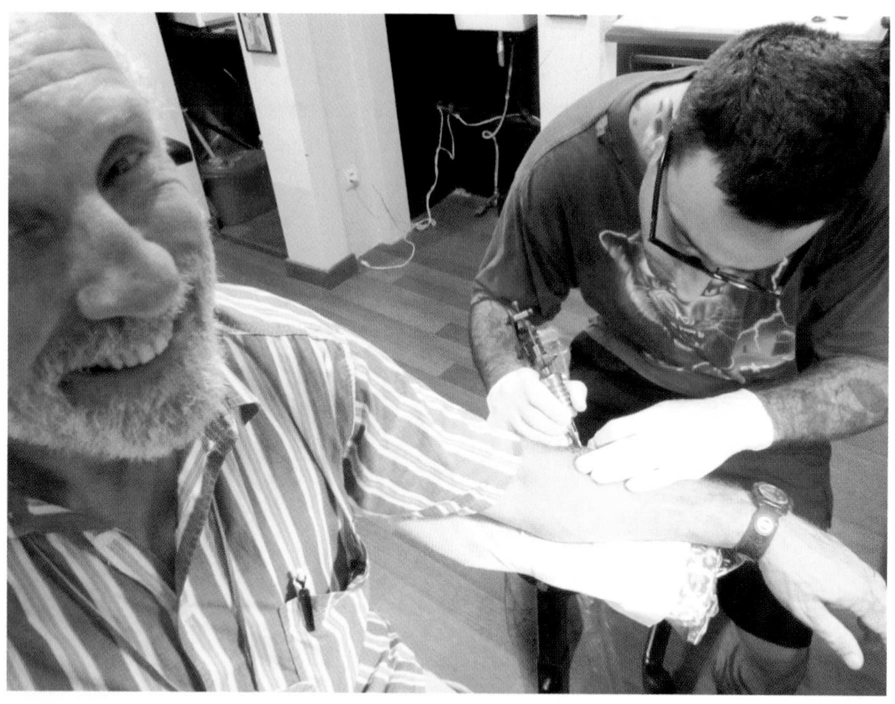

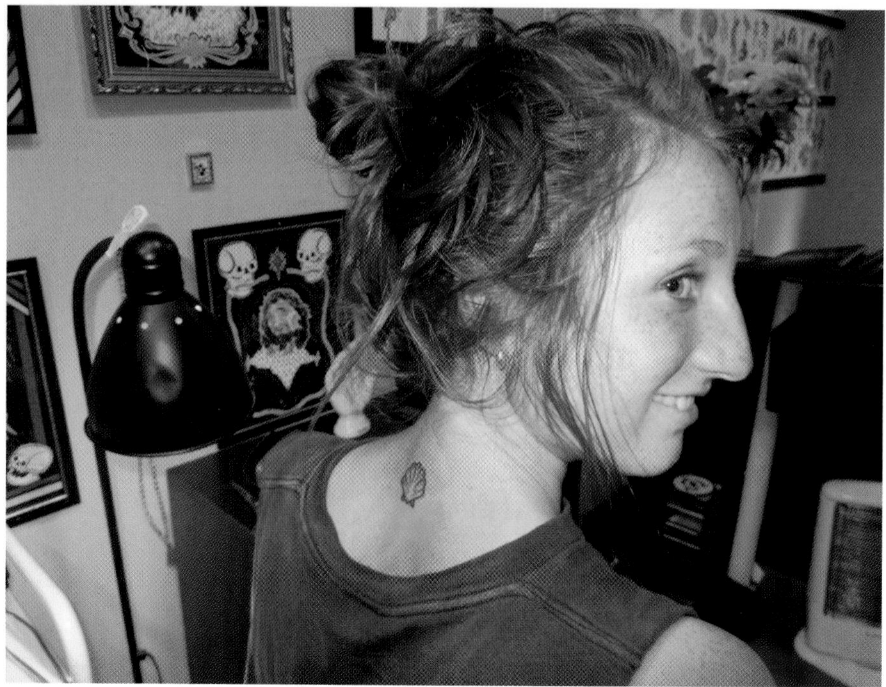

I just collapsed into a blubbering heap of tears and incoherence. I think I said, "Wonderful! Amazing!" I know I said thanks but then everyone around was cheering, laughing, clapping me on the back, pouring me wine. The camera, it seems, has been found in the church. Thomas's memory was accurate: I had indeed put it on the floor when I knelt to pray at vespers. It had been found there by Padre Augustine after the pilgrims had departed the church and he was checking if anything had been left behind. He and his colleagues were delighted with the turn of events when Elaine arrived in the monastery shop asking after a lost camera. They pointed to the sky and said "Santiago" with big smiles on their faces. Padre Augustine insisted that he have his photo taken in the monastery shop and the saga of the camera was the talk of the day among the monks. Padre Augustine gave Elaine a present of a book marker as she hurried away to call me.

Once I got myself together, I hurried off to tell Tash.

NATASHA: Today was a day of miracles. Looking back on it, I still can't quite believe what happened. The day began like any other Camino morning, but very quickly, and very suddenly, it turned into a horrifying, emotionally draining day.

We left Samos in the complete darkness of 5.30 pm. All of us walking together, along the main road, then slip down into the woods along the Camino. I find myself very tired this morning, and feeling like I have walked 730 kilometres. And once the darkness clears, I gradually fall behind everyone, with Andrew, who has a bad knee. We plod along the forest path casually, not a bother in the world, making regular and unnecessary pit stops. After about 10 kilometres my phone starts ringing; it's Dad.

"Hey Dad, how are you?" I answer.

"Tasha, where are you? I've lost the camera. I'm going back to Samos."

He spills everything out in one go.

"Oh my God. Do you want me to go back? I'm further behind you," I replied, trying to help.

"No, it's fine. I'm going to go to a main road and get a taxi to bring me, and then I'll get it back. Louise has your passport."

For some reason, I felt his voice was calm, and he appeared confident in the location of our camera. I just want to get to the next village where everyone is, so I can see Dad.

"What's happened?" Andrew asks, concerned.

"Dad's lost our camera," I say bluntly, with almost no emotion.

We walk a bit faster than before, wanting to find the others, and maybe catch my dad before he gets in a taxi. Andrew distracted me fairly quickly, and soon I found myself laughing. I don't think I really thought it was gone. I believed it was going to be in the *albergue*, waiting for Dad's return. I had complete faith at this stage.

We carried on walking for another couple of kilometres, and then a tiny village became vivid in our path. I could see a café and people sitting outside it. Everyone was sitting there.

"Where's Dad?" I asked immediately.

"He literally just hopped into a taxi," Louise said delicately.

She comforted me and told me Dad would find the camera. Reece assured me that St James was looking down on Dad and that he would get it. Nobody seemed to be that worried, so at this point it hadn't really hit me. But then I sat alone and started to think about it. Our whole trip was on that camera. We had nothing to go home with and show Mum and Patch. We had nothing for the book. We had nothing to look back on together and laugh about. Yes, we always have memories, but photos are what trigger the memories, or remind you of things you would have never remembered.

Dad told me he thought he left it on the bench where we had been drinking that night. If this was the case, there wasn't a hope for us. But I had a feeling it was in the bathroom, where Dad had packed his bag. If this was the case, chances were higher that we would retrieve it.

Dad said to go on with the others, and leave his bag in the café, and he would collect it when he was dropped back. I took out the netbook, charger and a book and put them in my bag to try and lighten his load. I left his bag in a storage room in the café. We all walk on. I'm quieter now, as I really begin to think about what this means, and the chances of Dad finding it. Everyone is trying to distract me but it doesn't work. Dad's next text only makes things worse. "Not in *albergue*, not at bench, not in church. This looks bad."

The last text I received is: "It's gone. This is a disaster."

I was devastated. I couldn't believe it. I started to cry. I told Andrew. He only said positive things such as "A pilgrim might have it, look at the photos and recognise you or your dad". I held onto that last bit of hope until I saw Dad. In the middle of all this, I received a text from the CAO.

It told me I had received a Round 1 offer, and that I could check it online. I presumed it was one of the ones far down on my CAO, one that I didn't want. I ignored it. I arrived in Sarria half an hour after receiving that text. We went into a shop and Louise asked me if I had heard anything. I told her it was gone. She hugged me and told me all the possible places it could be. I cried. I didn't know what we were going to do. I told them I was going to wait for Dad and that they should go on. Reluctantly, they left me.

To add to the bad news, I was hungry and needed food. I went to the ATM. There wasn't a penny in my account. Brilliant! I went back to the shop, which was on the Camino, so that Dad would see me. I was very tired. I sat down beside the shop door and found my head dipping in tiredness. Suddenly I woke up, 40 minutes later, dribble down my front, with pilgrims staring at me. I got up, and within five minutes my phone was ringing; it was Dad, arriving into Sarria. I saw him coming down the street. I walked towards him, not knowing what to say.

"I'm so sorry, Dad," I squeaked, and we hugged.

"I'm devastated. It was my Camino, our memories, all the wonderful pictures of you." He was unstable and couldn't stop crying. I felt so sorry for him. There was nothing I could do or say to calm him. We went into the shop where we got fruit and a drink. We decided to sit down somewhere and talk about our situation. Almost immediately after sitting down Dad asked me for my CAO form.

"Eh, it's in my bag. Do you really need it?"

"Yes," he said.

With that, I rummaged through my bag and took it out.

He pointed at my third option: DN012.

"What is this?" he asked.

"UCD; English and philosophy," I informed him, confused.

He broke down, again. "You've got it," he could barely speak.

My reaction was no different. I burst into floods of tears. I kept repeating no. I couldn't have got it. I couldn't believe it. It couldn't be possible. I thought I hadn't got it. We hugged and sobbed in an emotional overflow.

"Mum rang me and told me you had got an offer from this course, but she wasn't completely sure what it was," Dad said, after catching his breath.

I was so happy! I couldn't believe I was going to be attending university in September, studying all I have ever wanted to study.

It was now 11.20 am, and we had only done 15 kilometres. There was a thought in my head that we weren't going to see the others tonight. We were too far behind, and there were floods of pilgrims passing us, all unfamiliar faces, with tiny bags, looking fit as a fiddle. There wasn't a hope in hell we would get a bed if we walked on to where the others were. But we just walked for now. I quickly forgot about my good news, and I was brought back to reality by looking at Dad's face, head hanging low, looking at the ground, and walking with no motivation.

"Dad, we still have our Camino, and each other and all our memories," I broke the silence. "Louise and Tim said we could use their photos, and Gary said we could have his too. It's not that bad." But all Dad was saying was how it was his fault and how he should have backed the photos up. After a while he said that we should stop at the next *albergue*; otherwise we were going to find ourselves sleeping rough. We would catch up with the others in the morning. We walked and walked, through small clusters of houses in the middle of farmland, but there was never any sign of an *albergue*. Reece rang us, asking where we were. We told him we thought we were coming into a place called Ferreiros. He informed Dad that's where they were staying. We couldn't quite believe we had caught up with them that quickly, and that we were actually going to see them. That's when Dad observed our targets up ahead.

"Hey, that's Thomas and Sascha," he said.

"No way. I thought they were far ahead," I replied in shock.

It was them. And they thought the same, that we were far ahead of them. They knew the camera had not been found; the others had told them. Thomas had been speaking to people in Spanish, asking if they had seen a Canon camera, and if they did, could they call him. They were both very sorry for us. Dad then told them of my good news to lighten the mood; with it, he choked up, as did I. At this stage, anything set Dad and me off, we were so emotional. As we were in Galicia, we were just waiting for the day to come when it rained. The gods decided today was the day, and it started lashing. I didn't have any waterproof clothing. Dad offered me his, but I didn't want it. I just wanted to arrive in the *albergue*.

Finally, after marching the last five kilometres in hope of catching a bed, we arrived at a tiny crossroads, where a bar/*albergue* sat, with

Andrew looking out at us from a picnic area. "Go straight to the front. I don't know how many beds there are," he said. It didn't look hopeful.

Dad marched right around the corner and straight to the door. We were welcomed by a woman saying: "Completo." It was full. There were no beds. It had been raining and the ground was soaked. We went back around to where Andrew was sitting. There was a sheltered picnic area across the road. We agreed we would sleep there. To be honest, neither Dad nor I had the energy to care.

"For some strange reason, if that picnic area starts to fill up, put our bags over there," he said and off he went to get a large beer.

"Is he alright?" Andrew asked.

"No. He's in bits. I don't know what we're going to do. It's looking bad for us."

The very last hope we had was Dad's friend Elaine, who was arriving in Samos behind us. Dad had asked her to look in the church, a grocery shop and the monastery shop. I had lost most faith by now, and I didn't really believe she would find it. The chances were far too low.

I didn't really want to talk about it, I was so upset.

"Andrew," I said after a minute of silence.

"Yea?"

"I got offered my English and philosophy course in UCD." I looked at him and smiled.

"Seriously? Oh my god, that's amazing. You must be very happy!"

He gave me a big hug, which cheered me up. Louise came out 10 minutes later with a big smile on her face. Dad had told everybody the good news. They were all so nice. Again, I cried. I was tired and cold, and it only hit me then that Dad and I didn't have a place to stay. Andrew offered me his bed numerous times but I didn't want it. He then asked if I wanted to have a nap now, so I could get at least one hour's good sleep. I took him up on the offer and we walked down to the *albergue.*

I slept for what seemed like an hour, but was only 15 minutes. Looking around all the occupied beds I badly wished that I had one. I noticed there was a lounge area with a few seats. That would do Dad and me brilliantly. Sneaking in could be tricky, though. We sat on the bed for a while, just chatting. I couldn't take my mind off the camera.

"Tasha." I heard Dad's voice coming down from the other end of the room. I sat up and saw him walking briskly down the aisle. His eyes were red and he was crying, and then he smiled. I jumped down off the bed. I burst out crying, I knew it was about the camera, and I knew it was good news. "Elaine found it. She has our camera." He was hysterical at this point.

"I had completely lost faith, Dad."

"Never, ever, lose faith," he said.

I have never had such a surge of emotion as I did then. I was speechless and overwhelmed. I couldn't believe it. Andrew and Louise watched as Dad and I rejoiced.

"I was most upset about losing the photo of you in the sunflower field," he struggled to finish his sentence. I had never seen Dad cry this much.

This was a day that shows what happens when you're on the Camino. With the help of incredible people, amazing friends and pure faith, anything is possible.

PETER: At some late hour, we all snuck into the *albergue*—two more than there were beds. Gary insisted I take his bed; Louise gave him a camping mattress for the floor; she and Tim doubled up, giving Tash a bed. After a communal fit of the giggles, we all slept like babies.

In the morning there was some other bloke asleep on soft chairs in the dining area. I was glad he got in. What a day! No one deserved to be without some sort of bed after such trauma!

Ferreiros to Palas do Rei: 33 km in 5.5 hours

PETER: "This is the day the Camino changed," Sascha reflected after this day's walk. And he was right. Today was the day when a hierarchy emerged on the Camino. There are now some very marked differences between the pilgrims. This is because of what happens at Sarria, the consequences of which only really became apparent to us today.

Some years ago, in the 1980s, the church, in a quite arbitrary manner, ruled that anyone who travelled a minimum of 100 kilometres on the Camino was entitled to obtain a certificate, the much prized *compostelana*, testifying that pilgrimage had been undertaken and indulgences granted. What this has meant on the ground, as it were, is that the first major town 100 kilometres from Santiago has become the *starting* point for many pilgrims. Sarria is about 110 kilometres from Santiago and the two cities are linked by good road, bus and rail connections. And so now there is a considerable tourist industry bringing pilgrims to Sarria and nursing them along the Camino to Santiago where they overwhelm (in numbers at any rate) all other pilgrims, to whom they see themselves as equals.

"I didn't think I'd resent this," said Gary as our walk from Ferreiros progressed, "but I do, I really do."

Everything initially was fine when we began the day's walk at about 6.30 am. Yes, there had been a noticeable increase yesterday in numbers after Sarria but nothing really that would cause concern. This morning, after the Camino ambled its way through some characteristically lovely Galician woods and dales, including our first stepping-stone stream crossing just like the Clapper Bridge in Killeen near Louisburgh in Mayo, we got a shock. The Camino came to Portomarín, a strange, eerie holiday village above a reservoir. Part of the strangeness is due to the fact that Portomarín was built between 1956 and 1962, as the flood waters of a new dam drowned the original village. Even though major structures were removed as the waters rose and reassembled further up the side of the valley, Portomarín is almost just 50 years old and it has no heart, no soul. It is a dead, lifeless place, at least to this observer, and I have been there three times now.

With no reason to dally, we press on. After Portomarín, the Camino travels a good distance beside the road and it was then that we saw it. Up ahead of us, the Camino was black with people; it looked like Henry Street in Dublin on Christmas Eve. There were, quite simply, thousands of people, all walking in one direction, all needing a bed for the night.

The word pilgrim in Spanish is *peregrino.* Steve coined the word *tourisgrino* to describe most of these people. It is impossible for we who have walked such great distances to regard these walkers as pilgrim equals—they are having a week's walking in some rather pleasant countryside. All very fine in itself but not the same as what we have done. The resentment arises from the fact that we have walked almost 800 kilometres from the Pyrénées; we have carried great loads on our backs, experienced extreme conditions in terms of temperatures and the mountains we have scaled. Some of us have suffered bedbugs; we have all lived modestly; we have sought and treasured the quiet time granted us by the Camino for contemplation. We have earned our blisters and our sores and our sprained muscles, damn it. We have earned the right to be called a pilgrim.

Most of these people by contrast carry no bags, apart from little things like school satchels which contain a shower mac or something to drink. Their suitcases are ferried from village to village by a fleet of transit vans and buses. Tourist companies, who have booked beds in private hostels en masse, look after their every need. And they all come with their silly walking poles, or faux pilgrim staffs; they all have their scallop shell attached, often with the year, 2010, printed on them (their first souvenir!) and they amble along the Camino as though out for a Sunday afternoon stroll. They tend to stroll four abreast, chatting about this and that, like the Camino is just another holiday, albeit a slightly different one. I am sure many of these people have great faith and look forward to their moment in Santiago Cathedral. But I am sure also they are not our pilgrim equal and I don't care what rule the church has ordained.

So the hierarchy is thus. At the top in prime position, I place anyone who has walked, carrying their belongings as they go and staying in pilgrim *albergue*s, starting essentially anywhere east of Galicia. You have to scale at least one serious mountain range, and the peak at O Cebreiro will do as a benchmark. Next come pilgrims who do the same on horseback. Next come cyclists. Next are walkers who have some vehicular assistance—people whose bags are ferried ahead of them who at least walk substantial distances. Last come the tourists who coat tail the pilgrimage from Sarria.

Reece, Gary and Natasha and I get so miffed at these people cluttering the Camino that we break into fast walk after Portomarín to get past the hordes and cover seven kilometres in an hour and a bit. "Buen vacances!" we say as we pass them.

NATASHA: It was very frustrating. Our path was completely mobbed by the newbies—newbies with their bags being carried, and some even hopping on and off the Camino by taxi. The once empty, dusty path was speckled with every colour of the rainbow, for as far as the eye could see. It was ridiculous. It was so crowded that one could not simply pass another pilgrim out. There wasn't enough room; you have to say "Hola!" or "Excuse me," to get their attention, and then race by. In 500 metres this would happen 10 or 15 times. As a pilgrim walking from St-Jean-Pied-de-Port in France, it is incredibly frustrating to walk 30 kilometres and find the *albergue* filled by pilgrims who are getting help from transport. To pass people with no bags on their back strolling along the Camino, full of energy and often with no respect for the 'original' pilgrims. At one stage we were passing through a small village, and there was a pile of fresh-faced pilgrims, wearing clean clothes, normal trainers and with not a bead of sweat on their faces, bent over a fountain, complaining about the walk. I could have killed them, but I just stormed by. Reece quite rightly said they don't even deserve a "Buen Camino!"

Maybe it's us being sour and jealous of their cleanness, but unfortunately, it does take away from the last leg of the journey. When I wasn't thinking about how angry I was, my mind was on yesterday. I still couldn't quite believe the day we had been through, the luck we had had, and the generosity of all our friends. Then I thought about how excited I was to start university in September, studying what I want. I smiled every time I thought about it.

Because of the worrying number of people along the track, we had to walk extremely fast. Dad and I walked with Gary and Reece for a majority of the way. Within one hour I had pains in my shin from pushing myself this far, and I just wasn't enjoying the day. We couldn't stop for anything to eat, so I picked apples from any trees I saw along the way. We worked it out that we were walking seven kilometres an hour. This was the fastest we have ever walked. Andrew, with his bad knee, was nowhere to be seen. We presumed he was behind us. There was no way he was walking as fast as us. We were positive. I had no phone battery, so I couldn't text him. But Reece got a call from him, at around 11.30 am, saying he was in Palas do Rei. We couldn't believe it. It was almost impossible. Then again, after the day we had yesterday, anything could happen.

For the last eight kilometres we thought we had passed everyone out in our morning storm of 20 kilometres. I walked at a nice pace with a girl who we met in Ferreiros, named Maria. She was lovely and very interesting to walk with. We were having a nice conversation, walking along a tree-covered woodland path, when Reece came flying past.

"Andrew just called. The *albergue* is full, and the municipal one is filling. There are queues everywhere."

With that we marched right into the town. There were people everywhere. The whole area was completely jammed with pilgrims and other walkers. Lines of bags flooded the ground, and the worst part was most of them were new pilgrims, with small bags. We saw Andrew, still in disbelief he made it here before us, standing in the queue for the municipal *albergue.* Luckily, there were plenty of beds and we were going to make it. However, it filled within 15 minutes, as did the private *albergue* across the road. This led to the opening of the local sports hall, where mattresses were provided for around 200 people.

Tired, and rather overwhelmed by what we had seen on our journey, we all wanted some food in us. Andrew didn't look so good. He was pale, walking extremely slowly, and feeling dizzy. All he had eaten that day was a peach. We went straight to the nearest pizzeria and shared a margarita. He still didn't feel well, so we walked back to the *albergue.* He slept.

I wanted to get to a computer to apply for my rechecks. Even though I had got the course I wanted, for my own satisfaction I wanted to look over them and got Dad to come with me. We had all the information we needed in an e-mail sent from my history grinds teacher, Miss Leddy. It was all a bit complicated, and the pressure of the timer on the computer made me say, "Let's just forget it. I got what I wanted, and I don't want you to pay €80 for something that's not necessary." Instead, we signed onto the CAO website and I accepted my offer. I would be attending University College Dublin, studying English and philosophy! I couldn't believe it. I rang Mum as soon as we got back to the *albergue.* She was happy for me. We had a little teary moment as we told each other how much we missed each other. I couldn't wait to see her.

When I was writing later that evening, I was alarmed by Andrew's state. He looked really sick. Suddenly he got out of bed and walked to the bathroom. Next thing, there was a crowd of people around the cubicle, some of them being members from the Red Cross. Within five minutes he was being brought in a medical car to the doctor's clinic. It didn't seem good. Some thought it was food poisoning, but it couldn't have been, because we shared food the night before, and for lunch. Others suggested sun stroke. He was brought back after just over an hour, being told he had bad heat stroke, with instructions to stay inside, and not to walk tomorrow. He was delirious, and devastated that he was going to have to get the bus on his third last day walking.

Everyone went to dinner, but I stayed in bed writing, with Andrew beside me resting. It was awfully amusing. He was having full blown conversations with himself, curling into a little ball, and flapping his hands about. I bought a few drinks and snacks for him in the *albergue* opposite, to try and get something into him, but he wouldn't touch the food.

I didn't sleep well that night. Every movement he made, I worried he would either vomit across his bed, and in my face, or pass out.

Thankfully, the night remained vomit free.

Palas do Rei to Arzúa: 30 km in 6 hours

PETER: Today we head for Melide, the pulpo capital of Galicia (or so it has always seemed to me). Pulpo is octopus, boiled octopus to be specific, and, for the passing pilgrim, pulpo defines Melide more than anything else. How Melide, which is some 60 to 70 kilometres from the sea at Coruña, came to be so associated with boiled octopus is beyond me. But there it is: you walk into Melide and you are confronted with it fairly quickly—numerous pulperia (essentially, pulpo taverns) along the main street.

The first thing just before that, however, is the delightful medieval, four-arched bridge over which the Camino passes as it enters the village of Furelos, for all intents and purposes now really part of Melide itself. The Camino here is part of the old Roman road across northern Spain, the Via Traiana. A little to the south of here there are 2,000-year-old funeral barrows, some of which have been made of old Roman roof tiles. To me, it is amazing to contemplate that the places through which we are passing, the stones over which pilgrims walk, have been walked upon for some 2,000 years.

Across the bridge is the tiny chapel of San Juan, which I enter each time I pass. Inside there is always a kindly lady ready to stamp one's pilgrim passport and press a religious card into one's hand. On this occasion she gives me a prayer to St James. "I am here, as thousands of pilgrims have been all through the centuries," it begins, "offering Our Lord the tiredness caused by following the Way of St James." And it goes on to request for the pilgrim "a big and generous heart" so that he too may be an apostle of Christ.

In the meantime, a plate of pulpo will do nicely.

The pulperia last frequented by Natasha and me is on the left of the main street as one follows the Camino through the town. We remember it had great shining copper vats of boiling octopus, but this time these have been replaced, sadly, by rather characterless, utilitarian stainless steel pots. Other than that, though, the place remains much the same: a giant hall with, at the front on one side, the boiling vats of octopus and, on the other side, the bar. Stretching behind to the back of the premises are rows of benches and tables, a bit like a German beer hall, waiting for customers. It's just after 9.00 am and the pulpomeister hasn't really got the show on the road yet. But he's fast. We sit down, Natasha, myself, Reece and Steve and order three plates of pulpo and a bottle of house white (yes, the sun is hardly over the horizon but you cannot eat boiled octopus for breakfast and not wash it down with white wine). We ordered just the three servings because Natasha and I both recall that a small amount of pulpo goes a long way. In the event, we are pleasantly surprised: the servings—freshly boiled octopus tentacles, all purple, white and fleshy, garnished with paprika, rock salt and olive oil, and served on wooden plates—are delicious and are polished off in no time at all. We set off for our destination, Arzúa, with a spring in our step, though in my case the spring is tempered by an aching right foot and anxieties about getting somewhere to sleep tonight as the crowds are thickening once more.

By the time we reach Arzúa, the *albergue*s are indeed full but there is word about opening a sports hall. The local fire department has taken charge of an indoor basketball arena and is opening it to pilgrims for €3 a head. We arrive and already there is quite a queue. I flop onto the grass in the shade of a wall. The young Spanish man beside me has his iPod playing and asks if I mind. It's Dire Straits so the answer is a definite "No problem!" The slightly ethereal air of *Brothers In Arms* wafts about and sore feet begin to recede as the lyrics sink in …

There's so many different worlds
So many different suns
And we have just one world
But we live in different ones
Now the sun's gone to hell
And the moon's riding high
Let me bid you farewell
Every man has to die
But it's written in the starlight
And every line on your palm
We're fools to make war
On our brothers in arms …

Around 4.00 pm they open the sports hall. Within minutes 160 pilgrims have been admitted, each one taking a judo mattress from the gym storeroom and making a nest for themselves for the night. It is baking outside … and soon inside as well. Before long, all 200 available mattresses have been taken and some are accommodating two people each. There are, it seems, over 600 pilgrims in town for the night. I'm starting to think about Santiago, about walking into the city, going into the cathedral, what sort of emotions I will be feeling. And then Finisterre: walk or take the bus? It's another 85 kilometres or so and my feet really are reaching their limit. Both my little toes are now black with bruising and I fear I will lose both toenails. My left ankle where the front of my shin joins the foot, as it were, is swollen and grinds like the bearings are all crushed. And to top it all, Tash is unwell. It seems like too much sun but I hope she is not as sick as Andrew was and has to take a bus or hold back a day. We both want us all to walk into Santiago as a group.

Thomas hunts down a restaurant. Natasha comes along for the company but won't eat. In the event she can't manage to stay the course and I bring her back to the sports hall for an early night. I manage to hobble back and finish dinner. Everyone sleeps surprisingly well and, thankfully, Tash is fine in the morning …

NATASHA:

Dear Dad,

Today leaving Palas do Rei, I realised there wasn't a lot left to the journey. I was sad to think about it ending, yet excited to arrive in Santiago, after walking there for five weeks, and covering nearly 800 kilometres. I also thought about what I had learned along the way, and what I have gained from the walk so far.

Most definitely, the biggest gift the Camino gives to you is time. I am so grateful for the time I have been given on the Camino. I have come to realise and understand things I have never noticed, and all they needed was some time.

There is something in particular that I am referring to. Something that has been there all my life, and obviously I have appreciated and thought about, but walking the Camino this time, I thought so much deeper. It's about you, Dad. I want to write how I feel about you, and what I have come to realise. This is something I will never be able to say to your face, but I would also never let it go without you knowing it.

You wrote your letter to me earlier on the Camino and I am writing this now, because I have also just read what you wrote about Granny, and it was so wonderful. I wish she could read that. People have constantly been telling me how wonderful it is that I'm doing the Camino with my Dad. This I know. I knew it was special before we arrived here. A relationship like ours is not common. Nearly every person we have spent time with has told me what a wonderful person you are. And you are. You have taken care of many people on the Camino, whether it's their dinner, or simply taking the time to talk to the person nobody else will because their English is bad.

You appreciate the smallest things in life. I know I always laugh at you as you try to be a poet about your surroundings but the joy a beautiful field gives you is priceless. The things that many people wouldn't lift their head at, you stop and take it all in. This is something I hope I take on in life better.

There have been plenty of times in the past where I have been unable to understand why sometimes you get angry at me, or don't allow me to do something. It has all come with growing up; I understand I hurt you when I'm careless and your reactions are because you love me. I know this. And I am sorry for all the times I have made you think I'm dead in a ditch late at night.

When we were drinking in the albergue *in Burgos, you left to go to bed. As soon as you were out of sight, everybody started telling me how lucky I was to have such an amazing Dad. Andrew told me that the first thing he said to the guys when they met us in Estella was, "Wow, they are like a couple of best friends." You are a best friend to me.*

You probably know this, but someone else who was very proud of you was Granddad. He often told me how you made him feel. When he spoke about you and the things you have achieved in life, there was happiness and love in his face.

I want to thank you for everything you have done for me in life. I love you more and more every time I'm with you. I hope that I make you proud, and I hope that you know I will always love you and be there for you, no matter what.

When you are gone, I am completely positive that my best memories of you will come from the Camino. This has been the best thing in my life so far. You make me so happy, Dad, and it's a happiness that I will have for the rest of my life.

Thank you,

Love always, Your Daughter.

Arzúa to Pedrouzo: 22 km in 5 hours

PETER: Our second last day. The day before we enter Santiago. Tomorrow we will walk into the city of St James, exactly one calendar month to the day since we struck out from St-Jean-Pied-de-Port. It is hard to believe it but our Camino is almost over … but not yet! Today's walk is among the most pleasant we have had. This is partly because we have decided to take it easy, not to put ourselves under any great pressure to clock up good mileage. We are about 40 kilometres from Santiago and so today, 20+ will do nicely; leaving something over 15 kilometres for tomorrow for the march into the city.

In the meantime, however, my body has opened up a new front in the pain war. My right leg has made common cause with my left. While the pain in the ankle on the left is under control, thanks to doses of anti-inflammatory painkillers given to me by the lads from Belfast, a shin muscle on my right leg has kicked into action. The lads call the pain shin split and that's exactly what it feels like—like the front of your lower shin is bursting open. The pain is excruciating, and while painkillers help, they don't help sufficiently. What does work, however, is a bandage wrapped around my right calf muscle giving it support. I look like the walking wounded but who cares? I can walk again and the pain is at a low enough level to walk through it.

Our walk today is through yet more lovely Galician countryside and hamlets. Clusters of working farms, homes and out-buildings all made of Galician granite and gneiss; most have *horreos* in the farmyard. These are the distinctive, rectangular granite or timber buildings measuring about three metres in length by two metres high, by about a metre deep. Their sides are made either of red bricks with holes in them, or vertical timber slats with gaps between each upright. The buildings are usually built on the top of walls, or some other elevated position, or perched on granite legs. They usually have traditional Spanish red tile roofs. They are used for drying corn and are very much part of the landscape of rural Galicia. They are a delightful architectural/cultural feature that, for me, help define this lovely area. In many farmyards, there is evidence of rapid change: old wooden carts lying disused in barns, or wooden cart wheels that have become garden ornamental features.

The fields hereabouts may be divided by hedges of shrubs and brambles (the blackberries are now in their prime and are delicious) or by upright slabs. The fields themselves are given over to mixed farming—pasture for grazing cattle, maize and other domestic vegetables. In the half light of dawn there is something comforting about walking through these hamlets listening to the hum of the milking machines in the parlours. The roads (dirt tracks more accurately) are spattered with cow dung. This is the way so much of rural Ireland used to be up to perhaps 40 years ago and it is lovely to experience it again. The smells are familiar, the pattern and pace of life somehow comforting.

When we left the sports hall in Arzúa shortly after 6.00 am, there was a row of saloon cars outside. The phoney pilgrims were busy loading their bags into the back of them. Again, we all feel a mixture of sniffy superiority and anger towards them. But further along the trail, as we pass through eucalyptus and pine forests, deeply breathing in the lovely mixed aroma that comes from both, I come across four young Irishwomen who make me rethink.

"That sounds like a familiar accent," I say as I come up behind them. "Where are you from?"

"Dublin," says one.

"Yes," says I, "but where?"

"Northside; Donabate," says another. "Where are you from?"

"Rathfarnham originally but I live in Greystones in Wicklow now."

And so we fall into conversation. The four are Claire Collins and her sister Mary, Aoife Smeaton, and Aideen Kinsella. They are part of a group of 30, the oldest among them being John aged 72; and Aoife, at 19, is the youngest. They all began at Sarria and they have a hire car to ferry their belongings ahead of them to their next private hostel for the night. They fit the profile of the surge of walkers whom we have found annoying and on whom we look down.

"What do you think of it?" I ask.

"Oh, it's great," answers one, "really lovely."

"And what has you doing it?"

And they explain their story. They are all walking for an organisation named Casa, the Caring and Sharing Association, that has two respite homes, one in Swords, the other in Malahide. The homes are also known as break-out houses; they are places where families looking after a dependent relative can get some badly needed support that takes the pressure off them for a while. Each of the 30 people on the walk has raised €2,000, a total of €60,000, of which €40,000 is going straight to Casa—a fine sum of money for any charity.

Claire is studying general nursing in Louth; Aoife is doing science in UCD; Aideen is doing social science there as well; and Mary is doing arts at St Patrick's in Drumcondra with teaching in mind. We are chatting outside a café on the side of a busy road when a man passes. "How's that cross, Claire?" he says as he strides past. "Oh grand. I have it here," she says. I ask her about it and she opens her hand to show me a small, smooth wooden cross in the palm of her hand. What's this about? I ask.

"Each day, one of us carries the cross," says Claire. "I'm carrying it today because I had a friend in a band, the Liberty Kings, in a camper van in England and they were in a crash. They were on the hard shoulder of the motorway when a lorry went into them. Eoin from Inchicore died. My friend Brian Kelly was in a coma but he's fine now; he's making good progress."

I ask them how they raised the €2,000 each, because it's a lot of money.

"I had a birthday party," says Aoife, "and instead of presents I asked all my friends to sponsor me."

"We did bag packing and church collections and coffee mornings," said Aideen.

They ran a mini-marathon and cadged money from friends, said Claire and Mary.

"My Mam is in Casa," says Mary, "and for the last two years, we've gone to Lourdes to raise money, and so doing this is just another way of raising money for Casa."

We resume walking, myself and them for a kilometre or two, chatting about the Camino, why Natasha and I are doing it. They are knocked out at the idea that we began on Croagh Patrick and immediately start talking about doing the same thing, climbing the Reek in the night and then maybe doing some of the Camino, the Camino long before Sarria. And thinking about these smashing, lovely, generous, selfless and well-motivated young women later, I feel awfully guilty at having judged harshly all those people clogging the Camino. How many of them are also raising money for good causes? I certainly haven't been.

A little after parting company with the Donabate girls, there is a rather touching memorial set into a rough stone wall. It recalls the life of Guillermo Watt who, on 25 August 1993 while walking the Camino, collapsed at this very spot and died aged 69—just one day short of reaching his clearly cherished goal of Santiago. A plaque records his death, noting that he now 'lives in Christ'. A hollow in the wall contains a bronze cast of a pair of walking shoes, presumably his, and pilgrims have left touching messages, often relating to pilgrim friends who have also died, though not quite as the luckless Guillermo.

NATASHA: Last night was the worst night I've had on the Camino. The last five kilometres into Arzúa were in the blistering heat, and I could feel myself becoming dizzy. However, it wasn't until 6.00 pm that I really felt ill, and my symptoms were just as Andrew had described his. I was paranoid I was going to fall as ill as him, and be told not to walk the next day. But there wasn't a hope in hell I would get on a bus to Santiago, or anywhere else, after coming this far. Steve and I, and possibly Tim and Louise, are the only ones of the group who haven't taken any kind of transport yet, and I plan to keep it that way. At 7.00 pm, when it was time to go for dinner with everyone, including Thomas and Sascha, I felt worse, much worse. I was finding it hard to walk, talk and keep my eyes open. I ended up vomiting and going to bed dinnerless. I was worried what the morning would bring.

Thankfully, when I was woken this morning by Dad at 5.30 am, I felt okay. I have woken feeling better but I felt fine to walk. I think I just had a mild sun stroke or something like that. Walking out of the sports hall, we crossed the road to find our way back to the Camino. We happened to notice there was a small group of people huddled around a couple of cars with the boots open. As we get closer, we see the boots are filled with bags, and the people around the car are pilgrims. Newbie pilgrims—tourisgrinos. We march past them without interaction.

The first eight kilometres out of Arzúa were in the dark forests and difficult for me. I felt extremely weak and was sweating far too much. I felt completely drained of all energy. The Camino gradient was constantly changing, from ridiculously steep to being irritatingly down hill. Andrew still hadn't recovered fully, and the two of us plodded along behind the others, following the fading light of Louise's torch. Both of us were in silence, but grunting every so often. Finally, when a trendy little café popped out of nowhere, I dived right into a cup of tea, biscuits dipped into it and some fresh fruit. Almost instantly I felt better. My energy levels went up to their norm, and I was ready to finish the last 12 kilometres we had planned for the day. From the café onwards, Andrew and I, the patients, led the way. We overtook all the clean-smelling newbies with their clean trainers and their tiny fanny packs carrying essentials that couldn't be left with their bags in the car. Soon enough there was nobody in our path, and it felt like we were ahead of the whole pack.

The walk was enjoyable now my energy was back, and I was feeling normal again. A lot of the Camino today consisted of eucalyptus forest, separating small villages. The eucalyptus trees grew tall and straight and shot through the sky. They smelt fresh and minty, and made one feel clean in their presence. Their dried, dead leaves scattered the forest floor, looking like mini banana peelings. The sky was very like a sky seen in Ireland—grey, heavy and cloudy. We felt right at home. Thankfully it never bucketed down, only spat occasionally towards the end.

We had planned to do 21 kilometres, bringing us to Pedrouzo. Dad and I stayed here last Camino, so knew it was a good distance to leave for Santiago the following morning. The thought of arriving into Santiago tomorrow morning hasn't quite hit me yet. We have been walking for a month tomorrow, covering an average of 25 kilometres a day, all travelling to the one destination, and tomorrow we will arrive there. We will have covered around 800 kilometres.

It's crazy. I have such mixed emotions. Of course I am going to be happy to get there and see Santiago and be with everyone in celebration. But I'm also sad that it's the end. And with the end, come goodbyes. And some goodbyes are harder because deep down you feel you may never see that person again. It will be the end of our walk to Santiago, but I don't believe it will be the end of our Camino within us. It's going to be something I carry with me for the rest of my life, and share with everyone I did it with. It's going to live in the stories I tell and the memories I share. The photos I have will remind me of the small things, and the people I achieved it all with, the great moments we had together. The Camino will never die in you, unless you want it to.

We have 18 kilometres until we reach Santiago. I will walk a kilometre for every year of my life so far.

Pedrouzo to Santiago: 16 km in 3.5 hours

PETER: Just as the evening was winding down last night before we went to bed, we had one of those encounters that people who do the Camino treasure. It happened in the dining area of the *albergue*. Tim and Louise and Gary and Reece and I were chatting and downing a few glasses of wine before bed. We were all thinking of the great day to come—the day we would achieve our long-nurtured desire of walking into Santiago, into the cathedral to see the shrine of the saint and then, of course, enjoying some of the delights of a beautiful city and the comforts it offers after all our hard walking.

What happened is this. One of the people on the Camino who has been with us on and off for many hundreds of kilometres is an Italian man named Georgio. He is a very tall man with a huge smile and a friendly personality to match. And there is an almost saintly quality to him; his warmth is matched by a gentleness that we have all seen and is very much part of what makes him an attractive personality. Every time you see Georgio he hails you with an extravagant wave, a big smile and a "Ciao!" And of course the greeting is returned. The attractiveness is enhanced by the fact that Georgio is not a young man; there is a strong feeling—an assumption—that Georgio is in fact a wise old man, but sadly, although he is very friendly towards us all, because of the language barrier, contact does not progress much beyond the "Ciao!" stage. Nonetheless, Steve and the lads from Belfast have built around Georgio a character of mystical quality. It is a joke on him but played out with affection. There are ribs about how the sun always shines when Georgio is around; about how a light seems to radiate from him; about how unruly lads become instantly calm and personable in Georgio's presence and that bird song surrounds him as he strides along the Camino. The gag is good-natured fun, underpinned by real affection for the man. I was not wholly aware of what was going on until after the incident in Carrión de los Condes when I learned afterwards that the man whose feet were being bandaged by the nun was Georgio. In its own way, the incident confirmed for me that Georgio indeed had some sort of aura around him.

Anyhow. We're sitting there in the Pedrouzo *albergue* thinking about Santiago and down to half a bottle of wine between five of us when Georgio walks in and places two fresh bottles in the centre of the table, announcing his presence with his trademark big smile and "Ciao!" A present for us! We are all knocked out by this and immediately see that he is with three or four Italians. One of the Belfast lads grabs one of the Italians: "Can you speak English?" Yes comes back the answer and within no time we are sitting around chatting to Georgio through a young woman translator who is a diplomat from San Marino and about to begin (she hopes) work for the United Nations.

Georgio is wearing a loose-fitting basketball-style vest T-shirt, shorts and sandals; his hair is combed neatly, and despite the casual nature of his attire he looks as elegant as ever in the way some continentals seem to manage whatever the occasion. The first thing we do is thank him very much for his wine gesture. We ask, with the help of the San Marino diplomatic service, to hear his story—his reasons for walking the Camino and what it has done for him. He tells us that this is his fourth time doing the Camino. Previously, he walked with friends and did sections only. But this time he is alone and is doing the whole thing—St-Jean to Santiago.

"I have no problem with friends," he assures us, "but doing the Camino alone is an opportunity to reflect. Now I am 69 years old and I think about what I have done in the past and could have done. By walking in nature and watching life, I feel very free. In the city, people are conditioned by the way they dress ..."

It emerges that Georgio, who is Georgio Eligio and a happily married father of two grown children, has spent his working life in the Milan fashion industry, mostly selling women's lingerie—a detail that prompts a frisson of enhanced interest among his male listeners ... Georgio laughs. The fashion world is very superficial, he says.

"I like the early morning and being alone, such as in a forest. I don't like my way to be lit in the dark; I like to follow the light of the moon and the stars. This year, doing the Camino the way I am, I have the opportunity to feel that there was something in common with other people. But the problem is that you are too fast," he says, looking at me in particular and laughing. "What counts in life is communication and you can communicate without talking. What counts is being aware there are people close to you. This is the difference for me [doing the Camino] this year and this is why I am very happy."

I ask him what else he has learned doing the Camino this time.

"I found that you have to continue; you cannot stop. If I had stopped, it would have been a disappointment [to me]. This means that you can solve any problem in your life." The Camino is a call, he adds, to return to traditional values of self-reliance.

Are you religious? I ask.

"I am a believer," he says. "I go to church to pray but I am not a closed-minded Christian. My religion is about respecting other religions." And then Georgio says that he has been observing us as much as we have been watching him. So why did we do the Camino and what have we taken from it?

Reece says that he wants to be more spiritual as a person. Meeting people from different cultures has helped him make decisions about his life. Reece, who comes across as quite a private person and is by far the best walker among us, does not say what those decisions are but adds that meeting Georgio has helped him and given him great pleasure.

Gary says that the Camino has moved him more than he expected. He says he really isn't religious or spiritual. "But I realised that while I don't have faith in God, I have faith in people. I can see God in people. The Camino has taught me about the good and the bad in myself and why some people mean a lot to me."

Georgio: "The important thing is to be honest with yourself. My mistakes were my mistakes but I could not admit that. I can now."

Louise's turn comes around.

"I have done a lot of walks, but this time I wanted to do it with the man I love and I know I will be with for all time," she says turning to Tim and embracing him. "I didn't expect to meet so many wonderful people who have touched me. I too am an emotional person," she adds looking at me, tears rolling down her cheeks.

I give my reasons—time with Natasha, writing this book, the death of my father and before that my mother; and I mention my own absence of faith and internal debate between religion and spirituality. Georgio says he thinks I am a very determined person; he has watched me walking and sees me as very determined and he thinks my doubting and questioning is a good place to start. "I think you are a very wise old man," says one of the Northern lads. "Old yes," says Georgio, "Wise? I don't know." I ask what advice he has for us all.

"Be yourself and be determined," he says. "Even if you don't know what you want, you won't know if you are not determined. I have always been optimistic and believed in people. To trust yourself doesn't mean you are superior to other people but it means being honest with yourself."

Georgio says that at 69, instead of going to St-Jean and scaling the Pyrénées and walking over 700 kilometres to Santiago, he could have got a bus to a beach. "But one morning, seeing the light in the dark, that morning all pain and confusion passed." He says that, after Santiago, he is going on to Finisterre where he will "spend a day sitting on a rock next to the lighthouse".

I'll see you there with Natasha, I tell him. Next morning we all awake at about 5.30 am and Georgio has gone from the *albergue* dormitory. Determined, it seems, to get to Santiago ahead of us and have his enriching walk in the dark through the pine and eucalyptus forests. Soon we are after him, walking mostly in darkness, our way lit by a full moon, the silence broken occasionally by the sound of owls hooting in the distance or the hum of car and lorry engines in the world beyond, the world with which we shall soon reconnect.

Just before Santiago, there is a village named Lavacolla, a nondescript place which nonetheless is part of Camino history and lore. There is a stream there, and in the Middle Ages pilgrims would wash themselves before entering the Holy City. Specifically, they washed their genitalia, according to Aymeric Picaud's *Liber Sancti Jacobi.* We all agree we'll restrain our enthusiasm for living historical accuracy and keep the proceedings to hands and face. Gary, enthusiastic as ever, floats his walking shoes off downstream, glad to see that back of them. I splash water onto my face, head, arms and legs. It is cool, very cool, and unexpectedly refreshing. A few kilometres more and we reach Monte de Gozo, a hill overlooking the city where we get our first glimpse of the towers of the cathedral. The Monte itself is nothing to write home about save for two aspects. The first is the truly hideous monument; two complementary swirls of rusting metal and stainless steel sitting on top on an enormous square on the sides of which are amateurish bronze panels showing Pope John Paul II and aspects of devotion to Santiago. It is an awful edifice and hopefully one day will be done away with and replaced by something more subtle and uplifting.

The other thing of note is the Monte de Gozo *albergue.* As this is effectively the final stop before Santiago (it being 4.7 kilometres from the cathedral), it caters for the final surge of pilgrims—up to 1,000 people per night—in what looks like a Butlin's holiday camp. Mercifully, I have managed to avoid staying there every time I have passed!

NATASHA: Walking up the hill towards Monte de Gozo, I knew what was on the other side. The city we have all been waiting for, the city that we have been walking for—Santiago! I feel a cold sensation throughout my body. I feel a sense of excitement that is overwhelming. I feel my feet running away with themselves as I get a rush of energy.

There are crowds of people gathered on the hilltop, looking towards the city. Lovers embrace, parents hold their children, and friends simply share their moment together. I don't look until I am at the very top of the hill. I don't want to spoil any of it. I want the whole city in my complete view, in all its glory. So there I am, standing with the wind blowing in my face at the top of the hill where the statue sits, Santiago lying below me. My eyes immediately fill with tears and I phone Mum. I want to tell her that I've made it. I've finally made it to Santiago, with Dad by my side every kilometre of the way.

The atmosphere at Monte de Gozo is wonderful. For me, it's the first moment a pilgrim feels achievement, as the city is in sight for the first time. The cathedral spears through the morning sky with power and strength, marking the centre of the city. It is exactly 4.7 kilometres away. The first kilometre is on the road which goes straight down towards the city. I walk this with Dad, holding his hand. He jumps a step to be in sync with my walking. "You've been doing that since I was a little girl. You always do it," I told him, as I looked down at our feet, walking together.

"My Mum used to do it with me," he replied. I looked at him. His eyes were red and glassy.

—

SANTIAGO

NATASHA:The outskirts of the city is like any other; grungy apartment blocks, run-down little stores and a couple of filthy bars where people like Disgusting Man might hang out. Yet this time I love it. I love it all because they are Santiago grungy apartment blocks, run-down little stores in Santiago, and filthy bars in Santiago, home to filthy men from Santiago.

We all walked together—Tim and Louise, Andrew, Gary and Reece, Dad and I. We reach the old town quickly and the change is dramatic. The path turns to old cobble stones, and the streets are narrow. The shops are dominated by family-owned *panaderías* selling that morning's fresh bread, meat and cheese shops, and little boutique clothes shops. The aroma of the morning pastries fills the air.

The way is covered with fellow pilgrims who have also just arrived. We wave and smile at one another, in celebration of our pooled accomplishment. The beautiful thing about your arrival in Santiago is that you are surrounded by pilgrims you have never seen or met before, yet with whom you share something very special. No words are needed to be exchanged, as a smile from one pilgrim to another says it all.

Walking down off the main tourist street, towards the cathedral, Galician music dances through the crowds and echoes along the narrow streets. The sun is breaking through the clouds and the streets seem to glitter as light catches on things. As we get closer to the square in front of the main entrance of the cathedral, the crowds thicken. Our pace quickens with excitement to run up the stairs to the main door. Under an archway and down some little stairs we go, into the main square, turning the corner and there she is: the Cathedral of Santiago, standing brilliantly under the sun, looking like an ant's hill as the pilgrims flood up and down the main stairway.

Dad holds my hand and squeezes it tight. We look up to the top of the stairs where the balcony overlooks the square. And there, looking down on us, are Thomas, Sascha, and Tasmanian Steve. We run up the stairs as fast as we can, embracing one another when reaching the top. Congratulations right, left and centre. Tears are streaming down my face. I'm overwhelmed with emotion. So are many others, including Dad. That moment is unbelievable. The moment where you all reach the doors to the cathedral, full of happiness and excitement, and somehow you are met by your lost friends who you weren't sure when you were going to next meet. This moment lasts only a few minutes.

After this, we went straight to the pilgrim's office to get our certificates. We knew the queue would be massive, and we didn't want the day to slip away. Surprisingly, although the queue was indeed very long, it only took an hour for us to get our certificates. Of course in the queue, lots of familiar faces were seen, and people whom we had met only once along the way were recognisable.

While standing at the very front of the queue, waiting to be called forward by one of the people working behind the desk, I noticed something on the wall, a sheet of white paper with the clear writing:

Charlie Morris
Please telephone
Your family in
France

I pointed it out to Dad, wondering what had happened and Dad said, "Oh God, that's Charlie, as in English Charlie, the small fellow with the St Jude walking stick." This worried me. I hoped he and his family were okay. Charlie was the type of person who would wander the world for half a year without a plan, a phone and just €200 in his pocket. I couldn't stop thinking about where he could be.

PETER: The first time I walked into Santiago, the time Tash and I walked 300 kilometres from León, I was elated and emotional just like Natasha describes now. I loved the joyousness, the whooping and shouting from young people, as they rushed delirious into the great plaza in front of the cathedral. This time, however, it is a little different for me. Yes, I am happy and emotional to some degree and rushing up the steps of the cathedral holding Natasha's hand will be with me for a very long time. It was a beautiful moment and I am proud of our achievement; proud of her especially. But this time, on this Camino, for me the important thing has been getting there rather than arriving. The process of walking, of making friends of strangers, of talking and thinking—processing my feelings about the deaths of my mother and father and my relationship with Natasha; this feeling of straddling the generations and now, with Mum and Dad gone, there's only me left above my children; and all the thinking about faith and spirituality—all of that has weighed with me more than the actual arrival in Santiago, joyous and all as that it. I feel the residue of this Camino is something more solid, something more enduring. Perhaps time will reveal to me what it is … I certainly want to do it again, but before that I have business to do in Finisterre.

For now, though, I want to collect my certificate, my *compostelana*. In the entrance hall to the pilgrims' office where they are issued, there is a huge pile of discarded walking staffs, cast aside by pilgrims with an air of nonchalant triumph—"Won't be needing that again!" In the Middle Ages, pilgrims would walk straight into the cathedral and down to the crypt to gaze awestruck at the casket reputedly containing the remains of the saint. Today the relics are in a silver casket in an alcove under the altar, the public held at bay by iron bars. The casket sits on a white marble plinth on which are carved two peacocks, birds whose flesh was held, in pre-Christian times, to be immortal, hence their adoption as Christian symbols. Middle-Ages pilgrims would leave a token of their pilgrimage at the altar, a walking staff perhaps, or a scallop shell, a cross, a bell, candles or perhaps something more personal. Such was the mountain of discarded material in the Middle Ages that the cathedral authorities had a system of dealing with it. A 13th-century regulation declared that everything should be gathered up each day and sorted; anything that could be melted down and re-used, should be, and the rest dumped.

Once Natasha and I got to the head of the queue, getting our certificates, our *compostelana*, turned out to be a surprisingly serious business. There were half a dozen counters to which people were called from the head of the queue, one by one. When our turn came, Tash and I were called and stood side by side, being dealt with by two separate women. They examined both our pilgrim passports diligently. This was no cursory glance. Each stamp was looked at and the sequence.

"After Sarria, where did you stay?" I was asked.

I took me a while to recall that it was Ferreiros and that I did not have an *albergue* stamp because the *albergue* was full and we snuck in, courtesy of Gary and the lads. All I had was a stamp from the bar, under which I had written 'camera found!' I explained the illicitly obtained night and the young woman smiled knowingly. And then she noticed that the name 'M. Éireannach' on my pilgrim passport did not quite correspond to the Peter Murtagh name on my actual passport. I laughed and explained the mix-up in St-Jean-Pied-de-Port and said that I quite liked being known as Mr Ireland, the pilgrim. But oh no, that could not be allowed to stand! And so my real name had to be written onto my pilgrim passport. But thankfully she allowed the 'M. Éireannach' to stay, un-crossed out, before finally signing and issuing me with my *compostelana*. It is written in Latin.

> *CAPITULUM hujus Almae Apostolicae et Metropolitanae Ecclesiae Compostellanae sigilli Altaris Beati Jacobi Apostoli custos, ut omnibus Fidelibus et Peregrinis ex toto terrarum Orbe, devotionis affectu vel voti causa, ad limina Apostoli Nostri Hispaniarum Patroni ac Tutelaris* **Sancti Jacobi** *convenientibus, authenticas visitationis*

litteras expediat, omnibus et singulis praesentes inspecturis, notum facit: Dnum Petrum Murtagh hoc sacratissimum Templum pietatis causa devote visitasse. In quorum fidem praesentes litteras, sigillo ejusdem Sanctae Ecclesiae munitas, ei confero.

*Datum Compostellae die 27 mensis Augusti anno Dni 2010.**

And then, in her own hand, the young woman wrote 'Annus Sanctus' to show that my pilgrimage and resultant *compostellae* occurred in a Holy Year, as St James's Day 2010 fell on a Sunday. The certificate is rubber-stamp signed by the *Canonicus Deputatus pro Peregrinis.* The whole thing is framed by a Georgian-style border, a large scallop shell in the centre of the bottom, and vertical rows of scallop shells up either side. The top of the frame contains, within a circle, a drawing of St James, walking staff in his right hand, his cape sporting two scallop shells on his chest just below each shoulder.

After filling in a short form disclosing personal information, such as age and occupation, the woman keyed the data into a computer. "Can you tell me how many pilgrims have obtained *compostelana* since the start of the Holy Year?" I ask her. "Since 1 January?" she says. "Yes," I reply. She taps on the keyboard and, including Natasha and me, at that precise moment, 179,753 pilgrims were accredited for 2010 as having completed the journey to Santiago de Compostela by walking at least the minimum 100 kilometres from Sarria. (The statistics show a steady increase in the number of pilgrims over the past 40 years. In the Holy Year of 1971, just 471 pilgrims were recorded by the cathedral authorities as having completed the Camino. By the Holy Year of 1993, the number had grown to 100,000, an unprecedented number at that time. The numbers have tended to double in Holy Years which, with the 2010 figure heading for 200,000, suggests that around 100,000 are currently doing the Camino each 'ordinary' year. As a consequence of 2010 being a Holy Year, a full half of all my sins have been forgiven ... which still leaves a fair skip-load for Himself to get cross about.)

NATASHA: Once we had our certificates, we had our photograph taken at the cathedral doors, passports open showing all our stamps, and we then linked up again with the others and went for lunch together. Dad and I took them to a bar in Plaza de Fonseca, not far from

* See translation, page 234.

the cathedral, which we had been shown at the end of our last Camino. We had grown very fond of this place, and wanted to share it with our friends.

When Gary wants something, he often makes it his business to let everyone else know he wants it, and makes sure he gets it. Gary wanted steak, and had for a long time. He wanted a big juicy steak with pepper sauce and caramelised onions. So, when the menu was being observed, he of course ordered the steak. Gary would be content only when he had his steak. I ordered calamari, as this was the bar where I had the best in Santiago. Andrew, Louise and Dad had them too, while Tim had chorizo. Then finally the waiter comes, holding a large dish above us and pauses looking around the table to see where it was to be put. Gary watches eagerly, his eyes wide open. It was all very dramatic. And then slowly, the dish is lowered and placed in front of Gary. This is followed by a deathly silence, and then fits of laughter from all around the table. There, where a big steak should be sitting, was a large plate of salted tiny green peppers, probably the last thing on the menu that Gary would have eaten. The best part about the whole mistake was Gary's face—pure disappointment. He was not having as much fun as we were. To add to Gary's trauma, we probably had the best lunch of the trip. Of course Gary's no show steak remained the bottom of all jokes for the rest of the day.

After lunch everybody wandered and did their own thing for a while. Reece and Andrew went shopping, Tim, Louise, Dad, Steve and Gary met with Sascha and Thomas for a drink, and I went and got new knickers! Delighted with my buy, I went back to the hostel and had a shower to prepare for dinner all together at 7.00 pm.

Everyone was looking forward to this meal. Clothes that hadn't been worn before were taken out for the occasion. Louise had a pink floral maxi dress on, and a little black cardigan. She looked absolutely beautiful, and just when I thought she couldn't have looked better, she smiled. We all waited outside the hostel for every member of our Camino family to arrive. Gary was last but his entrance was about as dramatic as his steak's absence. He was geared out in new clothes: turquoise and black trainers and a white T-shirt with a huge picture Mr Spock of Star Trek fame. To match, he wore one of Gary's finest smiles. I learned later that, in the meantime, he had had his steak.

We dined at a seafood restaurant on Rúa do Franco, which is the main eating area of the historic district around the cathedral. It was the most expensive place we had eaten in the whole five weeks, but we deserved it. We were all there—Thomas, Sascha, Tim, Louise, Tasmanian Steve, Andrew, Gary, Reece, Dad and I. For starter, I had the house special salad which was lovely, and consisted of everything a salad could consist of. Then, Andrew and I had the paella for two. It was amazing; best meal of the Camino.

I wanted to have something from all of the family, something that I could always keep, in memory of them. I had noticed I had plenty of room in my pilgrim's passport for Finisterre and more. So, I split one of the pages into a grid, and in each square I asked everyone to write a message. This is what everyone wrote.

LOUISE:

Darling Natasha,
You are such an inspirational young lady and I'm so happy that I shared the Camino with you. My love always,
Louise x x

GARY:

I'm glad to have been on the Camino with our Camino family. We started out as friends but now we are all a lot closer than that. It has been the best,
Gary

DAD:

Natasha—
My daughter,
My friend,
Your Dad x x x

REECE:

So glad to have met you and your father on the Camino. I wish you all the best for your future, Natasha.
Reece

TASMANIAN STEVE:

Tash,
A real pleasure. I've been involved with a lot of people about your age in the past (not that I am extremely old) and there is a maturity, grace and style that sets you apart from most. I'm sure success is coming your way. Thank you for sharing the Camino with me.
Steve

SASCHA:

Dear Natasha,
The Camino wasn't only a way to find myself. It was the way to find this Camino family, too. Thank you very much for sharing the Camino with me. Looking forward to seeing you again, somewhere!
You know, you were the door opener.
Sascha

TIM:

Dear Natasha,
It's been an honour and a pleasure meeting you and walking with you.
Best Buen Camino ever!
Love Tim

THOMAS:

Thanks for walking,
Thanks for talking.
God bless you both.
Thomas

ANDREW:

Tasha,
I don't know how I can sum up all the memories and laughs we've had on the Camino. There are memories that I will never forget. I feel so happy to have had the opportunity to meet you. This is not goodbye. This won't be the last I see of you. Lots of love,
Andrew (Ox)

I never got a chance to thank everyone individually for their messages. So I'm thanking you now. Those little messages mean more to me than any stamp along the Camino. They are words I will keep forever and will read over every now and then. You have all changed my Camino experience and I thank you in a million different ways for everything you gave me. I wish all of you complete happiness and a life full of success and love.

The evening went long into the night, full of wine, beer and the odd shot of vodka. It also included a trip to my and Dad's favourite café in Santiago—Casino Café on Rúa do Vilar—where Thomas played the piano beautifully. A piece he had written himself. He had the whole café in silence. Reece, Andrew and I crawled to bed sometime in the early morning.

Thank you, Santiago, for a brilliant night.

PETER: The Camino de Santiago isn't over for me until I have attended a Mass in the cathedral and so at 9 am on the day after our arrival in the city, I made my way there.

It is an extraordinary building; a great lump of dark Galician granite whose many parts emerged between the 11th and 18th centuries. It is essentially Romanesque as opposed to Gothic. Its façades are festooned with statues of Santiago as pilgrim and, far from being a gleaming, bright structure, drawing the faithful towards it like a magnet, the cathedral can often appear dull and dirty, covered in lichen and sprouting weeds, fed by Galicia's typically inclement weather. The bells are wonderful and mark the passage of time throughout the day and night with great deep bongs! Wherever you are in the old city, whether strolling through chock-a-block narrow streets, idling away an hour outside a café or bar, or gazing at the many historic buildings, the cathedral makes its presence felt both by the sheer scale of its structure and because everything else evolved in place in relation to it. Simply put, the cathedral dominates old Santiago. Inside, it is a vast structure—87 metres long, 65 metres wide, and with a 32-metre high cupola, or small dome, above the crossing. It is a building designed to accommodate throngs of pilgrims walking around it, all seeking proximity to the relics of the apostle, in the belief that being close to the remains of St James brings closeness to God Himself.

The front of the cathedral overlooks the Praza do Obradoiro, a large, paved square whose buildings are dripping with history. Immediately opposite the cathedral is the Palacio de Rajoy, a neoclassical late-18th-century structure that today is the Casa do Concello, the seat of city government. On the left (or south side of the square looking at it from the cathedral) is the Colegio Mayor de Fonseca, which is attached to the university and opens onto my beloved little Praza de Fonseca. This was founded in 1525 by Archbishop Alfonso de Fonseca III and was a centre for studying humanities before becoming a university library. You can enter its cloistered courtyard and garden from the Praza de Fonseca and Rúa do Franco and it is a little pool of tranquillity in the bustling city. On a sunny day in spring it will be ablaze with flowering shrubs, but on any day it is worth a visit. Finally, on the north side of the Praza do Obradoiro there is the Hostal dos Reis Católicos which today is a Parador hotel where rooms for two start at around €275 a night and your every whim will be indulged … at a price. When it opened its doors in 1509, however, it was a hostel and hospice for pilgrims. Then, the staff included a doctor, a pharmacist and nurses, a cleaning woman and no less than three lawyers—presumably there to tidy up the affairs of the many pilgrims who expired on reaching their goal. Despite its current luxury status, the hotel still caters for pilgrims; with sufficient notice and proof of status, a handful are given accommodation and meals at pilgrim rates.

On the morning I attend Mass, several queues were already snaking across several squares around the cathedral at 9.00 am, each to different entrances to the building. In one queue, people lined up to visit the shrine of the saint; in another, they queued simply to enter the main building itself to inspect the nave, aisles and transepts. There is a special entrance, the Puerta de Perdón, reserved for accredited pilgrims in the Holy Year and so I was able to go there, flash my pilgrim passport and walk straight into the south transept where all the pews were still empty. But the central aisle was already packed. Some 15 of the 25 rows of pews on either side of the aisle were filled by parties of Spanish pilgrims, church and community groups mainly, all wearing coloured neckerchiefs.

From where I was sitting in the front pew of the transept, I had a near perfect view of the altar and crossing. My little silver box was with me—Mum and Dad would have liked to be there—as was my Mesolithic (maybe) Clew Bay scallop shell, now hanging around my neck instead of off my rucksack. In the centre of the cupola high above the crossing, an all-seeing eye, a strange almost Masonic-like representation, peered down from inside a triangle. Immediately below it is the complex mechanism from which is suspended the *botafumeiro*, an 80-kilogram, 1.6-metre tall silver-plated censer attached to a thick rope. Usually, but not always, at the end of the daily pilgrim Mass at noon, the censer is lowered by a group of men known as *tiraboleiros* so that incense may be placed inside it and lit. Then, as the giant organ with its vertical and horizontal pipes on either side of the main aisle lets rip, the *botafumeiro* is hoisted aloft and given a slight push towards one of the transepts. The special mechanism high in the crossing allows the *tiraboleiros* tug the rope in such a way as to accentuate the swing between the transepts. Soon, clouds of incense join the organ music filling the air as the *botafumeiro* sheers through the crossing at great speed, higher and ever higher until it almost touches the ceilings of the transepts. As the censer surges higher and higher, belching incense, so the organ music also seems to rise. It is a suitable crescendo to one's Camino—a great uplifting and theatrical event that never fails to thrill the congregation.

While the *botafumeiro* undoubtedly dominates the closing moments of the Masses in which it is used, the cathedral itself is dominated by what is immediately behind the altar, a huge Baroque structure built mainly in the mid-17th century. And what an extraordinary sight this is.

A metre above the level of the altar in the central niche is a Romanesque painted stone bust of St James, crowned like a king and sandwiched between two pillars of silver. Unseen by the congregation, pilgrims climb hidden stairs to a point behind the bust while on their way to the crypt containing his reputed remains. As they come to the bust, they are permitted to hug it, and almost everyone does. As the Masses proceed, every few seconds you can see a set of arms emerging from amid all the silver and gilt and gold surrounding the saint to embrace him.

Above this image of James is a massive baldachin, an ornamental canopy or ceiling, a giant platform held aloft by two rows of huge, oversized angels, four on either side, their flesh-coloured limbs flying through the air as though they are part of a synchronised swimming team.

On top of the baldachin, there is a statue of James as pilgrim. And above this, at the very peak of the structure, there is James on horseback, riding out into the congregation, smiting his enemies with raised sword as he goes. Surrounding all of this, on either side of the complete display, are slomonic columns smothered in vines and grapes, all gilded and shining bright.

It is an extravagant, utterly over the top display and it is totally wonderful!

Half a dozen priests from the college of clerics attached to the cathedral are there to say Mass. Their vestments are a creamy white with a single gold tabard-like panel down the front on which is embroidered the dagger-like cross of St James. They are supported by a similar number of assistants and a young tenor with a strong, firm voice. As the Mass proceeds, I am joined by Gary who soon is crying—Gary, the pilgrim who, like so many, myself included, has a very ambiguous relationship with God, is caught by the emotion of the occasion. It is very hard not to be; this, after all, is the culmination of over 30 days' hard walking; it was for this moment that we all pushed ourselves through exhaustion and pain to be here, right now, for this rich display of faith and devotion—even if we (I) do not entirely believe it all.

Both Gary and I take communion and, the Mass over (sadly no *botafumeiro* on this occasion), stroll to the rear of the cathedral, to the Portico de la Gloria, the Romanesque portal main entrance to the cathedral high above the Praza do Obradoiro. The portico has been described (by the art historian Kingsley Porter) as "the most overwhelming monument of medieval sculpture" in Europe and heavily influential on subsequent compositions in cathedrals in Chartres and Rheims, Lausanne and York. It was built between 1168 and 1188 and depicts several aspects of pre-Christian Old Testament history; the condemnation and redemption of human souls; and, in the centre, the resurrection of Christ. The Saviour is crowned as king and is surrounded by the four evangelists, eight angels, 40 saved souls and 24 musicians. On either side of this great, busy, semi-circular panel, are a series of wonderfully carved statues, several showing distinct, individual expressions. One, on the left as you enter from the Praza, is glancing at another statue and has a leering grin. It is said that the smile was carved onto his face by the stone mason to reflect the fact that the object of his gaze was a voluptuous bosom on a female statue. Wouldn't you just know that some spoilsport cleric later had the bosom chipped away.

A central pillar, or mullion, supports a lintel holding up the semi-circular panel. This pillar is the first object that pilgrims would have seen entering the cathedral via the Portico de la Gloria. On it is depicted the Tree of Jesse, the genealogy of Christ, but it is St James and not Christ who tops the pillar, smiling benignly to welcome pilgrims, staff in one hand, an open scroll in the other, and a bejewelled halo behind his head. For many centuries it was a tradition that pilgrims entering the cathedral here would fall to their knees at the Tree of Jesse and place their open hand near its base, at long last able to touch a piece of the cathedral itself. Today, one can see the smooth, shiny outline of a palm and fingers on the pillar, the result of millions upon millions of open palms landing on the spot. For some years the pillar has been protected by a low railing designed to prevent pilgrims placing their hand on it.

"I'm not leaving here without putting my hand there," says Gary. And, in front of group of pilgrims, he vaults the barrier to place his open hand on the spot. "Feck it, me too," I say, following him. And as I bounce back over the barrier, hugely pleased with myself, an elderly lady askes me where I'm from.

"Ireland," I say. "And you?"

"Glasgow," she replies. "Have you walked?"

"Yep!"

"How far?"

"Eight hundred kilometres, give or take," I say, even more pleased with myself.

"Oh," says she, "let me shake that hand!"

And with that, Gary and I exit the portico, down the magnificent double stairs into the Praza do Obradoiro. Sinners still, for sure, but with maybe a little redemptive credit now in the bank.

Finisterre—Day 1: Santiago to Negreira; 21 km

NATASHA: As we all met in the plaza in front of the cathedral in Santiago for our Camino family photo, we waited for the last two to arrive: Tim and Louise. I sat alone in the shade watching all the people in the plaza. There must have been a few hundred. Some were newly arriving pilgrims, some were pilgrims who had arrived the day before and were leaving, and some were simply people hanging around to enjoy the atmosphere. Andrew, Gary and Reece had their bags with them, ready to head to the airport, along with Tasmanian Steve who had booked a flight back to Ireland with them for a little extended trip.

PETER: It was great to get the group photograph. The Belfast boys, Andrew, Gary and Reece, were there; so too Thomas and Sascha; and Tim and Louise; but we also had Elaine, the hero of the lost and then found camera and Georgio from Milan and Johanna, the lovely Peruvian girl studying in Switzerland. Everyone promises to stay in touch and I think we will. There is more than a passing interest in the fact that Natasha and I are writing a book about our Camino and the people we meet along the way.

And a little while after the photo, we ran into Gloria whose Italian fan club has clarified to single person membership. He is Giancarlo Enna, an elegantly handsome and quiet man who lives near Milan, a place to which Gloria hopes to be travelling very often from now on! Giancarlo is an estate agent having previously had a career in the Italian navy. He and Gloria are blissfully content in each other's company and are planning a future together. Gloria seems changed: she is happy and relaxed and has even given up smoking. Before we leave Santiago, we also run into Aran Han, a delightful young woman from Korea who is living in Galway where she is learning English. She was with us on and off through much of the Camino. She always has a smile and giggles like a delighted schoolgirl at the slightest encouragement.

NATASHA: Goodbyes along the Camino are always sad. It's very hard to explain to someone who hasn't done the Camino, the strong connection you build with people you meet along the way. People presume it's just like any other holiday friendship. But the Camino isn't a holiday, it is a journey you take in life, where you learn and grow, all the while, with the people you walk and talk with. It is an experience, a wonderful, beautiful experience. And to share that with someone means a lot more than a 'holiday bond'.

This time, the sadness I had for the boys' departure was brief, as I knew I would see them again very soon. It wasn't a goodbye; it was a "See ya later". Andrew and I have arranged to see each other when I get back. And I'm guaranteed to see him on the 22nd, as he's coming to my debs with me!

What was bothering me was Finisterre. I wasn't completely sure if I wanted to walk there. There was a part of me that felt Santiago was where the walking should stop; it's where the ceremony is, and where about 90% of pilgrims normally stop. Only about 10% of pilgrims go onto Finisterre, and most go by bus. It only takes two hours, and is often just a day trip, whereas walking the 85 kilometres is another three days. I felt that continuing the walking beyond Santiago would be walking away from the Camino and away from everything the Camino is. I thought it would be like walking an unknown path, one that led me away from everything the Camino was for me. I felt it would be a lonely journey.

I couldn't have been more wrong. Walking out of Santiago this morning was a little sad but about two kilometres along the way something hit me, and seemed to have hit every other pilgrim who decided to walk on: the Camino was back. The path had never been more beautiful, and there isn't a soul in sight. It is all mine. The tranquillity and peace I felt I had lost along the last 100 kilometres, I have found again.

I was walking alone through the eucalyptus forests, towering all around me, looking like leaved pilgrims' staffs and my mind was completely clear. The more I walked, the louder the birds and the insects got, and the quieter the roaring of the trucks got. The gradient often grew closer to my face and challenged me but I didn't mind. There was nobody around me, passing me out, or sitting on my tail, setting a pace for me, or rushing me. I walked how I walk.

A lot of the path looked like something out of the film *Jurassic Park*. The path was 'U' shaped and the banks went high, sometimes up to eye level. The ground was soft and easy on my feet. A slight, cool breeze whispered through the forest and moved the leaves of the eucalyptus trees, looking like shoals of fish, swimming high above my head.

In the early morning I was incredibly tired. I think my body had given in and presumed the end had come after a day of rest in Santiago. I suppose the late night out didn't help either. But I didn't know how I was going to make 25 kilometres. Now, walking through the forest, I had forgotten what that tiredness had felt like.

When I wasn't in the forest, I was walking along farm roads, through tiny little towns, usually on a slight downhill. I passed lots of fruit trees. Tiny little yellow, peach-type fruits hung delicately on the tips of branches, looking like mini suns. Then there were huddles of ripe, juicy red apples that weighed down the boughs of the tree, low enough for me to pick and enjoy. I walked with such a rhythm, simply given to me by the joys that surrounded me. I could have walked all day. On arrival in Negreira, I was surprised I had walked over 20 kilometres—it felt like 10.

I could have kept going, but it was nice to relax without necessarily dying for it. I booked in both Dad and myself, and waited for him to come.

Unfortunately, there was sadness to the day. It was the last day Sascha was going to be with us. Because of his tight schedule, he had to walk a further 30 kilometres. I've been told there is a place for me in Berlin any time I want. And then, he was gone. The evening finished with a meal with Tim, Louise, Thomas, Elaine, Dad and Roman, our Spanish friend who pops up every now and then. It was an early bed for me, in preparation for the next leg of our journey.

PETER: Before saying goodbye to Sascha, I asked him whether he had found all the keys he was seeking on his Camino. Yes, he said, and with typical Germany efficiency, he paused to enumerate them.

"One," he said, "you must trust that what happens to you in life is okay—if not now, then later. Two, don't worry—what happens, happens. Three, the basis of all is God. Four, the Camino analogy: in your backpack you carry a lot but what do you really need to carry? So, in life carry only the things that you and your family need."

And off he went, vowing to walk two full days in one, a total of 54 kilometres, arrive in Finisterre before us and then get to Santiago airport on time for his flight to Germany where he will present his wife Julia with the complete diary of his Camino. Later that night, Sascha texted to say that he'd made it!

Finisterre—Day 2: Negreira to Olveiroa; 33 km

NATASHA: I had hoped the walk today would be just as enjoyable as yesterday. I walked quickly early on, just to get ahead of the others. Not because I didn't enjoy their company but because I wanted to be alone. I feel that these three days to Finisterre are for thinking. They are the last hours I have of complete time to myself, in inspirational surroundings. I wanted to think about every possible thing I could.

The way didn't disappoint, and again, it was wonderful. It began with woodland paths through fairytale scenery. Then it led onto straight dust roads with tall pine trees guarding me on either side. Then came a few country trails, with blackberry bushes in the hedgerows. A lot of it looked like the little roads around our house in Doughmakeon in Co. Mayo.

I was thinking about what it was going to be like coming home. Things were going to be so different. I started thinking about Andrea, and what she was up to. I felt like a little chat, so I texted her telling her I was going to ring her later. Last time I was talking to her, she brought good news. She got an offer from Dublin Institute of Technology to study business and Italian. I was happy for her as she originally hadn't been happy with her results; she too thought she had missed out on everything. To her surprise this offer came in the first round, and of course she accepted. Business and Italian is what Andrea wanted to do the most and it's what she will be doing in September. I was also relieved that she was going to be studying in Dublin as I didn't want us to be separated.

For some reason the walk today seemed much further than it was. I was exhausted after 20 kilometres. The sun was extremely hot which probably didn't help. Last night in the *albergue* in Negreira, Tim and Louise had seen advertisements for an *albergue* that provided tents for anyone who wanted them, and all the equipment needed. They thought this sounded like fun so rang them up and reserved places for themselves, Dad and me, Thomas and Roman. I was looking forward to this.

Dad's leg was really swollen and causing him a lot of pain so he was going to walk slowly with Thomas and Elaine who is leaving us today because she has to fly home to Dublin. At around 12.00, I came to a bar, the first in about two hours. I was wrecked and hoped this was where I was meant to stop. Looking at my map, I realised I had another 13 kilometres to go, nearly three hours walking. I didn't have a penny on me either, so a cold Coke wasn't available to cool me. I rang Dad to see how he was getting on, and let him know where I was. He wasn't in pain, but was just feeling tired, like myself. I informed him of the bad news, and wanted to make sure it was safe to go on. We didn't actually have the option to stop anywhere earlier than Olveiroa, as we had to make it to Finisterre in three days. Reluctantly, I got up from my seat under the shade outside the bar, and carried on towards the exposed route of the Camino.

Thankfully, the beautiful scenery was there to distract me. I found myself walking along what reminded me of small Irish country roads, cutting through tiny farm villages. I then walked parallel to a large pine forest, which at times provided me with shade, but only briefly. I had been walking on a slight gradient, curving around the perimeter of the forest when all of sudden I saw something I thought I hadn't seen in five weeks—water. A huge mass of water, carved right into the land down in the distance ahead of me. Could it be the sea, I wondered to myself. It had to be it. What else could it have been? With a rush of excitement I threw my bag onto the road and rummaged for my phone. I rang Dad.

"Dad! I can see the sea! I can see the sea right in front of me!"

Dad laughed at my excitement. He was pleased and told me he would see me soon enough. Using this image of the water as motivation, I put my bag on quickly and carried on walking. I was walking for about two kilometres, heading straight towards the water. I was thinking about what I was going to do when I got to the *albergue.* Should I put my bag in our tent and unpack, or should I just head straight for the sea for a swim? Just as I was in my thoughts of how good this swim was going to be, the Camino went off the road, and a yellow arrow pointed me down a dusty road, in the complete opposite direction to the water. I stood there in confusion for about five minutes. This couldn't be right. There's no way God would allow this water to be in a pilgrim's view, and then snatch it away! Later that day, I discovered my excitement over 'the sea' was rather ridiculous. It was most definitely not the sea and was in fact just a lake.

At around 3.00 pm I came to a village named Ponte de Olveiroa. To me, all that seemed to be there was a strange, triangle-shaped, trendy looking bar, and nothing else. I thought this couldn't be where we were staying as there wasn't an *albergue* in sight. I rang Dad telling him where I was and that I must be near Olveiroa. He and Thomas were just at the point were they could see the stretch of lake. He told me he would see me in a couple of hours. I carried on walking. Finally, three kilometres later, I came to Olveiroa, and went straight to the *albergue.* There was no sight of camping though, and there was only one *albergue* here. I asked in the bar if there was anywhere to camp here but the lady knew nothing of the kind. Too tired to care I went to the *albergue* reception.

The *albergue* was wonderful. It was made of three medium-sized buildings scattered on either side of a small lane in the village. The buildings were separated into the reception, cooking and cleaning building, and then the other two buildings were where the bedrooms were. The buildings were made out of pale grey stone, and the wooden doors and windows were painted a gorgeous blue. There was a notice in the reception saying there would be someone here at 6.00 pm for the pilgrims to pay €5, but for now, just go and pick a bed. I picked a bed in one of the two bedroom buildings, and had a shower. The only person I recognised was Giorgio, and he was sleeping right opposite me. I then napped.

I was woken by my phone ringing. It was Dad.

"Hi, where are you? I'm at the camp."

Flustered and confused, as I had just been woken, I groaned: "What? Where? What campsite. There is no campsite. I'm in the *albergue*!"

After a minute or so, we realised the strange looking, triangle-shaped bar I had passed three kilometres back was in fact the campsite I was meant to be sleeping in tonight, along with the others; disaster. Dad suggested I walk back to him and Thomas, but I told him I had already showered and picked a bed. He wasn't so sure he was going to be able to make it here as Thomas's dodgy knee had just packed in, and Dad was feeling fairly wrecked himself. Pulling out the sulking teenager card, I told him it was fine and that I would just stay here alone tonight. With that I got a text saying he would be there in half an hour.

When Dad eventually made it here, followed by the brilliant Thomas, he really liked it. I was relieved as I didn't want to be bombarded with complaints about the place, resulting in me feeling rather guilty. I was a little disappointed that we were going to miss out on camping, but I got over it soon enough as the *albergue* was so lovely and we were that small three kilometres ahead of the others.

While Dad and Thomas hit the bar, I rang Andrea. I hadn't spoken to her since Foncebadón, and was looking forward to catching up. She was in Co. Clare with a few people from school, so I got to have brief chats with some of them, before getting all the gossip from Andrea. She asked me a lot about what I was up to; she finds it all so curious. We spoke about college, and our different new beginnings, and what all the other girls were doing. One of my best friends, Ciara, had got into Trinity to study business and German; this was brilliant. Another had gotten sociology and another, speech therapy. I also learned I wasn't going to be alone in UCD, as a large crowd from my school was also going there. I was glad as I was getting rather scared of being alone. I asked her about her birthday, what she had gotten up to and what presents she had got. I still hadn't fully planned her present, and I really needed it to be special. Talking to her made me realise how much I missed her. I couldn't wait to see her when I got home.

Our evening ended with a very satisfying meal in the bar opposite the *albergue*, and an early night for me, in preparation for our last day walking the Camino.

Finisterre—Day 3: Olveiroa to Finisterre; 30 km

PETER: The walk today, our final day walking after 31 days and covering close to 900 kilometres, is filled with excitement and expectation. We will see the sea—the Atlantic Ocean—for the first time since leaving Ireland. And thankfully, it turns out to be a beautiful walk. A further bonus is the fact that my leg is holding up well—the bandage is holding everything together, literally.

Soon after leaving Olveiroa not long after 6.00 am, we are up into the Montes de Buxantes, a ridge about 300 metres above sea level that we must cross to get to Finisterre. The walk traverses what is essentially open moorland, carpeted by heather and gorse and bracken and pine. The dawn breaks behind us and the day is strangely quiet; there's very little bird song and almost no wind. In a small valley we come upon a tiny church, the Capela da Nosa Señora das Neves, where a few people have gathered just before 9.00 am. The church sits among leafy plane trees and is made of rough granite and has a red tiled roof. There's a small belfry and a little shrine at the side of the church where passing pilgrims have left messages—the usual motley collection of words and pictures and trinkets. The people have gathered, it seems, for a funeral, or maybe prayers for someone who has died. Inside the building there is a small *retablo* and a statue of St James on his horse, putting those dreadful Moors to the sword once more.

We leave before whatever ceremony that is about to take place starts and rise again back up onto the moorland. There has been a forest fire here, perhaps last year, and all that is left of the young pine trees are their blackened trunks standing naked against the skyline. As we walk, a lone crow sitting at the top of one burnt stump calls "ka-ka-ka" as we pass. He pauses for a few moments before repeating himself—"ka-ka-ka." He seems to follow us for about a kilometre. "Ka-ka-ka" and again, "ka-ka-ka." It's quite eerie: the black crow on the burnt stump amid a small forest of dead trees, his ka-ka-ing the only sound around.

After a while, Natasha, who is leading our walk, gets excited—"The sea! I can see the sea," she cries and immediately telephones Moira to tell her. And yes, there it is, over to our left—this time it is not a lake! I call back to Thomas to tell him the good news. And a little further on, the full panorama of Finisterre, and what the Galicians call the Costa da Morte, the coast of death, presents itself to us. We are on Mont Brens, 255 metres above Cee, a medium-sized coastal town with what looks like a smelting plant on one side of its bay. On the far side there's a pretty seaside resort, Corcubión. In the further distance, on the left side of a finger of land pointing out into the ocean, lies Finisterre with, a few kilometres beyond, its famous lighthouse.

Thomas is elated. He walks to the edge where he has the best view and raises his staff over his head in triumph. There's a huge smile on his face. And then he sits down to telephone his wife, Ulrika. I think he is quite overcome by the moment. He has spent eight years walking, by his own estimation, some 2,800 kilometres from his home in Germany. And now the end is in sight—literally—to something that has been a huge part of his life. Natasha and I leave him to his thoughts and descend to the tiny beach in Cee where there is a café promising coffee and Spanish omelette and a huge plate of parma-style ham—for the paltry sum of €4.50.

"Where are you from?" asks the café owner in unexpectedly good English. "England?"

"No. Ireland, but we speak English," I say.

"Ah!" he replies, his eyes open with delight as he rushes to the rear of the café. He grabs a football and plonks it down on the counter in triumph. It has FAI stamped all over it. Then he rushes back and returns with a little woolly sheep.

"I have friend from Cork," he says. The friend apparently walked the Camino as far as Finisterre and came back to buy several apartments. They have all become friends and the café owner and his wife are looking forward to visiting Cork. We have a long discussion about airports and routes before asking him, in a moment of weakness, whether it would be possible to get a ferry from Corcubión around the headland to Finisterre. We have reached the sea, damn it, and that would be a very stylish way to come to the end of the earth—by sea! But there is no ferry; the fishermen of Corcubión are also not interested in taking us around, and so we must walk the final 16 kilometres.

NATASHA: Waking up this morning I couldn't quite believe that it was our last day walking, and that we were going to the sea for the first time in nearly five weeks. Back at home in Wicklow I open my blinds every morning to the sea. I had so many emotions running through me, none of which I had control over.

The walk began very early; we were all excited and eager to get out. It was a warm, dark morning, and remained dark for a good bit. We had been warned by Sascha of a difficult climb today, and after every slight hump in the path, I would turn to Dad and say in a hopeful tone, "Ah, that must have been the difficult part Sascha was talking about." Unfortunately it came when I was least expecting it.

Extraordinarily, at 5.45 am, in the complete darkness of the morning, a light shone in the near distance; a café, open. We couldn't believe it, how wonderful, and sitting outside was Thomas, with a cup of coffee and a chocolate doughnut. Inside the café were signs warning pilgrims that there wasn't another café for 15 kilometres. We chose not to buy food, as in 15 kilometres it would only be lunch time, and we figured we would reach another café in time.

The walk was beautiful, as the Camino generally had been for my whole experience. It was also quiet. Dad, Thomas and myself walked a little apart, as it was a time for oneself. It was the last time you had to think, before ending your Camino. I felt it was important to have that time alone.

Without really noticing, we had been walking gradually upwards, and were now walking along the top of a small mountain ridge. I was walking ahead, not a soul in front of me, Dad a little behind, and then Thomas a little behind Dad. My head was busy with thoughts about Andrea's present when I suddenly stopped walking. I was looking out to the horizon and noticed a boat floating along what I had thought was the sky, but was actually the sea, which was the exact same colour as the sky. I squinted my eyes, trying to look for the horizon separating the sky and the sea. It was definitely the sea, and there was definitely a boat sailing along it. I couldn't believe it. With the realisation of the sight of the sea, a stream of tears came down my face. I turned around and waved at Dad, shouting his name.

"The sea! I can see the sea!" I was pointing ahead. This time it really was the sea. I would actually like to take this moment to point out that I saw it first! I couldn't stop crying, and thinking about it now, I'm not entirely sure why I was crying. I suppose it was a surge of happiness over realising what Dad and I had just achieved. For me, the sight of the sea for the first time was the peak of ending the Camino. For me, it meant we had made it; we had made our journey, Dad and I together the whole way. It was incredible.

The walk down into Cee was lovely, as bay after bay appeared, each one harbouring little cafés and restaurants. The whole coast was like a tropical holiday resort. It was just beautiful. When we finally got down into Cee, we had a lovely lunch down in a small café right on the beach. Dad and I had both thought we had about five kilometres to go until we reached Finisterre, and we were utterly shocked and rather disappointed when we were informed it was actually another 16 kilometres. We had spent a little over an hour at our lunch spot, and had sort of got into our relaxation mode. And of course, the difficult part Sascha had warned us about was just about to hit us, coming up out of the bay of Cee and down into Finisterre.

Every time we came into another small village after leaving Cee, I would hear a loud curse from Dad behind me, as he passed the sign for the name of the village, which wasn't Finisterre. It got to a point where the beautiful little bays we were walking through were evil demon villages, part of the torment that was the 16 kilometres into Finisterre.

Finally, after what seemed like 10 hours, we reached Finisterre; the end of the world, and the end of our Camino. It was incredible. Every step, every tear, every blister, every 5.00 am start, every thirsty, hot kilometre, every café stop and every unexpectedly extended journey was worth it, just for the feeling I had right then and there. What Dad and I had just achieved was so wonderful I can't quite put it into words.

The ocean had never looked so beautiful; I wanted to run straight in. I couldn't believe the walking was over. I didn't have to put my boots on in the morning, or get up earlier than 8.00 am. The journey of the Camino was officially over, but for me the Camino itself will never be over. For me the Camino had been everyone I have met along the way, the feelings I have felt and that have grown, the things I have learned and seen, and of course my Dad. And those things will come with me along whatever other journeys I take in life. The Camino is part of me, and part of who I have become. It's the best thing I have done in my life so far, and will be one of my biggest achievements in life.

DAD

PETER: I learned from my Dad how to tie a fisherman's knot. It's a simple and very practical knot but a real finger twister for a child. You loop the fishing gut twice through the eye of the hook, then wrap the end of the line around itself several times before threading it back under the wraps and pulling it tight. The wraps slip down the line, thus tightening the knot down upon itself. If you are lucky enough to get a bite, the pull of the fish will only make the knot tighter. Well, that's the theory and, for my Dad and me fishing from Dun Laoghaire pier or off the rocks around Dingle, it worked often enough. We caught plenty of pollock and mackerel and dogfish. Dad also taught me how to swim. In Blackrock Baths he would place one hand under my tummy, the other under my chin, as he coaxed me to lie forward, kick with my feet and doggy-paddle with my hands. The hope was that I would eventually achieve buoyancy and move off the ground and through the water. It worked—eventually—and I swam.

When I was 18, Dad bought me my first serious motorbike—a Kawasaki 90SS. It replaced a Honda 50 and it went like a hot snot, as we said in those days. It was an odd thing for him to do. He was not a biker, nor was he the adventurous type, and it would have scared the bejazus out of him had he ever come on the back of it with me. More in character, he also introduced me to music, to Tchaikovsky's *1812 Overture* and *Serenade for Strings*, and I still think of him whenever I hear either. Music—Gilbert and Sullivan and light classical—was a companion throughout his life.

Dad was quite handsome and dapper, a snappy dresser with a great sense of occasion, theatre even, and always ready with a clever one-line quip that raised a smile on others. He drew on all these qualities during his brief TV career when late in life he did an antiques slot during an afternoon magazine programme.

I remember his hands. Some people have short, stubby, sausage-like fingers. Dad's were lean and long and he had prominent knuckles. The veins on his hands and forearms also bulged in a way that was somehow attractive; distinctive anyway. His arms were quite hairy and his skin tanned very easily. I have his hands and nose and Natasha has mine; it's funny that, when you are in the middle of three generations, you can sometimes see the threads that link. I remember as a child the smell and the feel of Dad's cheeks against mine—his were leathery and spiky when he had a little stubble and I loved the feel of them. Dad shaving was quite a ritual. He always used a wet razor when I was a child. He would fill the washhand basin with warm water and extend the life of his Gillette blade by rubbing the cutting edge rapidly along the side of the basin as though it were a whetstone. Barbers used to do the same with their cut-throat blades on a leather strap; I can still see them in Mason Prost's, the old-world barbers on St Stephen's Green and in Suffolk Street—all marble basins and work tops, and complex leather shaving chairs that went up and down and were operated by men in aprons.

Dad loved—adored—Dublin city. He loved its characters and its dirt; and he loved standing outside his tiny shop in Dawson Street watching the world go by, master of the little universe he had created for himself. His Dublin was the Dublin of the Jews of Clanbrassil Street, just down the road from his beloved St Patrick's Cathedral, where as a child he was a choir boy. In later life, many members of the Jewish community were his associates in the jewellery and antiques business and his friends also. His Dublin was replete with wits—like the butcher who, on the eve of some solemn pronouncement from the Catholic Church during which he would be closed, placed a notice in his window that read: *No Meat For The Dog Ma.* It was the Dublin of places like Kiss Arse Hill, the name he and his pals gave to a particularly treacherous, steep road somewhere around Thomas Street and the Liberties; it was the Dublin that had a shop with a big sign over the door proclaiming *Cigars Divan*, a place where gentlemen could go and have a smoke lying on a chaise longue but which he thought was run by a Mr Cigars Divan. It was the Dublin of Bang Bang, the harmless madman who used to shoot at buses with a pretend gun that was actually a big old key, while simultaneously providing his own sound effects. It was the Dublin of the woman outside Our Boys shop on Wicklow Street who plucked on the strings of a big harp and collected pennies that passersby dropped in a giant, glistening sea shell she placed on the pavement. It was the Dublin of tenement buildings, of Gur Cake and Crubeens; the Dublin of a particular type of 19th-century inner-city poverty that crept into the 20th and included his kind—the Protestant working class—before they were wiped out by a combination of time and circumstance and abandonment as a new order asserted its supremacy. The Protestant middle class protected itself by closing rank, by living in certain areas—such as Dundrum and Rathfarnham—where critical mass supported schools and youth clubs and parents had a reasonable prospect that their children would marry one of their own. And they channelled their young men into safe jobs in Protestant businesses, the likes of Guinness or Dockrells or Drummonds Seeds or, best of all, the Bank of Ireland.

Dad emerged from his background and gradually entered this world, a world further up the social scale than the one into which he had been born, the son of a gardener in Merrion Square. When he left St Patrick's Cathedral school, he got a job in West & Sons, the huge jewellery, silver and antique shop at the bottom of Grafton Street, long since gone. And thus he grew into another Dublin world that he also came to love—the world of lah-de-dah toffs and would-be toffs; of rogues and rascals and chancers who made the hucksters shops and antique auctions places of magical theatre and opportunity. When he opened his own small shop in the mid-1960s, few things gave him more pleasure than picking up a bargain and selling it next day at a handsome profit. But he never gouged; he was happy with a decent whack; I never knew him take advantage of someone …

After Mum died and Dad was left living with us, life quickly settled into a routine. His new home, a former garage at the bottom of our garden which previous owners had turned into a lovely cottage-style granny flat, had everything he needed: a bedroom, living room, bathroom and kitchenette all on one level. It was warm and bright, and even with his near complete blindness he could find his way around and largely look after himself. At 84, he still took pride in his appearance when dressing himself and was still able to walk to the post office to collect his pension and buy a bottle of whiskey on the way home. He soon became well known in the community. Each morning I would call into him, usually to make him his cup of tea and see that he was rousing himself and not sinking into bad habits like staying in bed all day. In the early years he could even make his own evening meal—or at least stick a ready-made one into the microwave. In the evenings when I came home, I would drop down to him to set out his tablets for next morning and we'd share a glass of whiskey and roll over the day's events. I came to loathe radio phone-in programmes, platforms for an endless parade of whining complainers whose often distorted world became Dad's window on current events.

As the years slipped by, he became more and more dependent on everyone around him. His health was largely stable; his doctors and the day care help from our health centre were excellent. But his capacity to bounce back from infections grew less and less until eventually he was reduced to a wasting-away wreck of what he used to be. As I looked at the increasingly helpless creature withering before my eyes, I'd wonder where was my Dad? Where was the big, handsome man of the strong hands and bulging veins; the dapper dresser with the yellow rose button hole and Prince of Wales check suit and brogues? The man who could no longer wash or dress, or at times feed himself, became totally dependent on me and Moira and Patrick and Natasha, on Nigel and Jane and on Carol, his devoted home help. He reached the point where he just wanted to die, wanted to be with Mum.

And so it came about. On 1 January 2010, four months after going into a nursing home, he stopped breathing. We—Nigel, Jane and I—were waiting by him in relays, knowing the end was near. Death stalked him from the feet up. They went first, ceasing to move and growing cold; it advanced up his body to his abdomen and chest and finally his head, his brain saying it had had enough and was shutting down. He was three days short of his 91st birthday. You can't complain after a life that long but I still miss him, still feel I owe him. He's been with me all the time on the Camino, him and Mum.

I guess this is a lot of what Finisterre is about for me—the completion of a journey that is about saying goodbye while sitting at what the ancients thought was the end of the earth and watching the sun go down.

Sunday, 20 June 2010. We will scatter Dad's ashes that day, suggests my brother. The evening before, we will all be in Dublin for a family occasion and we can do the scattering the next day. Only later, much nearer the date, do we realise that 20 June is Father's Day. The old ham would be pleased; it's the sort of thing he would have suggested had he thought of it himself.

His only instruction regarding his ashes was that they should be scattered in Merrion Square, a place to where memories of his childhood drew him increasingly in his later years. He never said much about the place other than that the family home had been a cottage in the city centre park where his father had been a gardener. The 1911 census has the family duly recorded: Arthur Murtagh, head of family; Mary Murtagh (née Hunter) etc etc etc. But no Dad because he hadn't yet arrived in this world. Date of birth: 4 January 1919; the Gardener's Cottage long since gone.

We knew nothing about the place of Merrion Square in his life until, some time in my late 20s, he gave Nigel and me each a large, framed, hand-coloured print showing a drinking fountain set into the railings of Merrion Square West, opposite the National Gallery of Ireland. "To her Grace Mary Isabella, Duchess of Rutland, this plate is most humbly inscribed by her devoted Servant, J Blaquiere," says an inscription on the print. Below this the story is told of the Duke of Rutland, "the late and much lamented Lord Lieutenant of Ireland", and how the fountain was erected in his honour "for the use of the poor of the City of Dublin" following his premature death.

"That's where I was born," said Dad when he gave us the print. "In a cottage behind that, behind the Rutland memorial," he said, indicating where a cottage once stood but which is not in the print and was certainly not there during the life of us, his children. Nineteenth-century maps confirm, however, that he was not making it up. There was indeed a Gardener's Cottage more or less where he indicated.

20 June 2010 in Merrion Square turns out to be the final day of the rather grandly titled World Street Performance Championship, the culmination of four days during which a motley collection of contortionists, magicians, break dancers, jugglers, troubadours and fast-talking comedians, most of whom seem to be American, take over the park and streets around the square for a brash, noisy and thoroughly fun-filled family time. It's a really bright, sunny day and up to 150,000 people are expected … along with Dad's ashes. Wisely, we resolve to get there a little early.

The Street Performance carnival starts at 12 noon. We're in place before then, assembled inside the park, behind the Rutland memorial, my brother and I trying to figure out where the Gardener's Cottage might have been. Not over there, not near the children's playground. Noisy, scampering children and Dad didn't mix. Eventually we settle on the beds of shrubs that surround a square cobblestone plinth behind the memorial. Around it are some well-maintained benches where people doubtless come and sit for a moment's reflection amid the dappled sunlight and quiet, away from the madding crowds of the city. A little in the distance but visible nonetheless is the corner of the park dedicated to Oscar Wilde, whom Dad once mimicked on the Gaiety Theatre stage during his years with the Rathmines and Rathgar Musical Society. A better place for his ashes could not be found. It is perfect.

The three of us, his children Nigel, Jane and I, take turns to plunge into the shrubbery, tipping out ash from the green plastic container. There's a bit of Mum in there as well, a handful of her ashes kept from her scattering on the Little Sugar Loaf Mountain in Wicklow in 2003. They'd have both liked this—the idea of them being spread about together, their individual specks of dust, one indistinguishable from the other, sprinkled around the undergrowth and onto the soil of Merrion Square park. We do our bit and then the grandchildren present take over—Siún and Duncan, Eoin and Stephen, and Natasha (my son Patrick was away). Somewhere through the trees in the centre of the park, a Gospel Choir begins to belt out *Oh Happy Day!* Why not? It's Sunday, there are loads of people around and it's a beautiful day. A middle-aged man with a camera is watching the scattering; the grandchildren cough and swot clouds of ash away from their faces as they shake and empty the container. The man with the camera looks on, curious. My brother, who can be more anxious and fretful at times than is good for him, feels the need to explain the situation. A big smile crosses the photographer's face. "Oh, that's lovely," he proclaims, "lovely! And the house was here? And you are all here for this! How wonderful! How old was he?"

Just then, one of the street performers, John Paul the puppeteer, arrives, pulling behind him a large wooden box on wheels. He's from Florida. He's wearing a silly-looking, plastic pork-pie hat and he exudes that typically American, ever so slightly excessive cheeriness that either grates or is infectious, depending on one's mood when at the receiving end.

"Hi guys!" he says, bustling through us and making his way to the centre of the plinth to set up his puppet show as we brush bits of my father off our clothes.

"Are you guys here for Man in the Box Productions?"

FINISTERRE

After Dad's death, we divided up his few possessions according to his wishes. A long life, well lived and now reduced to 'things'. One was his collection of Georgian and Victorian silver snuff boxes. He treasured them so much that in recent years he kept them hidden away rather than on display. We drew lots in turn and one of the boxes that I got was the one I have been carrying with me all the time on my Camino. A signature, JG Stokes, is engraved on the lid. I have no idea who JG Stokes was but I like his little silver box. It was made in London in 1788 by WS and Dad would probably have been able to tell me off the top of his head who WS was.

After we have been in Finisterre for a few hours and caught our breath, I suggest to Natasha that we go to the town's main beach, a beautiful, long, sandy expanse known as Praia Langosteira.

"Is it time?" she asks without elaborating because she knows what I want to do.

"Yep, I think so," I reply.

And so we stroll there from our *albergue* in the harbour, my right calf killing me after our 30-kilometre walk, the final, absolute end of our Camino. On the beach the water is crystal clear; the sky is blue and waves break gently on the sand. I stand surveying the scene for a few minutes. Mum and Dad would like it here, alright. This little bit of the end of the earth says summer holiday, relaxation, time off for a nice salad and glass of chilled white wine sitting in the shade.

I wade out into the sea, feeling a strange, unemotional detachment. I feel like an actor in my own movie. I have done this so many times in my head since climbing Croagh Patrick and then all the way across the Camino from the Pyrénées that somehow, right now, I don't feel a part of what I am doing. In some weird way, I am here but not really here at all. I dive into the water, cool, clear and clean, and stay swimming under it for a few metres. There is nothing below me except white sand and sparkling crystal twinkling in the sunlight through the water. When I open the little silver box held tightly in my left hand, nothing happens at first until I dig my finger inside. Then, with a silent underwater puff!, the last of Mum and Dad's ashes explode into the sea, a small gray cloud floating a little at first but then settling slowly and gently on the sand beneath me, the sand of Finisterre. I'm not sure what Dad would make of this but I know Mum would approve. She would understand, I think, the connection to ancient rites, to the idea of resting finally where the sun sets, in the place where the souls of the dead have gone.

Up at the lighthouse, pilgrims and others are gathering to watch the sun set. Thomas is here, so too are Johanna from Peru and Tasha and me and others we recognise from various stages of the Camino. The lighthouse building is huge, and just beyond it, almost at the very edge of the peninsula, is an aerial of some sort to which pilgrims have attached various items, a bit like the Cruz de Ferro but not quite that festooned. You simply can't go any further now: a Camino milestone with the familiar blue and yellow tile showing a scallop records the distance left to travel—'0,00 K.M.' Down below us, waves crash on the rocks. Around us, firemen continue to douse the earth, scorched by an afternoon blaze, probably caused by a pilgrim burning their clothes. Many do this at Finisterre, a symbolic act, like bathing, signifying a break with the past. After the bush fire, there'll be none of that tonight, though.

When Decimus Junius Brutus led his Roman legions into Galicia in 136 AD, his restless troops feared crossing rivers they believed divided their world from Hades, the ancient underworld of the dead. Brutus was the first Roman general to reach Finisterre and he was fascinated by the Celtic sun cult practised there, the Ara Solis, or altar to the sun. The clothes burning is something of a continuation of the rites performed at Ara Solis. All around the lighthouse, many of the rocks are scorch-marked from small pilgrim fires. The sun dies nightly in the west but is reborn again the next day, giving life to all who bask in her warmth. My guess is that the people who carved those swirling circles in the Boheh Stone by Croagh Patrick and elsewhere believed they owed the sun special attention for its life-giving properties. Sometimes, it's not hard to see from where the early Christians took some of their ideas ... Of course the church does not like the whole business of Finisterre, *finis terra*—the medieval, indeed pre-Christian, end of the earth. The church authorities in Santiago say the Camino ends in the cathedral, the final resting place, they say, of the apostle James. The church regards Finisterre as being a place of esoteric practices detrimental to the pilgrimage. But for many pilgrims, a minority for sure, their Camino ends in Finisterre where some feel they connect with a Celtic past redolent with pagan rites of passage. That sun, which has been on our back all along the Camino, rising above our heads as each day unfolded before setting facing us in the west, drawing us on, finally goes to sleep beyond Finisterre, in the great vastness of the sea stretching out into the Atlantic Ocean. In ancient times there was a belief that the sun was the ultimate giver of life. And if New Age sun worshippers feel the same way today and want to pay homage in Finisterre, what harm?

As the sun inches closer to the horizon, Thomas is thinking of his mother. She died aged 84 after enduring Alzheimer's for seven years. Before that, she was widowed aged just 34. "Did she find love again after that?" I ask Thomas. "Yes," he says, "I think she did." Natasha prances about on the rocks and I take her picture against the setting sun, as Thomas talks of his own daughter, Johanna, a little miracle in his and Ulrike's life. She was a little unexpected, it seems. They already had two sons, Jacob and Johanas, when one day Ulrike fell and knocked her head. When doctors examined her, x-rays showed slight internal bleeding and so she was given powerful drugs to prevent a brain haemorrhage. Then it was discovered she was pregnant and the doctors said they could not guarantee that the foetus was unharmed by the other treatment.

"I said to my wife, 'it's your decision but I will not do it. I will go with whatever you decide'. And so she decided to keep the pregnancy and this was my daughter," said Thomas, his eyes glistening.

Johanna is now 23 years old and she and Thomas sing and play together at weddings and funerals. "She gets paid and I play the organ for nothing!" he says with one of his great laughs. Thomas clearly loves his daughter as I love mine.

"What are you going to do now?" I ask Thomas as he removes the bandages, now signed by us all, from his knee and sticks them to the lighthouse aerial.

"Jerusalem," he says. "I'll start walking to Jerusalem next year," he says.

Later I text to ask can I join him. "Deal!" he replies.

Finally, at 9.14 pm, the sun goes down. Not the most majestic display of nature I expect Finisterre has seen but good enough for me after 900 kilometres. Tomorrow it will rise again, warming us all and making the plants grow.

"Tash!" I call as the last of the sunset, a thin sliver of bright red, dips below the far horizon.

"Yes, Dad?"

"Time to go home?"

"Yes, Dad," she says, "I think it's time to go home."

AND THEN ...

Gary McCartan, Andrew Lee and Reece Connolly returned to Belfast to resume their studies in nursing. Gary wants to remain within the healthcare system in Northern Ireland; Reece wants to do some more travelling before joining the British Army; Andrew is hoping to become a paramedic, but in the meantime he and Natasha spend a lot of time together, shuttling between our home in Greystones and his in Saintfield near Lisburn in Northern Ireland.

Steve Gill flew from Santiago to Dublin and spent a few days in Belfast with Gary, Andrew and Reece. He saw Down beat Kildare in the all-Ireland senior football semi-final in Croke Park, before touring the country and spending a weekend in Mayo where he climbed Croagh Patrick. After that, he went to Venice and Munich's Oktoberfest before going to London to seek work as a chartered accountant to save money for his next backpack foray.

Tim Hesse and Louise Tilley went to Portugal and from there returned to Glasgow before flying home to Melbourne in Australia. They are back living with their respective parents. Louise has started work in a private hospital and they are looking for a home of their own.

Sascha Thieme is back in Berlin. He gave his Camino diary to his wife and they fell in love with each other all over again.

Thomas Reiss returned to Ulrike and their children and his various choirs. He resumed teaching music and preparing the choirs for their Christmas concerts. He is also planning the first stage of his walk to Jerusalem in 2011, starting with the Westweg, a walking trail through the

Black Forest. "Finding out new ways to walk is my strategy to not think about the Camino," he says. In 2012, he hopes to come to Ireland with one of his choirs.

Elaine Byrne resumed her career teaching politics in Trinity College, Dublin, and analysing political events in Ireland.

Gloria Baizan and Giancarlo Enna have visited each other in Milan and Barcelona and are very happy together.

Johanna, whose full name is Johanna Perea Verdi, is studying chemistry and chemical engineering at the Ecole Polytechnique Fédérale de Lausanne in Switzerland. She hopes to do a Masters in environmental engineering and to improve her English by spending time in Ireland.

The notice in the pilgrim office asking Charlie Morris to contact his family in France related to the death there of his 27-year-old sister, Octavia, in an accident on 21 August. Efforts to contact Charlie have proved unsuccessful at the time of submitting this manuscript for publication.

Claire Collins has resumed nursing in Dundalk; Aideen Kinsella is in UCD in her second year of Social Science; Mary Collins is in second year in St Patrick's in Drumcondra studying Geography and English; Aoife Smeaton is in her first year in UCD, hoping eventually to specialise in zoology.

The Hungarian hussars, Ádám Barnabás and Pál Mike Bugnics, rode their horses for 68 days and arrived back on Hungarian soil on 20 September, wearing full dress uniform. Their reception party included officials from the Hungarian ministry of defence and army, plus a troupe of Hungarian musicians and folk dancers. Their unusual, 3,500-kilometre journey from Lisbon ended officially at the gates of Buda Castle on 15 October 2010.

Peter Murtagh is back working at *The Irish Times*. Natasha Murtagh is studying English and philosophy at UCD.

Before they left Santiago, they went to a tattoo parlour ...

SELECT BIBLIOGRAPHY

A number of books were consulted before we embarked on our Camino and several proved invaluable sources for us. We have used information from some and acknowledge that here.

Frey, Nancy Louise; *Pilgrim Stories On And Off the Road to Santiago—journeys along an ancient way in modern Spain*; University of California Press, Berkeley and Los Angeles; 1998. Began life as Ms Frey's doctoral dissertation in anthropology which, happily, she turned into a rich volume exploring why people undertake the pilgrimage, much of the explanation being in their own words.

Gitlitz, David M. and Davidson, Linda Kay; *The Pilgrimage Road to Santiago—the complete cultural handbook*; St Martin's Press, New York; 2000. A superb companion, filled with a wealth of useful and interesting information on the pilgrimage, local history, church by church detail and occasional forays into geography, geology, flora and fauna.

Hackett, Edel; *Clew Bay Archaeological Trail—exploring* 6,000 *years of Mayo's heritage*; 2003. Practical guide to 21 places of archaeological interest around Clew Bay, dating from between 4000 BC and 1900.

Hughes, Harry; *Croagh Patrick—a place of pilgrimage, a place of beauty*; The O'Brien Press, Dublin; 2010. A fine and well-sourced guide to the mountain, its history and contemporary appeal.

Melczer, William; *The Pilgrim's Guide to Santiago de Compostela*; Italica Press, New York; 1993. The first English translation of Aymeric Picaud's *Codex Calixtinus/Liber Sancti Jacobi* with excellent, and detailed, explanatory introduction exploring the origin of pilgrimage, the significance of relics and mythology associated with the cult of St James.

Moore, Fionnbarr; *Ardfert Cathedral—summary of excavation results*; Department of the Environment, Heritage and Local Government, Dublin; 2007. Detailed results of the 1989 and 1998 excavations carried out by the National Monuments Service.

Morahan, Leo; *Croagh Patrick, Co. Mayo—archaeology, landscape and people*; The Croagh Patrick Archaeological Committee; 2001. Exceptionally detailed and illustrated record of the 1996–1998 survey of the area around the mountain.

Murphy, Anthony, and Moore, Richard; *Island of the Setting Sun—in search of Ireland's ancient astronomers*; The Liffey Press, Dublin; 2008. Stimulating and beautifully produced exploration of pre-Christian practices in Ireland.

Sayers, Dorothy L. (trans); *The Song of Roland*; Penguin Classics, New York; 1957. The complete epic poem with useful introduction by Ms Sayers.

Thomas, N.L.; *Irish Symbols of 3500 BC*; Mercier Press, Dublin; 1988. Useful guide to reading Irish pagan rock art.

POEMS AND SONGS QUOTED

Page 21: *The Anastasis* by Sophronius (550 AD–638 AD); translated from the ancient Greek original by John Wilkinson (Jerusalem Pilgrims before the Crusades; Middle East Studies; 1977).

Pages 23–5: *The Song of Roland* (c.1140–1170), translated from the French by Dorothy L. Sayers (1893–1957).

Page 37–8: From *Devotions upon Emergent Occasions* (1624), a series of reflections in 23 parts written by the metaphysical poet, John Donne (1592–1631). Each of the parts is further divided into a Meditation. Meditation XVII contains the poem, *No man is an island …*

Pages 62: *Thank Heavens For Little Girls* (1958) by Alan Jay Lerner (1918–1986) and Frederick Loewe (1901–1998), from their 1958 musical *Gigi*; popularised by the French singer Maurice Chevalier.

Pages 68–9: *Hello Mary Lou*; lyrics by Gene Pitney (1940–2006) and Fr Cayet Mangiaracina (1935–); hit single 1961 for singer Ricky Nelson as B-side to his A-side record, *Travellin' Man*. Unlike Pitney,

Fr Cayet is alive and kicking and is chaplain at the Holy Ghost Catholic School in Hammond, Louisiana. He is a member of the Dominican Order which is grateful for the annual royalty cheques it receives for *Hello Mary Lou.*

Pages 70–71: *All Things Bright And Beautiful* (1848) by Cecil Frances Alexander (1818–1895), from *Hymns for Little Children* (1848); believed to have been inspired by *The Rime of the Ancient Mariner* (1798–1798) by Samuel Taylor Coleridge (1772–1834). Born in Dublin as Cecil Frances Humphreys, Mrs Alexander was a prolific writer of hymns and was married to the Church of Ireland Bishop of Derry, William Alexander, afterwards Archbishop of Armagh.

Page 106: *Imagine* (1971) by John Lennon (1940–1980); from the album *Imagine* (1971).

Pages 129: From *Ulysses* (1842) by Alfred, Lord Tennyson (1809–1892).

Page 186: From *Brothers In Arms* (1985) by Mark Knopfler; from the album *Brothers In Arms* (1985) by Dire Straits.

English version of the Latin text [on pages 201–2] of the *compostelana*, the certificate awarded to pilgrims by the Cathedral authorities in Santiago:

The Chapter of this Holy Apostolic Metropolitan Cathedral of St James, custodian of the seal of St James' Altar, to all faithful and pilgrims who come from everywhere over the world as an act of devotion, under vow or promise to the Apostle's Tomb, our Patron and Protector of Spain, witnesses in the sight of all who read this document, that: Petrum Murtagh has visited devoutly this Sacred Church in a religious sense.

Witness whereof I hand this document over to him, authenticated by the seal of this Sacred Church.

Given in St James de Compostela on the 27 August 2010

[signed]
Deputy canon for pilgrims

Translation provided by the Delegación Diocesana de Peregrinaciones, Rúa do Vilar, Santiago de Compostela

For anyone interested in doing the Camino, there is a wealth of detail available online, both from information-led websites and from blogs. Among the more useful sites are:

www.stjamesirl.com: the site of the Irish Society of Friends of St James.

www.csj.org.uk: the site of the UK-based Confraternity of St James.

www.caminosantiagocompostela.com: a site dedicated to helping people thinking of walking the Camino Francés, the main Camino that starts in St-Jean-Pied-de-Port.

www.caminodesantiago.me.uk: a site run by an individual enthusiast living in Ireland.

www.spanishsteps.eu: a commercial site with a lot of practical information on the various Camino routes in Spain and travel companies that will get you there.

www.onfootinspain.com/home: a site run by Nancy Louise Frey (see bibliography) and José Daniel Placer dedicated to educational hiking tours in northern Spain, particularly along the Camino, and Portugal.

www.theway-themovie.com: the site for *The Way*, a Camino film due for general release in the spring of 2011. Directed by Emilio Estevez and starring his father, Martin Sheen, and, among others, the Irish actor James Nesbitt, it tells the story of a father carrying the ashes of his son from St-Jean to Santiago.

www.caminodocumentary.org: the site for a documentary film, *The Camino Documentary*, being produced by Future Education Films of Portland, Oregon. The documentary follows the progress of six pilgrims from diverse backgrounds as they traverse their way to Santiago.

Buen Camino!

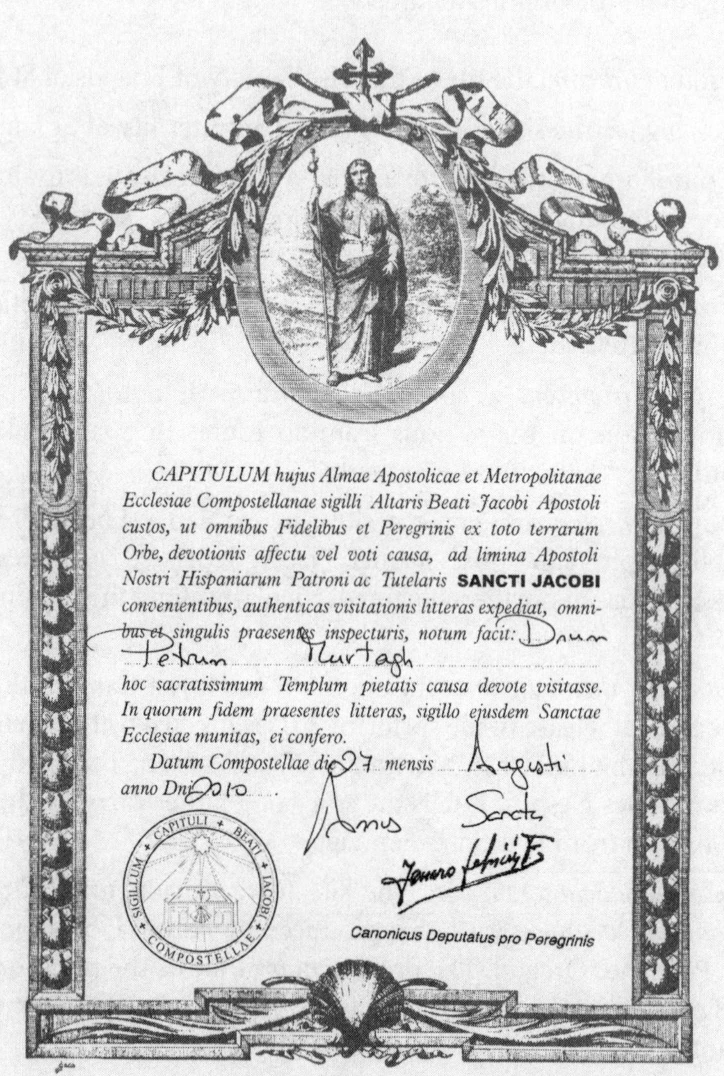

CAPITULUM hujus Almae Apostolicae et Metropolitanae Ecclesiae Compostellanae sigilli Altaris Beati Jacobi Apostoli custos, ut omnibus Fidelibus et Peregrinis ex toto terrarum Orbe, devotionis affectu vel voti causa, ad limina Apostoli Nostri Hispaniarum Patroni ac Tutelaris **SANCTI JACOBI** *convenientibus, authenticas visitationis litteras expediat, omnibus et singulis praesentes inspecturis, notum facit:* Dnum Petrum Murtagh *hoc sacratissimum Templum pietatis causa devote visitasse. In quorum fidem praesentes litteras, sigillo ejusdem Sanctae Ecclesiae munitas, ei confero.*

Datum Compostellae die 27 *mensis* Augusti *anno Dni* 2010

Annus Sancti

Canonicus Deputatus pro Peregrinis

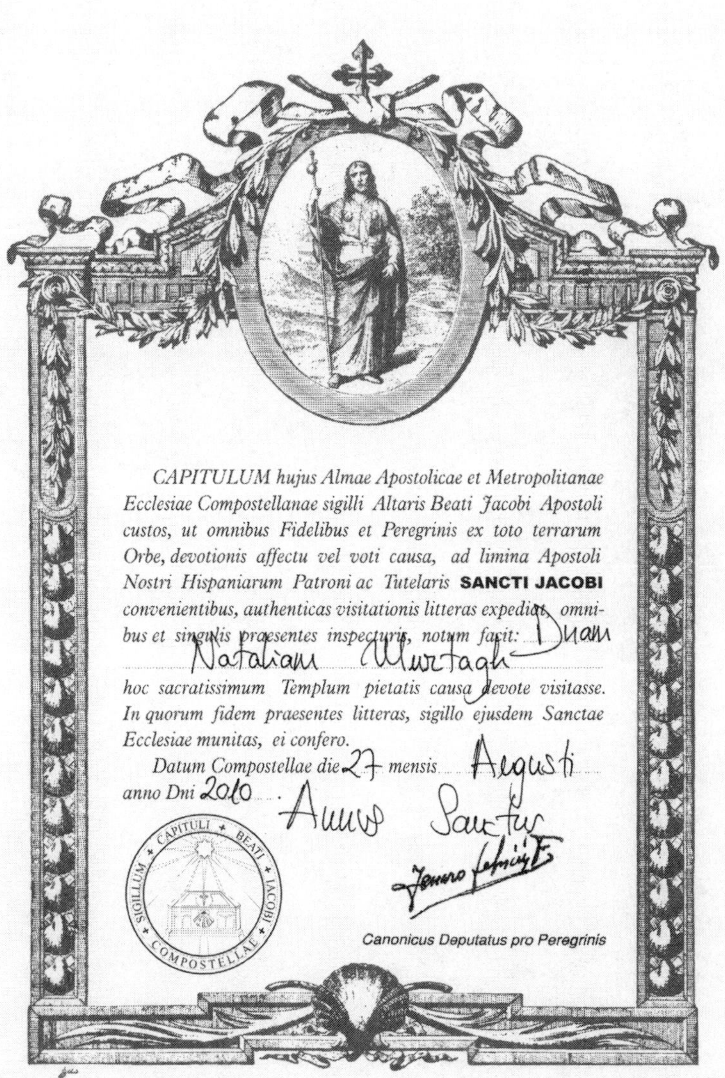

CAPITULUM hujus Almae Apostolicae et Metropolitanae Ecclesiae Compostellanae sigilli Altaris Beati Jacobi Apostoli custos, ut omnibus Fidelibus et Peregrinis ex toto terrarum Orbe, devotionis affectu vel voti causa, ad limina Apostoli Nostri Hispaniarum Patroni ac Tutelaris **SANCTI JACOBI** *convenientibus, authenticas visitationis litteras expediat, omnibus et singulis praesentes inspecturis, notum facit:* Dnam Nataliam Murtagh *hoc sacratissimum Templum pietatis causa devote visitasse. In quorum fidem praesentes litteras, sigillo ejusdem Sanctae Ecclesiae munitas, ei confero.*

Datum Compostellae die 27 *mensis* Augusti *anno Dni* 2010

Anno Sanctus

Canonicus Deputatus pro Peregrinis